Enabling Occupation II:
Advancing an Occupational Therapy Vision for Health, Well-being, & Justice through Occupation

Official practice guidelines for the Canadian
Association of Occupational Therapists

Researched and written for
Canadian Association of Occupational Therapists

Primary Authors

Elizabeth A. Townsend, Ph.D., OT(C), OT Reg. (NS), FCAOT

Helene J. Polatajko, Ph.D., OT(C), OT Reg. (Ont.), FCAOT

Published by
CAOT Publications ACE
Ottawa, Ontario

Copies may be purchased from:
Canadian Association of Occupational Therapists,
CTTC Building
3400-1125, Colonel By Drive,
Ottawa, Ontario K1S 5R1

Tel: (613) 523-2268, ext. 242
Fax: (613) 523-2552
E-mail: publications@caot.ca

And at our on line store: www.caot.ca

Disponible en français sous le titre :
Promouvoir l'occupation II : l'avancement d'une vision de l'ergothérapie en matière de santé,
bien-être et équité à travers l'occupation

Statistics Canada information is used with the permission of Statistics Canada. Users are forbidden
to copy this material and/or redisseminate the data, in an original or modified form, for commercial
purposes, without the expressed permission of Statistics Canada. Information on the availability of
the wide range of data from Statistics Canada can be obtained from Statistics Canada's Regional
Offices, its World Wide Web site at http://www.statcan.ca, and its toll-free access number
1-800-263-1136.

CAOT PUBLICATIONS ACE

ISBN: 978-1-895437-76-8   Printed in Canada

Dedication

To my parents, whose whims of iron taught me about enabling occupation.
To Harry, Jean, and Kelvin, for your amazing support.
And to my Dalhousie colleagues, whose challenges
and encouragement are my lifeline. ~ E. Townsend

To my parents, Theresa and Miron Polatajko, who, each in their own way,
taught me the true importance of occupation in creating
a meaningful and happy life.
To my husband, Walter C. (Pete) Howell, who always supports
my occupations fully with love and caring, frequently
sacrificing his own. ~ H. Polatajko

Primary authors

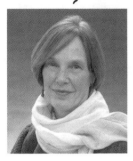

Elizabeth A. Townsend,
Ph.D., OT(C), OT Reg. (NS), FCAOT

Liz Townsend graduated with a Diploma in Physiotherapy and Occupational Therapy, and a B.Sc. (OT) from the University of Toronto, and with an M.Ad.Ed. from St. Francis Xavier, and a Ph.D. from Dalhousie University. Liz is Professor and Director, and a founder of the School of Occupational Therapy at Dalhousie University. Her involvement in *Enabling Occupation II* extends her participation in all eight Canadian guidelines publications, starting from the first meeting in 1980. She is registered with the College of Occupational Therapists of Nova Scotia.

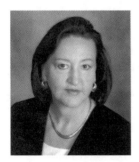

Helene J. Polatajko,
Ph.D., OT(C), OT Reg. (Ont.), FCAOT

Helene Polatajko graduated with a BOT from McGill University and an M.Ed. and Ph.D. from OISE/University of Toronto. Helene is Professor and Chair, Department of Occupational Science and Occupational Therapy and Graduate Department of Rehabilitation Science, and Professor, Department of Public Health Sciences and School of Graduate Studies, University of Toronto. She is registered with the Ontario College of Occupational Therapists.

Liz and Helene were invited to volunteer, as members of the Canadian Association of Occupational Therapists (CAOT) to conceptualize, organize, and write the book. They used an iterative writing and peer review process to integrate national contributions that have greatly enriched the book.

Contributing authors: Chapter co-authors, case and text box writers

Bice Amoroso, M.Sc. (candidate), OT Reg. (Ont.) Occupational Therapist & Clinical Education and Training Coordinator, Centre for Addiction and Mental Health, Toronto, Ontario

Catherine Backman, Ph.D., OT(C), OT Reg. (BC), FCAOT, Associate Professor, School of Rehabilitation Sciences, University of British Columbia and Research Scientist, Arthritis Research Centre of Canada, Vancouver, British Columbia

Sue Baptiste, M.H.Sc., OT(C), OT Reg. (Ont.), Professor, School of Rehabilitation Science, McMaster University, Hamilton, Ontario

Brenda Beagan, Ph.D. Associate Professor, School of Occupational Therapy, Dalhousie University, Halifax, Nova Scotia

E. Sharon Brintnell, M.Sc., OT(C), FCAOT, CDMP, Professor, Department of Occupational Therapy, University of Alberta, Edmonton, Alberta

Jocelyn Brown, M.Sc. (OT – Post-Professional), OT(C), OT Reg. (NS), Assistant Professor, School of Occupational Therapy, Dalhousie University, Halifax, Nova Scotia

Debra Cameron, Ph.D., OT Reg. (Ont.), Assistant Professor, Department of Occupational Science and Occupational Therapy, University of Toronto, Partner, Reach Therapy Services, Toronto, Ontario

Noémi Cantin, M.Sc., Ph.D. (candidate), OT(C), OT Reg. (Ont.), Graduate Department of Rehabilitation Science, University of Toronto, Toronto, Ontario

Josiane Caron Santha, M.Sc. OT (Post-professional), OT(C), erg., OTR, Occupational Therapist Private Practice, Boucherville, Québec

Jo Clark, M.A., OT(C), OT Reg. (BC), Regional Allied Health Practice Director, Vancouver Coastal Health Authority, Vancouver, British Columbia

Lynn Cockburn, M.Ed., OT(C), OT Reg. (Ont.), Assistant Professor, Department of Occupational Science and Occupational Therapy, University of Toronto, Toronto, Ontario

Anne M. Connor-Schisler, M.Sc., OTR/L, Occupational Therapist, Aging With Flair, LLC, Simpsonville, South Carolina

Janet M. Craik, M.Sc., OT(C), OT Reg NB, Project Manager, *Enabling Occupation II*, Peer Review Coordinator, OTJR: Occupation, Participation and Health

Jane A. Davis, M.Sc., Ph.D. (candidate), OT(C), OT Reg. (Ont.), OTR, Lecturer, Department of Occupational Science and Occupational Therapy, University of Toronto, Toronto, Ontario

Randy Dickinson, B.A., CM Executive Director, Premier's Council on the Status of Disabled Persons, Fredericton, New Brunswick

Susan E. Doble, Ph.D., OT(C), OT Reg. (NS), Associate Professor, School of Occupational Therapy, Dalhousie University, Halifax, Nova Scotia

Catherine Donnelly, M.Sc., OT(C), OT Reg. (Ont.), Adjunct Assistant Professor, School of Rehabilitation Therapy, Queen's University, Kingston, Ontario

Hilary Drummond, B.Sc. (OT), OT(C), OT Reg. (BC), Certified Executive Coach and Associate Certified Coach, C.E.C., A.C.C., LEAP Coaching/Creative Therapy Consultants, Oliver, British Columbia

Claire-Jehanne Dubouloz-Wilner, Ph.D. OT(C), OT Reg. (Ont.), Associate Dean and Director School of Rehabilitation Sciences, University of Ottawa, Ottawa, Ontario

Parvin Eftekhar, M.Sc. (candidate), OT(C), OT Reg. (Ont.), Toronto Rehabilitation Institute, Toronto, Ontario

Mary Egan, Ph.D., OT(C), OT Reg. (Ont.), Associate Professor, School of Rehabilitation Sciences, University of Ottawa, Ottawa, Ontario

Andrew R. Freeman, M.Sc., Ph.D. (candidate), OT(C), OT Reg. (Ont.), Rehabilitation Sciences Program, The University of Western Ontario, London, Ontario

Continued ...

Andrew Harvey, Ph.D., Professor, Department of Economics, St Mary's University, Halifax, Nova Scotia

Brenda Head, M. Sc. (OT – Post-Professional), OT(C), OT Reg. (NL), Memorial University, St. John's, Newfoundland & Labrador, Research Capacity Building Transition Coordinator, Dalhousie University, Halifax, Nova Scotia

Michael Iwama, Ph.D., OT(C), OT Reg. (Ont.), Associate Professor, Department of Occupational Science and Occupational Therapy, University of Toronto, Toronto, Ontario

Jennifer Jarman, Ph.D. Assistant Professor, Department of Sociology, National University of Singapore, Singapore

Lyn Jongbloed, Ph.D., OT(C), OT Reg. (BC), Associate Professor, School of Rehabilitation Sciences, University of British Columbia, Vancouver, British Columbia

Bonnie Kirsh, Ph.D., OT(C), OT Reg. (Ont.), Associate Professor, Department of Occupational Science and Occupational Therapy, University of Toronto, Toronto, Ontario

Terry Krupa, Ph.D., OT(C), OT Reg. (Ont.), Associate Professor, School of Rehabilitation Therapy, Queen's University, Kingston, Ontario

Zofia Kumas-Tan, M.Sc. (OT– Post-professional), Project Associate, Center for Health Policy and Research, University of Massachusetts Medical School, Shrewsbury, Massachusetts

Debbie Laliberte Rudman, Ph.D., OT(C), OT Reg. (Ont.) Assistant Professor, School of Occupational Therapy, The University of Western Ontario, London, Ontario

Jennifer E. Landry, M.Sc., Ph.D. (candidate), OT(C), OT Reg. (Ont.), Department of Public Health Sciences, University of Toronto, Toronto, Ontario

Mary Law, Ph.D., OT(C), OT Reg. (Ont.), Professor and Associate Dean (Health Sciences) Rehabilitation Science, McMaster University, Hamilton, Ontario

Nancy Lin, M.Sc, OT(C), OT Reg. (Ont.), Clinical Redevelopment Transition Manager, Centre for Addiction and Mental Health, Toronto, Ontario

Lori Letts, Ph.D., OT(C), OT Reg. (Ont.), Associate Professor, School of Rehabilitation Science McMaster University Hamilton, Ontario

Lili Liu, Ph.D., OT(C) Associate Professor and Associate Chair, Department of Occupational Therapy, University of Alberta, Edmonton, Alberta

Mary Manojlovich, M.Ed., OT(C), OT Reg. (NL), Professional Practice Consultant, Occupational Therapy, Eastern Health St. John's, Newfoundland & Labrador

Pat McKee, M.Sc., OT(C), OT Reg. (Ont.), Associate Professor, Department of Occupational Science and Occupational Therapy, University of Toronto, Toronto, Ontario

Daniel K. Molke, M.Sc., Ph.D. (candidate), OT(C), OT Reg. (Ont.), Occupational Science Field Health and Rehabilitation Sciences Program, The University of Western Ontario, London, Ontario

Patricia Moores, B.Sc., OT(C), OT Reg. (NL), Occupational Therapist, Captain William Jackman Memorial Hospital, Labrador City, Newfoundland & Labrador

Wendy Pentland, Ph.D., OT(C), OT Reg. (Ont.), CPC Associate Professor, School of Rehabilitation Therapy, Queen's University, Kingston, Ontario

Huguette Picard, BSc., erg., FCAOT, Directrice de l'enseignement clinique, Programme d'ergothérapie, Université de Montréal, Montréal, Québec

Lisa Purdie, M.Sc. OT, erg., Occupational therapist, West Island Health and Social Services Center, Lakeshore General Hospital Pointe Claire, Québec

Judy Quach, M.Sc. OT, OT(C) Regional Manager, Occupational Therapy, Peace Country Health, QE II Hospital, Grande Prairie, Alberta

Susan Rappolt, Ph.D., OT(C), OT Reg. (Ont.), Associate Professor, Department of Occupational Science and Occupational Therapy, University of Toronto, Toronto, Ontario

Patty Rigby, M.H.Sc., OT(C), OT Reg. (Ont.), Assistant Professor and Graduate Coordinator, Department of Occupational Science and Occupational Therapy, University of Toronto, Toronto, Ontario

Continued ...

Annette Rivard, Ph.D.
(candidate), OT(C),
Assistant Professor,
Department of Occupational
Therapy, University of
Alberta, Edmonton, Alberta

Amy Sedgwick, B.Sc. (OT),
OT(C), OT Reg. (Ont.),
Occupational therapist,
Toronto, Ontario

Robin Stadnyk, Ph.D., OT(C),
Reg. (NS), Assistant
Professor, School of
Occupational Therapy,
Dalhousie University, Halifax,
Nova Scotia

Lynn Shaw, Ph.D., OT(C),
OT Reg. (Ont.), Assistant
Professor, School of
Occupational Therapy,
The University of Western
Ontario, London Ontario

Debra Stewart, M.Sc., OT(C),
OT Reg. (Ont.), Assistant
Dean, School of
Rehabilitation Science,
McMaster University,
Hamilton, Ontario

Lynn Stewart, B.Sc. (OT),
OT(C), OT Reg. (Ont.),
Professional Practice Leader,
Occupational Therapy,
St. Joseph's Health Care,
London, Ontario

Rachel Thibeault, Ph.D.
OT(C), OT Reg. (Ont.),
Occupational Therapy
Programme, School of
Rehabilitation Sciences,
University of Ottawa,
Ottawa, Ontario

Barry Trentham, M.E.S.,
OT(C), OT Reg. (Ont.),
Assistant Professor,
Department of Occupational
Science and Occupational
Therapy, University of
Toronto,Toronto, Ontario

Louis Trudel, Ph.D., erg.
Professor, Department of
Rehabilitation, Laval
University, Québec, Québec

Joan Versnel, Ph.D., OT(C),
OT Reg. (NS), Assistant
Professor, School of
Occupational Therapy,
Dalhousie University,
Halifax, Nova Scotia

Claudia von Zweck Ph.D.,
OT(C), OT Reg. (Ont.),
Executive Director,
Canadian Association of
Occupational Therapisits,
Ottawa, Ontario

Daniel, Zimmerman,
M.Sc., OT(C), OT Reg.
(Ont.), Occupational
Therapist,TSR Clinics,
Toronto, Ontario

Table of Contents

SECTION II

SECTION III

SECTION IV

PRACTICE CASES and EXEMPLARS

FIGURES

TABLES

TEXT BOXES

Acknowledgements

From CAOT

CAOT has a long history of working together with members to provide a vision for the conceptual grounding, processes and outcomes of occupational therapy in Canada. In the 1980s this vision was first articulated in the *Guidelines for Client-Centred Practice*. This publication was followed in 1997 with the introduction of *Enabling Occupation: An Occupational Therapy Perspective*. These publications have been integral to guide Canadian occupational therapy practice and as well, are now used in many countries around the world. Over the past 2 1/2 years, CAOT has been actively engaged in the process of developing this new publication that is complementary to these current CAOT documents and provides a vision for the future of occupational therapy practice and education in Canada. CAOT is pleased to bring you a document that reflects the changes that have occurred in the context of occupational therapy practice in the past decade with shifts in Canadian health and social policy, increased emphasis on evidence and accountability and new language and models of health.

CAOT would be remiss if we did not recognize the tremendous time and effort donated by the primary authors and editors, Elizabeth Townsend and Helene Polatajko. Their guidance and vision were instrumental in the development and completion of this truly collaborative effort. Aside from authoring new material, both primary authors devoted numerous hours towards the fusion of contributions from occupational therapists across Canada in order to bring you this coherent vision of enabling occupation.

In addition, the work and ideas of the over 60 contributing authors are sincerely appreciated for providing a truly national and collaborative perspective for this new publication.

From the Primary Authors

The authors are grateful to the many individuals who supported the creation of *Enabling II*. In addition to thanking the Contributing Authors for the generous sharing of their expertise, we wish to acknowledge and thank all those who contributed to the creation of *Enabling II*. This book would not have been possible without the generosity of the contributing authors, the vision and support of the CAOT, the dedication and skill of the Project Manager, the sage advice of the National Advisory Panel, the critical reflections and expertise of the peer reviewers, the keen eye of the readers and the capable work of the research assistants and publication team.

The Canadian Association of Occupational Therapists, in its efforts to promote excellence in occupational therapy in Canada and internationally, showed vision and leadership in initiating this project and bringing it to fruition. Dependent on the voluntary work of the primary and contributing authors, the national advisory panel, the readers, and the peer reviewers, this project would not have been possible without the generosity of the CAOT. Their funding and support provided the infrastructure necessary to enable the completion of this ambitious and important project. In particular, a special mention of gratitude is extended to Kathy Van Benthem, CAOT Professional Education Manager and Claudia von Zweck, CAOT Executive Director.

Project Manger

Many thanks to our Project Manager, Janet Craik. Janet managed the complex coordination of over 60 national contributors with multiple pieces of writing and ongoing submissions. Her superb organization of webconferencing with CAOT and the National Advisory Panel, and her research, as requested by the primary authors, helped the Primary Authors to manage the project with CAOT on time and on budget.

National Advisory Panel (Listed from west to east)

Jo Clark, M.A., OT(C), OT Reg. (BC), Regional Allied Health Practice Director, Vancouver Coastal Health Authority, Vancouver, British Columbia

Lyn Jongbloed, Ph.D., OT(C), OT Reg. (BC), Associate Professor, School of Rehabilitation Sciences, University of British Columbia, Vancouver, British Columbia

Lili Liu, Ph.D., OT(C), Associate Professor and Associate Chair, Department of Occupational Therapy, University of Alberta, Edmonton, Alberta

Bonny Jung, M.Ed., OT(C), OT Reg. (Ont.), Assistant Professor, School of Rehabilitation Science McMaster University, Hamilton, Ontario

Andrew R. Freeman, Ph.D. (candidate), OT(C), OT Reg. (Ont.), Rehabilitation Sciences Program, The University of Western Ontario, London, Ontario

Barry Trentham, M.E.S., OT(C), OT Reg. (Ont.), Assistant Professor, Department of Occupational Science and Occupational Therapy, University of Toronto, Toronto, Ontario

Terry Krupa, Ph.D., OT(C), OT Reg. (Ont.), Associate Professor, School of Rehabilitation Therapy, Queen's University Kingston, Ontario

Louis Trudel, erg., Ph.D., Full Professor, Department of Rehabilitation, Laval University, Québec, Québec

Randy Dickinson, B.A., C.M. Executive Director, Premier's Council on the Status of Disabled Persons, Fredericton, New Brunswick

Christel K.A. Seeberger, B.Sc. (OT), OT(C), OT RegNB, OTR, Occupational Therapist tOTal ability, Saint John, New Brunswick

Robin Stadnyk, Ph.D., OT(C), OT Reg. (NS), Assistant Professor, School of Occupational Therapy, Dalhousie University, Halifax, Nova Scotia

Peer Reviewers

Consumer

Shawn Jennings, MD
Retired family physician, brainstem stroke survivor, and author of *Locked In Locked Out*, Rothesay, New Brunswick

International

Gail Whiteford, Ph.D., Professor and Chair, Occupational Therapy Charles Sturt University Albury, New South Wales, Australia

National

Thelma Sumsion Ph.D., OT(C), OT Reg. (Ont.), Director, School of Occupational Therapy, The University of Western Ontario, London, Ontario

Sandra Bressler, M.A., OT(C), OT Reg. (BC), FCAOT, Clinical Assistant Professor, School of Rehabilitation Sciences, University of British Columbia, Vancouver, British Columbia

Francophone

Louis Trudel, erg., Ph.D., Professor, Department of Rehabilitation, Laval University, Québec, Québec

Line Robichaud, erg., PhD, Professor, Occupational Therapy, Department of Rehabilitation, Laval University, Québec, Québec

Chantale Marcoux, erg., Lecturer, Occupational Therapy, Department of Rehabilitation, Laval University, Québec, Québec

Manon Boucher, erg. MSc., Lecturer, Occupational Therapy, Department of Rehabilitation, Laval University, Québec Québec

Geneviève Pépin, erg., PhD, Assistant Professor, Occupational Therapy, Department of Rehabilitation, Laval University, Québec, Québec

Monique Carriere, erg., PhD, Associate Professor, Occupational Therapy, Department of Rehabilitation, Laval University, Québec, Québec

Readers

Brenda Beagan, Ph.D., Associate Professor, School of Occupational Therapy, Dalhousie University, Halifax, Nova Scotia

Walter C. (Pete) Howell, Ph.D., Professor Emeritus, The University of Western Ontario, London, Ontario

Zofia Kumas-Tan, M.Sc. (OT–Post-professional), Project Associate, Center for Health Policy and Research University of Massachusetts Medical School, Shrewsbury, Massachusetts

Research Assistants

Helena DeZoysa, B.Sc. (OT) (candidate), Dalhousie University, Halifax, Nova Scotia

Becky Sittler, B.Sc. (OT) (candidate), Dalhousie University, Halfax, Nova Scotia

Publication Team

Lauren Klump, Copyeditor, Ottawa, Ontario

Lyne St-Hilaire-Tardif (LYNE'S WORD), Editing/Proofreading /Translating Services, Ottawa, Ontario

Lauraine Teodoro-Goyette, Senior Translator and Copy editor, Promo Texte, Rockland, Ontario

Danielle Stevens Peak, Graphic Design Coordinator, Canadian Association of Occupational Therapisits, Ottawa, Ontario

Doug Porter, Virtual Image Productions, Halifax, Nova Scotia

Kathy Van Benthem, Professional Education Manager, Canadian Association of Occupational Therapisits, Ottawa, Ontario

Foreword

The quality of life and participation of all persons are significantly influenced by the occupations they engage in every day. Indeed, participation in occupation is essential, as much as food to eat, clothes to wear, and air to breathe. Occupations are complex and change over a person's life course. Participation in the daily occupations such as self-care, work, play, education, and leisure sustains our health and well-being.

Occupation is the context in which people develop skills, express their feelings, construct relationships, create knowledge, and find meaning and purpose in life. Yet, for many citizens in Canada and indeed, worldwide, occupations are not easily undertaken. For those who are marginalized because of chronic illness, disability, or life circumstances, participation in daily occupations is all too often restricted.

Occupational therapists in Canada are committed to enabling occupation for all citizens, whether individuals, groups, or populations. This book, *Enabling Occupation II: Advancing an Occupational Therapy Vision for Health, Well-Being, & Justice through Occupation* is an important reflection of this commitment. *Enabling Occupation II* is Canada's eighth publication of national guidelines for client-centred enablement focused on occupation and occupational performance (CAOT, 1991, 1993, 1997a, 2002; DNHW & CAOT, 1983, 1986, 1987).

Drawing on the experience and research of over 60 Canadian authors, *Enabling Occupation II* advances the core concepts of occupation and enablement and their application in practice, education, and research. Within the book, a new definition of occupational therapy is offered. *Occupational therapy is the art and science of enabling engagement in everyday living, through occupation; of enabling people to perform the occupations that foster health and well-being; and of enabling a just and inclusive society so that all people may participate to their potential in the daily occupations of life.*

Enabling Occupation II is a sequel and companion to *Enabling Occupation: An Occupational Therapy Perspective* (1997a, 2002). *Enabling Occupation II* continues the goal of increasing our understanding of approaches and methods to enable individual and social change. The book is organized into four sections – the core domain of concern, the core competency, practicing occupation-based enablement, and positioning practice. An expanded Canadian Model of Occupational Performance and Engagement (CMOP-E) locates the focus of practice in occupation, occupational performance, and beyond.

This book challenges assumptions held about occupational therapy in Canada and broadens the focus of the profession. I have no doubt that ideas within this book will encourage lively discussion, support occupational therapy education, and lead to innovative developments. Fostering our leadership in enabling occupation within Canada is clearly articulated. Congratulations to Elizabeth Townsend and Helene Polatajko, to contributing authors, and to the profession of occupational therapy on advancing a Canadian vision of health, well-being, and justice that engages Canadians as participating citizens in their everyday occupations.

Mary Law, Ph.D., FCAOT
Associate Dean and Director
School of Rehabilitation Science
McMaster University
Hamilton, Ontario

Prologue

The Canadian journey toward client-centred occupational therapy has a very rich history. We took our first tentative steps in the early 1980s when a national group of occupational therapists and medical representatives joined to develop the *Guidelines for the Client-centred Practice of Occupational Therapy*, published in 1983. That was a pivotal moment in our history, and we have never looked back. A committed group of therapists continued to move the work forward through the development of many subsequent documents that have shaped our practice, and reminded therapists to ensure that the client is a key player in our actions and interventions. Our thinking, and the theoretical underpinnings of our work, have continued to develop over the intervening 24 years and have culminated in the production of this milestone publication. Many knowledgeable and talented therapists have contributed to this document that will lead our practice for many years. This work greatly clarifies both the development and use of relevant models to guide our interventions. It also provides clarity on many complex concepts and introduces new concepts to challenge our thinking and ways of applying a client-centred approach. My sincere thanks to the primary authors and contributors who have ensured that Canada will continue to lead the campaign for client-centred occupational therapy.

Thelma Sumsion, Ph.D., FCAOT
Director
School of Occupational Therapy
The University of Western Ontario
London, Ontario

Introduction

Vision

To herald an era of occupational enablement for occupational therapists and their clients.

Purpose

To honour our past, affirm our present, and profile a future that is focused on occupation-based enablement.

Objectives

- To publish the sequel and companion to Enabling Occupation: An Occupational Therapy Perspective (Canadian Association of Occupational Therapists [CAOT], 1997, 2002);
- To extend our understanding of the concepts of occupation and enablement introduced in *Enabling Occupation* (CAOT, 1997a, 2002);
- To profile occupation as the core domain and enabling as the core competency of occupational therapy;
- To explicate the practice mosaic that is occupation-based enablement, describe a process for examining occupational issues and a practice framework for addressing them, and provide exemplars that illustrate the breadth of occupational therapy with its diverse clients in diverse contexts;
- To honour and affirm Canada's 25 years of occupational therapy leadership, and to profile occupation-based enablement supported by scholarship, evidence, accountability, funding, and workforce planning in multiple systems and multicultural contexts;
- To present a glossary of terms, references, and keyword search strategies associated with occupation-based enablement.

Intro.1 A watershed book with a national perspective

Enabling Occupation II: Advancing an Occupational Therapy Vision for Health, Well-being, & Justice through Occupation is a watershed publication by the Canadian Association of Occupational Therapists, the national professional body for occupational therapy in Canada. The book honours the past, affirms the present, and profiles a future for occupational therapy focused on occupation-based enablement. The book advances the transformation of occupational therapy from being a profession focused on the therapeutic use of activity, to one dedicated to enabling all people to be engaged in meaningful occupation and to participate as fully as possible in society.

Enabling Occupation II advances the core concepts of occupation and enablement, and their application in practice, education, and research. Benefiting from the contribution of over 60 authors in Canada, *Enabling Occupation II* raises complex sociocultural issues, such as diversity, individualism and collectivism, language, economy, and regulation. Cultural and linguistic variations, growing evidence from occupational therapy journals, texts, and conferences indicate that the concepts and practice of enabling occupation resonate with occupational therapists, other professionals, and society across Canada and worldwide. An occupational perspective is an idea whose time has come. Practical strategies for advancing a vision of health, well-being, and justice, through occupation have high potential to serve societies everywhere.

With its focus on occupation as the core domain and enablement as the core competency, this book addresses the age-old question, What is occupational therapy? We offer an updated response to this question in the book's new definition of occupational therapy.

> *Occupational therapy is the art and science of enabling engagement in everyday living, through occupation; of enabling people to perform the occupations that foster health and well-being; and of enabling a just and inclusive society so that all people may participate to their potential in the daily occupations of life.*

Consultative strategies gave the book a national perspective through:
- formation of a 11-member, national advisory panel, which generally met bimonthly to provide input on content and the national, consultation process, representing:
  - diverse practice: clinical, management, consultation, education, research;
  - consumers;
  - Health Canada;
  - CAOT staff.
- direct invitations to individuals from across the country, based on expertise, to become contributing authors: chapter co-authors, case writers, or text box writers;
- a multi-step, peer review process: each chapter was reviewed by contributing authors and the book was reviewed by consumer, national and international experts;
- extended sessions at the 2005 and 2006 national CAOT conferences;
- topic-specific focus groups with national and international audiences;
- a public discussion board on the CAOT Web site with updates and an invitation for comments.

Intro.2 Primary authors' perspectives

Enabling occupation is a dream shared by the CAOT and this book's two primary authors, Elizabeth Townsend and Helene Polatajko. The primary authors are both long-time advocates of occupation-based enablement from different perspectives.

Townsend, an occupational therapist with a Ph.D. in adult education, takes a social perspective on enabling social justice. In her *Muriel Driver Memorial Lecture* (1993), she critically analyzed client-centred practice and proposed that occupational therapy is based on a historic, implicit social vision of justice in everyday occupations:

> *Occupational therapy has tremendous unfulfilled potential ... critical analysis shows that occupational therapy's vision is to promote social justice by enabling people to participate as valued members of society despite diverse or limited occupational potential ... this is an enabling rather than a treatment type of therapy ... The use of everyday occupations is fundamental ... we have a vision of society beyond individualism ...We are challenged to fulfill our activist heritage ... and take our place on a world stage* (Townsend, 1993, pp. 174-184).

Polatajko, an occupational therapist with a Ph.D. in educational theory, takes an individualistic perspective on enabling people to be fully occupationally engaged. In her *Muriel Driver Memorial Lecture* (1992), she highlighted the importance of framing our profession in occupation and advocated for the adoption of an enablement perspective. Subsequently, she argued for the elaboration of our understanding of occupation and enablement:

> *With our new enablement perspective, our challenge is to learn to fully understand the occupational human and the nature of enablement, to push forward a science of occupation in conjunction with a science of enablement. If we do this well, our opportunity and our privilege will be to enable the occupation of all people, to go beyond the medical mission of preserving life to the occupational mission of enabling living (adapted from Polatajko, 2001, p. 207).*

Intro.3 Values and beliefs for enabling occupation

Enabling II is entrenched in the values and beliefs that guided the development of the original *Enabling Occupation* (CAOT, 1997a, 2002). With *Enabling II* these values are reaffirmed and adapted to reflect the new content presented here. Accordingly:

About occupation, we believe that:
- Occupation gives meaning to life;
- Occupation is an important determinant of health, well-being, and justice;
- Occupation organizes behaviour;
- Occupation develops and changes over a lifetime;
- Occupation shapes and is shaped by environments;
- Occupation has therapeutic potential.

About the person, we believe that:
- Humans are occupational beings;
- Every person is unique;

- Every person has intrinsic dignity and worth;
- Every person has the right to make choices about life;
- Every person has the right to self-determination;
- People have some ability to participate in occupations;
- People have some potential to change;
- People are social and spiritual beings;
- People have diverse abilities for participating in occupations;
- People shape and are shaped by their environments.

About the environment, we believe that:

- The environment includes cultural, institutional, physical, and social components;
- The environment influences choice, organization, performance, and satisfaction in occupations.

About health, well-being, and justice, we believe that:

- Health is more than the absence of disease;
- Health is strongly influenced by having choice and control in everyday occupations;
- Health has personal dimensions associated with spiritual meaning and satisfaction in occupations, and it has social dimensions associated with fairness and equitable opportunity in occupations;
- Well-being extends beyond health to quality of life;
- Justice concerns are for meaningful choice and social inclusion, so that all people may participate as fully as possible in society.

About client-centred practice, we believe that:

- Clients are experts regarding their own occupations;
- Clients must be active partners in the occupational therapy process.

(Adapted from *Enabling Occupation*, CAOT, 1997, 2002, p. 31)

Intro.4 Background of Canadian guidelines development

In 1997 the CAOT produced *Enabling Occupation: An Occupational Therapy Perspective* (CAOT, 1997a), reprinted in 2002 with an updated Preface (CAOT, 2002, pp. xvi-xxxi). By describing occupational therapy as enabling occupation, the 1997 Guidelines made explicit, occupational therapy's intention to reinstate *occupation* as central to practice; both as means (therapeutic medium) and ends (outcome) (Townsend, 2002). During most of the 20th century, occupational therapy was described as the *therapeutic use of activity* (Polatajko, 2001). By publishing the *Occupational Performance Model* (OPM), adapted from Reed and Sanderson (Department of National Health and Welfare [DNHW] & CAOT, 1983, p. 8), in the first national guidelines, Canadian occupational therapy signaled the renaissance of occupation as a core concept for occupational therapy (CAOT, 1991; DNHW & CAOT, 1983). Further, by naming *enabling* as the profession's primary *modus operandi* in 1997, the profession encompassed what was described in the 1980s guidelines as the *teaching-learning process*, with recognition of the worth of the individual and respect for holism (CAOT, 1991, pp. 15-19).

Enabling Occupation II: Advancing an Occupational Therapy Vision for Health, Well-being, & Justice through Occupation is Canada's eighth publication intended to serve as national guidelines for client-centred enablement focused on occupation and occupational performance (CAOT, 1991, 1993, 1997a, 2002; DNHW & CAOT, 1983, 1986, 1987). The development of the *Canadian Occupational Performance Measure* (COPM) (Law et al., 2005; Law, Steinwender, & Leclair, 1998) was a direct outcome of the 1987 guidelines, *Toward Outcome Measures in Occupational Therapy* (DNHW & CAOT, 1987). *Occupational Therapy Guidelines for Client-Centred Mental Health Practice* (CAOT, 1993) were the only targeted guidelines. Their purpose was to broaden the definition of client-centred practice and give prominence to the "concept of enabling, which has been fundamental to occupational therapy philosophy" (CAOT, 1993, p. v).

A study of occupational therapists' perceptions of the guidelines (Blain & Townsend, 1993) found that they provided a unified view of the core concepts of practice. Given the growth of practice, graduate education, and research, the study recommended that new guidelines develop the *Occupational Performance Model* (OPM), and include illustrations for integrating the concepts across the scope of practice. To follow up, CAOT sponsored a national consultation that resulted in publication of the 1997 guidelines with the new *Canadian Model of Occupational Performance* (CMOP).

Since their publication in 1997, the guidelines for enabling occupation have sparked important discussions. Key points of critique, which were raised in the 2002 preface to *Enabling Occupation* and elsewhere, have influenced *Enabling Occupation II*. The main developments that distinguish the books are captured in table Intro.1.

Intro.5 The Canadian context

The context of Canadian practice is affected first and foremost by Canada's sociocultural diversity. The broad cultural mosaic that is Canada offers a complex and challenging context for making practice relevant and effective. Our diversity in Canada calls on us to enact an occupational therapy that is inclusive, equitable, just and truly enabling, and to develop a more progressive mandate in the broader global context. We are reminded to pay attention to the existence of diverse world views, and the fundamental effect of such views on the understandings of the form, function, and meanings of occupation (Iwama, 2003).

In light of Canada's sociocultural diversity (Association of Canadian Occupational Therapy Regulatory Organizations [ACOTRO], Association of Canadian Occupational Therapy University Programmes [ACOTUP], Canadian Association of Occupational Therapists [CAOT], & Professional Alliances of Canada [PAC], 2006), occupational therapists are being spurred toward a deeper appreciation for the complexity of occupation and enablement. *Enabling Occupation II* addresses the issue of sociocultural diversity in numerous ways. The book has been written with consideration for diverse people, practice settings, and systems in the cases and language used throughout. Reflections on diversity issues are inserted to set a tone of critical reflection as a hallmark of occupational therapy. Such attempts to articulate consciousness of culture and diversity may encourage Canadian occupational therapists to pursue equitable and socially progressive practice. It may be our Canadian contribution toward advancing the profession to maintain relevance and meaning for our clients in an increasing global world.

Table Intro.1 Distinguishing the 1997 and 2002 guidelines from *Enabling Occupation II*

Concepts and critiques of the original *Enabling Occupation*	Treatment in *Enabling Occupation II*
Occupational performance: Occupational therapy is concerned with more than performance, for instance: occupational transformation, occupational meaning, occupational identity, occupational engagement, occupational justice, and occupational balance.	Section I, which focuses on occupation, discusses occupation *beyond performance* and captures the importance of this extension by renaming the CMOP as the CMOP-E.
CMOP with the person in the foreground: The implication is that occupational therapy's primary concern is with persons, not occupation.	Section I introduces a trans-sectional view or *side slice* of the CMOP-E showing occupation both as the core domain of concern and also as the concept that delimits concerns for persons and environment.
CMOP with the person in the foreground: The implication is that occupational therapy is only concerned with the individual.	Occupational therapists have historically worked with individuals, families, groups, communities, organizations, and populations as clients. Section II introduces a client pyramid to illustrate the diversity of occupational therapy clients
CMOP with environment at the back: The implication is that the environment, being at the back, is external to occupations and persons and is of secondary concern.	The CMOP-E *side slice* shows the environment larger than persons in relation to occupation, and it depicts occupation, persons, the environment, and spirituality as interconnected.
Person-Environment-Occupation (PEO) Model: Many have wondered about the relationship between CMOP and PEO, and have confused the PEO for the "Canadian model." The PEO illustrates a transactional view of occupational performance at the intersections of person, environment, and occupation, without making spirituality or the focus on occupation explicit.	*Enabling Occupation II* introduces the CMOP-E which makes explicit the focus on occupation and the inclusion of spirituality. While the PEO is referred to, it is not specifically included in this book in order to avoid confusion.
Occupational Performance Process Model (OPPM): The OPPM was developed primarily for working with individuals (CAOT, 1997a, pp. 57-94; Fearing & Clark, 2000). The OPPM omits important stages of the occupational therapy process, such as *enter/initiate, set the stage,* and *conclude/exit.*	*Enabling Occupation II* emphasizes practice with a range of clients and diverse practice in management, consulting, policy, education, and research contexts. A new Canadian Practice Process Framework (CPPF) is based on client-centred enablement, is evidence-based and occupation-based to allow for application in diverse practice contexts, is goal driven, and applies to the full scope of clients engaged in processes of occupational enablement.
Enabling: Enabling Occupation contains relatively little discussion of the specifics of the concept and practice of enabling. The term is simply defined as "more than client-centred practice," and is followed by a detailed discussion of client-centred practice.	Section II focuses on enabling (verb) and enablement (noun) as the core competency of occupational therapy, consistent with the definition of competencies in the updated *Profile of Occupational Therapy Practice in Canada* (CAOT, 2007).

Intro.6 Learner-centred practice guidelines

Enabling Occupation II is a sequel and companion to *Enabling Occupation* (CAOT, 1997a, 2002). Descriptions of the Canadian Model of Occupational Performance (CMOP), the Person-Environment-Occupation (PEO) model, and the Occupational Performance Process Model (OPPM) published in *Enabling Occupation* (1997a, 2002) are not republished in *Enabling Occupation II*.

Instead, learners are presented with scholarship and evidence to firmly ground occupational therapy in occupation and enablement. Learners will find a *triple model framework* to guide occupational therapy: the Canadian Model of Occupational Performance and Engagement (CMOP-E), which portrays an occupational perspective that includes and extends beyond occupational performance; the Canadian Model of Client-Centred Enablement (CMCE), which portrays a spectrum of enablement skills based on enablement foundations (beliefs, values, assumptions, concepts) to alert practitioners to the core competence and power relations in occupational therapy's client-centred practice; and, the Canadian Practice Process Framework (CPPF), which portrays eight action points and alternative pathways in the process of practice with clients who may be individuals, families, groups, communities, organizations, or populations.

The authors have taken a learner-centred approach both in structure and language. The cases and exemplars are drawn from actual people, places, situations, or practice conditions. Professional reasoning on occupation and enablement, practice cases and exemplars, and strategies for positioning the profession for leadership in occupation-based enablement are interwoven to prompt experiential, competency-based, case-based, or problem-based adult learning styles, beyond rote learning. Theory is illustrated to guide practice just as practice continues to inform the evolution of occupational therapy theory. Reflective practice, attending to diversity and context, not standardized practice based on fixed protocols, is emphasized. These are not technical guidelines for specific procedures. Rather, the book offers practice guidelines for the broad and complex application of the profession's core concepts.

Intro.7 Voice and audience

The first *Enabling Occupation* (CAOT, 1997a, 2002) was written about occupational therapy in the third person. This version is written in the first person *with* and *for* occupational therapy students and practitioners — from front-line clinicians to consultants, administrators, researchers, academics, and support personnel — who address the occupational issues of various types of clients in diverse practice contexts.

We welcome occupational therapy allies, partners, consumers, employers, governments, business, and the public to read the book. We encourage you to learn about modern occupational therapy. As Dr. Shawn Jennings, a reviewer for the book, stated, "*Enabling Occupation* opened my eyes to a new understanding about the mission of occupational therapy… [and to] occupation as a health benefit."

Intro.8 Organization of the book

Enabling Occupation II: Advancing an Occupational Therapy Vision for Health, Well-being, & Justice through Occupation is organized into four sections; each begins with a statement of vision, purpose, objectives and practice implications.

Section I addresses occupation and describes its centrality to our domain of concern, giving an overview of the key characteristics of human occupation and positioning it in the science of occupation. The introduction of an expanded Canadian Model of Occupational Performance and Engagement (CMOP-E) locates the focus of practice in occupation, occupational performance, and beyond. A transverse view of the CMOP-E clarifies that occupation is our primary concern and that person and environment are points of analysis to inform an occupational perspective.

Section II addresses enablement as our core competency, giving an overview of key enablement foundations, client-centred relationships, and enablement skills. The Canadian Model of Client-Centred Enablement (CMCE) identifies the key skills for enabling individual and social change. The range of ineffective to effective client-centred enablement is portrayed on an Enablement Continuum.

Section III integrates the two core concepts of occupation and enablement to describe the rich practice mosaic of occupation-based enablement. It gives shape and form to the theoretical foundations for enabling change and introduces a Canadian Practice Process Framework (CPPF) for use with various clients in diverse settings. The CPPF is illustrated with practice cases and exemplars of occupation-based enablement of individual and social change.

Section IV addresses the enablement of the profession itself, and the positioning of occupational therapy for leadership in enabling occupation. It positions the profession's occupational perspective within the context of scholarship, evidence-based practice, accountability strategies, policy and funding, and workforce planning.

SECTION I

Occupation: The core domain of concern for occupational therapy

Introduction

Occupational therapy, in the broad sense of the term, has become the most serious problem before the statesmen of every nation in the world at the present time. All over the civilized globe, the widespread disease of unemployment, (lack of occupation), is monopolizing the attention of national parliaments and world conferences. Everywhere the effort is being made to remedy human dissatisfaction and mental unrest by providing daily tasks in order to occupy minds, so that bodies may be healthy, and the means of sustenance may be found (Howland, 1933, p.4).

As reflected by the words of Goldwin Howland, first President of the Canadian Association of Occupational Therapists, Canadian occupational therapy has been concerned with occupation from its inception. Occupation as a core concept has been rediscovered at various points throughout the history of our profession, culminating in the 1997 publication of *Enabling Occupation: An Occupational Therapy Perspective* (CAOT), which named occupation as a core concept of occupational therapy.

This section will focus on the concept of occupation. It will name occupation as the core domain of concern for occupational therapy, describe the evolution of its central role, and present the most current understandings we have of the concept. The section will draw on the literature from occupational therapy, occupational science, and relevant disciplines to specify the concept and present the key characteristics of human occupation. Organized into three chapters: chapter 1 will specify the concept and its centrality for the profession by drawing on our history; describe the evolution of the primacy of the concept bringing some clarity to the language of occupation; and, present the major models that have been created to explicate the concept. In chapter 2, the key characteristics of human occupation will be discussed, including how occupations develop across important life stages, how occupation changes, and how occupation affects and is affected by context. Finally, chapter 3 will position occupational therapy relative to occupational science and present information from key Canadian occupational scientists whose work provides evidence of the social significance of occupational therapy's occupation-based practice.

Vision

To embrace *human* occupation as the core domain of concern for occupational therapy.

Purpose

To present our best understanding of human occupation as it relates to occupational therapy.

Objectives

- To identify occupation as our core domain of concern;
- To reflect on the evolution of our occupational perspective;
- To introduce language frameworks and models that address occupational performance;
- To project our scope of concern beyond occupational performance;
- To describe the state of the art in our understanding of human occupation;
- To situate occupational science in occupational therapy;
- To describe the implications of selected occupational science topics for occupational therapy practice.

Practice implications

Section I allows you, as a practitioner, to reflect on the implications that embracing occupation as our core domain of concern has for your practice. It invites readers from outside occupational therapy to recognize the centrality of occupation in our lives. The section promotes an appreciation of the full breadth of human occupation and facilitates the adoption of an occupational perspective in viewing the world. In reading and using the research presented in Section I, you are encouraged to adopt an occupational perspective — as a clinician, an educator, researcher, administrator, manager, consultant, or other type of practitioner, or as a reader who is not an occupational therapist. Immerse yourself in the language, frameworks, and models that will help organize your thoughts. Explore the learning that occupational science offers, and articulate your understanding and appreciation of occupation.

Chapter 1

Specifying the domain of concern: Occupation as core

Helene J. Polatajko
Jane Davis
Deb Stewart
Noémi Cantin
Bice Amoroso
Lisa Purdie
Daniel Zimmerman

CASE 1 Bonnie Sherr Klein: Doing my real work

Bonnie Sherr Klein, an accomplished filmmaker, author, and disability activist, has written and spoken extensively about her recovery from a debilitating brain stem stroke, and her experience of being a disabled person in a world that is not really ready for the disabled. In her keynote address at the 1995 annual conference of the Canadian Association of Occupational Therapists, while speaking on the theme of *Partners in Practice*, Bonnie recounted a particularly poignant story. But first, the context!

In August 1987, at the age of 46, Bonnie was in the midst of *Mile Zero: The SAGE Tour*, when she suffered two catastrophic strokes caused by hemorrhaging of a congenital malformation in her brain stem. She became quadriplegic, required a respirator to breathe, and experienced panic attacks and locked-in syndrome. Having survived an extremely delicate and high-risk operation, Bonnie began a long and arduous process of rehabilitation that lasted over 3 years. Bonnie was determined to finish her film, and during the early stages of her rehabilitation she devoted all her weekends to that goal.

During the keynote she recounted:

> "I would work during my weekend off and return exhausted. I was often scolded for wearing myself out on the film. I felt as if I was cheating on my rehabilitation work ... when I was doing my real work of filmmaking. It was not until after the film was finished and released nearly one and a half years after the stroke that I realized myself that this was my occupational therapy (as occupational therapy was probably meant to be). It required all my previous skills and experience, plus many new adaptations: it was going to be useful; it reconnected me to the wide world outside my body; it forced me to 'come out' and be seen in public; and it brought me validation as a productive person. I regained a sense of myself" (CAOT, 2002, p. viii-ix).

Mile Zero: The SAGE Tour was released in 1988.

Data sources: CAOT (2002)
and Library and Archives Canada (2006)

1.1 Introduction

As Bonnie Sherr Klein noted, recovery from stroke, enabled by engagement in meaningful occupation, is occupational therapy as it is meant to be. From its very beginning, occupational therapy has been concerned with occupation and its role in health and well-being. As early as 1919, Dunton established this in his credo:

> *Occupation is as necessary to life as food and drink*
> *Every human being should have both physical and mental occupations*
> *All should have occupations which they enjoy, or hobbies*
> *Sick minds, sick bodies and sick souls may be healed thru occupation.*
> *(Dunton, 1919, p.10)*

However, as the *Ottawa Charter for Health Promotion* (WHO, 1986) makes clear, the emphasis on health should not be overstated; occupation has value in its own right as a resource for everyday life.

> *To reach a state of complete physical, mental and social well-being, an individual or group must be able to identify and to realize aspirations, to satisfy needs, and to change or cope with the environment. Health is, therefore, seen as a **resource for everyday life**, not the objective of living. (WHO, 1986, p. 1).*

1.2 The evolution of our occupational perspective: Occupation as the core domain

Over the course of the profession's history, the concept of occupation has evolved, as has the centrality of its role. In 2001, for the 75th anniversary issue of the *Canadian Journal of Occupational Therapy*, Polatajko traced this evolution by reviewing all the issues of the journal from 1933–2001. She concluded that the path has been **from the provision of diversional activity, through the use of therapeutic activity, to enablement through meaningful occupation.**

Initially occupation was essentially conceptualized in terms of work – not necessarily paid work, but work nonetheless. Polatajko's (2001) review noted that the term "occupational therapy" was first coined by George Barton, an American architect, who championed the idea of curing by means of work. The pervading belief at the time was that work, or occupation, was essential to health, well-being, and happiness.

> *Our greatest happiness in life does not depend on the condition of life in which chance has placed us, but is always the result of good conscience, good health, occupation, and freedom in all just pursuits (Thomas Jefferson).*

Thomas Jefferson (1743–1826) stated "it is neither wealth nor splendor; but tranquility and occupation which give you happiness." And, more importantly for occupational therapy, as the quote from Howland at the outset of this paragraph suggests, the absence of work leads to a general deterioration of the human spirit.

Accordingly, the initial aim of occupational therapy was to provide opportunities for occupational engagement, (a.k.a. work), in order to occupy individuals during their convalescence: "… to provide the patient with a well-balanced day, as nearly approaching normal as is possible in an institutional set-up" (LeVesconte, 1935, p. 6). It was assumed that this diversional use of work would not only prevent deterioration, but promote recovery instead.

> *The objective [of occupational therapy] is two-fold. First, to keep occupied, during at least part of the long, tiresome period of invalidism, the minds of those who are temporarily swept aside from healthy living by the ravages of disease and of those who are permanently unable to live normal lives with normal people. Second, to adapt the methods of treatment to the needs of the individual so that, by active occupation, maimed limbs and minds may be once more restored to health (Howland, 1933, p. 4).*

That occupation has the potential of therapeutic value was a central tenet of practice from the inception of the profession in Canada. However, from the 1940s onward, the curative potential of occupation was no longer referred to in terms of occupation; rather, it was captured in a number of other concepts including work (e.g., Martin, 1941) and arts and crafts (e.g., Robinson, 1942). The most longstanding among these was the concept of therapeutic activity, which was given prominence by Howland in his writings in 1944.

> *Occupational therapy is based on the principle that since voluntary activity is a normal function of every organ and structure, then, when injury or disease has resulted in an impaired activity, amelioration or recovery may be greatly assisted, on the one hand by physical exercise of the disabled member, while, on the other hand, the patient's mind is kept preoccupied with some diversional occupation such as art, music, crafts or recreation (Howland, 1944, pp. 32-33).*

With Howland's statement, the profession was defined in terms of therapeutic use of activity for the next 50 years. There seemed to be no need for a focus on occupation.

The emphasis on **therapeutic use of activity** notwithstanding, literature in the 1950s began to describe ever-broader roles for occupational therapy. In 1953, Hossack noted that occupational therapists should assist people in carrying out their occupational roles. By the 1960s, it was suggested that therapists should help their patients "participate more effectively in our society" (Roberts, 1962, p. 5); that the role should go beyond the restoration of function and "… seek to help him grow and develop, to make use of all of his abilities and thus more effectively realize his potential" (Jantzen, 1963, p. 23); to live, not merely exist (Cardwell, 1966), engaged in activities that are meaningful to them (Shimeld, 1971), in their own environments (McKay, 1974).

The evolution of our perspective on occupation is evident in the Canadian literature — from the use of diversional activity through the therapeutic use of activity, to enablement through meaningful engagement in occupation. We now recognize that "the vital need served by occupational therapy is man's need for occupation" (Woodside, 1976, p. 12). The concept of occupation was revived in occupational therapy by the American occupational therapist Mary Reilly (1962), one of the most influential writers in the profession in the latter part of the last millennium. Reilly reintroduced the focus on occupation and extended the profession's scope beyond the medical/curative model to an occupational model. In 1992, Polatajko suggested that the profession embrace this occupational perspective and name and frame itself as *enabling occupation*. In 1993, Townsend, echoing that vision, extended it beyond the individual to include a social mission. The 1997 publication of *Enabling Occupation: An Occupational Therapy Perspective*, entrenched the centrality of occupation as our domain of concern in stating that, "This primary role of enabling occupation constitutes a necessary and sufficient condition for the practice of occupational therapy" (CAOT, 1997a, p. 30).

1.3 Specification of an occupational perspective: Our language

Definitions

In broadening the role of occupational therapy from occupying the invalid to enabling occupation with diverse clients, the concept of occupation was broadened. As defined in *Enabling Occupation* (CAOT, 1997a), the term *occupation* refers not only to work, paid or unpaid, but to all manner of human doing be it self-care, productivity, or leisure.

> *Occupation refers to groups of activities and tasks of everyday life, named, organized, and given value and meaning by individuals and a culture. Occupation is everything people do to occupy themselves, including looking after themselves (self-care), enjoying life (leisure), and contributing to the social and economic fabric of their communities (productivity) (CAOT, 1997a, p. 34).*

Broadening the definition of occupation in Canada was in keeping with international trends. For example, in 1983, Reed and Sanderson defined occupation as, "activities or tasks which engage a person's time and energy; specifically self-care, productivity and leisure" (p. 247). Christiansen, Clark, Kielhofner, and Rogers (1995) defined occupation as the ordinary and familiar things that people do every day. Kielhofner's (1995) definition specified that occupation included doing culturally meaningful work, play or daily living tasks in the stream of time and in the contexts of one's physical and social world. Perhaps the most widely cited definition was that offered by Yerxa and her colleagues (Yerxa et al., 1990) who stated that occupation refers to "specific chunks of activity within the ongoing stream of human behaviour which are named in the lexicon of the culture" (p. 1).

These definitions ascribe a meaning to occupation that is not only broader than that understood by occupational therapists in the early days of the profession; the meaning is broader than that understood by the general public. In general day-to-day parlance, the primary understanding of the term *occupation* is "a person's usual or principal work or business, especially as a means of earning a living; vocation" (Merriam-Webster, 2003). This day-to-day parlance notwithstanding, Merriam-Webster (2003) cites as the first definition "occupation: an activity in which one engages (pursuing pleasure has been his major occupation)."

A taxonomic code for occupation

Occupational therapists' rediscovery of the concept of occupation does not mean that other concepts, in particular the concept of activity, no longer have a place in the profession. Rather, it means that the profession has to specify the use of these terms and their relation to each other (Polatajko et al., 2004). Indeed, many of the current definitions of occupation do just that; for example, occupation refers to groups of activities and tasks (CAOT, 1997a, 2002); doing culturally meaningful work, play, or daily living tasks (Kielhofner, 1995) activities or tasks (Reed & Sanderson, 1983); "specific chunks of activity" (Yerxa et al., 1990, p. 5).

The relationship between occupation, activity, and task is not consistently defined; in some instances definitions are contradictory. In the absence of consistency, members of the profession and those who read our literature are left with considerable confusion. The term occupation is applied to all manner of human doing, regardless of the degree of complexity. For example, accountancy (Hagedorn, 2000), report writing (Law, 1996), and tea-drinking (Hannam, 1997) have all been given equal status as occupations in the occupational therapy literature. This situation leaves the profession at risk. Occupational therapy is in the awkward position of not yet having an agreed upon vocabulary to address the complexity of its domain of concern. With increasing interest in occupation in occupational science and occupational therapy, we may be poised to develop a consistent language for easy and clear communication with clients and their families, the public, other health professionals, service providers, governmental agencies, and third-party payers.

The lack of vocabulary to describe our core domain is not a new problem for the profession. In 1933, Dunlop wrote, "From those early days until the present, occupational therapy has suffered almost continuously from a misunderstanding…" (p. 7). Polatajko (2001) argues that it is the lack of specification of our language, in a manner that was easily understood by the public, that lead to the disappearance of the term *occupation* from our literature. She notes that the term disappeared from use early in our history. Except for its continued use in the title of the profession, it was essentially absent from the Canadian literature throughout the 1940s, 50s, 60s, 70s and 80s, being replaced by such terms as activity, task, work, and function (Polatajko, 2001).

A remedy for lack of vocabulary is a taxonomy, that is to say a clear and consistent system for differentiating among the levels of occupation and the relationship of terms to each other. A taxonomy is a hierarchical ordering of related concepts that enables the specification of concepts and their placement in relation to each, allowing for more in-depth understanding (Bloom, Engelhart, Furst, Hill, & Krathwohl, 1956; Krathwohl, Bloom, & Masia, 1964). A number of occupational therapy scholars have proposed that a taxonomy would allow for the breakdown of an occupation into its various levels of complexity (Christiansen & Baum, 1997; Hagedorn, 2000; Johnson, 1996; Levine & Brayley, 1991; Pierce, 2001; Polatajko et al., 2004).

In Canada, Polatajko and colleagues (Polatajko et al., 2004) propose use of the Taxonomic Code for Occupational Performance (TCOP) to specify the language of occupation. Developed over a two-year period, through a process involving literature reviews, affinity mapping, scholarly discourse and debate, and evaluation of communicability and comprehensiveness, the code proposes seven levels of complexity. Subsequent investigations of the validity of the TCOP both from the perspective of international experts and of novice student occupational therapists (Purdie, Zimmerman, Davis, & Polatajko, submitted) indicate that the TCOP is a useful and usable instrument to categorize the various levels of complexity of occupational performance and place them in relationship to each other. While the TCOP is relatively new and in need of further professional discourse, the TCOP is unique among existing classification systems in occupational therapy, being the only one that has been subject to validation. Thus, it is currently the best available method for organizing the language of occupation.

The revised TCOP consists of five levels, with each level having one more dimension of complexity and subsuming all the characteristics of the levels below it (see figure 1.1). Occupation appears at the top of the hierarchy. As in the rules of taxonomy (Bircher, 1975; Bloom et al., 1956; Kerlinger, 1979, 1986; Krathwohl et al., 1964; Reynolds, 1971), occupation subsumes all the levels below it: occupations are composed of a set of activities: composed of a set of tasks, composed of a set of actions, composed of a set of voluntary movements and mental processes. Using the examples listed above, accountancy is an occupation and report writing is an activity, as is tea drinking.

Figure 1.1   The Taxonomic Code of Occupational Performance[1] (TCOP)

Level of complexity	Definition	Example
Occupation ↑	An activity or set of activities that is performed with some consistency and regularity, that brings structure, and is given value and meaning by individuals and a culture	Accountancy
Activity ↑	A set of tasks with a specific end point or outcome that is greater than that of any constituent task	Financial report writing
Task ↑	A set of actions having an end point or a specific outcome	Printing the report
Action ↑	A set of voluntary movements or mental processes that form a recognizable and purposeful pattern (such as grasping, holding, pulling, pushing, turning, kneeling, standing, walking, thinking, remembering, smiling, chewing, winking, etc.)	Folding, remembering the meaning of numbers
Voluntary movement or mental processes	A simple voluntary muscle or mental activation (such as flexion, extension, adduction, abduction, rotation, supination, pronation, blinking, memory, attention, focusing, scanning, etc.)	Flexing, attending

[1] All levels of performance are subserved by *cognitive*, *physical*, and *affective* performance components. *Spirituality* pervades.

       (adapted from Polatajko et al., 2004; and Zimmerman, Purdie, Davis, & Polatajko, 2006)

As expected of a taxonomic hierarchy, the number of possibilities increases with each level of the TCOP. At the lowest level, there are relatively few possibilities (the human is only capable of performing a very finite number of voluntary movements), while at the highest level there are almost limitless possibilities (Wikipedia alone lists over 1,000 occupations). Correspondingly, the lower levels add to the higher levels. This makes it possible to predict performance in a large number of occupations from knowledge of performance on a relatively fewer number of activities and, in turn, relatively fewer tasks, actions and voluntary movements, and mental processes. Knowing that a person has limited flexion at the hip or poor attention, for example, allows prediction of performance on a large number of actions, tasks, activities, and occupations. The TCOP can, thus, direct practice to the most appropriate level to maximize occupational enablement. We can communicate the reasoning for choosing tasks, activities, or occupations as therapy with our clients to ensure that the relevance of our choice is not lost on them, as it was on Bonnie Sherr Klein (see case 1):

> The occupational therapist worked with humiliating seriousness. We played shuffleboard, and ping-pong, but no one explained that they were to practice our balance and I was too out of it to understand. Everything seemed random and irrelevant (CAOT, 1997a, 2002, p. viii).

1.4 Specification of an occupational perspective: Our assumptions

After saying that "everything seemed random and irrelevant," Bonnie Sherr Klein continued:

> We did pre-kindergarten puzzles with large wooden pieces, carnival games with clown face targets, and uninspired paint-by-number crafts. My partner devoted herself to a pre-fabricated wooden nativity scene for Christmas, while I made potholders ... as it happens I was in the middle of making a film (not potholders) when I had the stroke (CAOT, 1997a, 2002, p. 34).

All professions have some basic assumptions that, by definition, are not questioned, but rather are held to be true. They are changed only when there is a large accumulation of prevailing evidence to suggest that the assumptions are no longer tenable. That the earth was the centre of the universe or that the world was flat were long standing assumptions held to be true until it was demonstrated otherwise (some still hold these to be true). Basic assumptions are necessary to guide the art and science of a profession.

Occupational therapy holds a number of basic assumptions about human occupation (see figure 1.2). Dunton (1919) proclaimed two primary assumptions in his credo: that occupation is a basic human need; and, that occupation has the potential to be therapeutic. These have guided our art and our science since the inception of the profession and have led to the articulation of further assumptions as our occupational perspective evolved.

Fundamental to the practice of occupational therapy is the conceptualization of the **human as an occupational being** (Wilcock, 1996, 1998a, 2006; Yerxa et al., 1989; Yerxa, 1998), for whom occupation is a basic need (Dunton, 1919). Accordingly, occupational therapy views engagement in occupation as a basic human need. Opportunities and resources to engage in occupation should be available to all people (Wilcock, 1993) because occupation is required for survival, health, and well-being (Fidler & Fidler, 1978; Polatajko, 1992; Wilcock, 2006). Dunton (1919) proclaimed this assumption when he said that occupation is as necessary to life as food and drink. The assumption of human needs has been echoed in the occupational therapy and occupational science literature across the decades (Reilly, 1962; Rogers, 1983; Wilcock, 2006). By extension, anything that reduces a person's ability to engage in occupation has the potential to negatively affect the health and well being of the individual, even to generate pathology (Duxbury, Higgins, & Johnson, 1999; Fidler & Fidler, 1978). Conversely, anything that overextends a person's need to engage can result in occupational

Occupation: The core domain of concern for occupational therapy

Figure 1.2   Basic assumptions

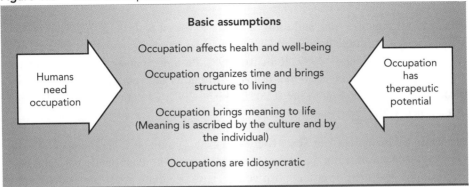

Basic assumptions

Humans need occupation

Occupation affects health and well-being

Occupation organizes time and brings structure to living

Occupation brings meaning to life
(Meaning is ascribed by the culture and by the individual)

Occupations are idiosyncratic

Occupation has therapeutic potential

imbalance and negatively affect health, increase stress, and may actually result in depression (Duxbury et al., 1999).

The corollary of the first primary assumption is the second; that **occupation has potential therapeutic value**; in the words of Dunton (1919), "sick minds, sick bodies and sick souls may be healed through occupation." (p. 10). This second assumption has prevailed in our profession since the beginning and can be seen repeated in our literature throughout our history. In 1933, Howland wrote, "by active occupation, maimed limbs and minds may be once more restored to health" (p. 4); and still later, Fidler and Fidler (1978) wrote on purposeful action and self-actualization based on the idea that doing is the remedy. That occupation should have therapeutic value is explained by the further assumptions we hold about it.

Occupation brings meaning to life. Occupation is deeply seated in human existence (Clark, 1993, 2000), so much so that in our culture people identify themselves by what they "do," making "occupation … the crucible in which our identities are formed" (Polatajko, 1998). Occupations contribute to one's social and self-identity (CAOT, 1997a; Unruh, 2004; Yerxa et al., 1990). Occupations connect us to people (Rowles, 2000) and our past, present, and future (Laliberte Rudman, Cook, & Polatajko, 1997). They allow us to explore and learn from the environment, to master skills, to express our individuality, and to sustain life.

The meanings ascribed to occupation have two sources: the culture, and, ultimately, the individual (CAOT, 1997a, 2002). As an occupational being, the person has interests and intrinsic motivation to choose and engage in particular occupations (Yerxa, 1998). The motivation to persevere with occupations is influenced by individuals' values, interests, and exercise of choice (Kielhofner, 1997). Ultimately the meaning associated with an occupation is personal and cannot be understood by observation alone; each occupation is uniquely experienced by the individual engaged in it (CAOT, 1997a, 2002). However, humans are "not decontextualized entities"; rather, they "act on and interact with a myriad of environments, using occupation" (Yerxa, 1991b, p. 200). According to Yerxa, engaging in occupation enables individuals and groups to participate in society, as well as to find meaning through occupations and to place themselves within their own culture. Yerxa (1998) reinforced the idea of occupation being context dependent. People are self-organizing, responding and adapting to diverse environmental challenges as they engage in occupations throughout their lifetime.

Occupations organize time and bring structure to life; it is through engagement in occupations that people bring a rhythm to their days and organize their time (CAOT, 1997a, 2002; Kielhofner, 1997; Rebeiro, 1998). Prolonged and consistent occupational engagement can lead to the formation of habits and routines, which provide structure and organization to life (CAOT, 1997a, 2002; Christiansen & Baum, 1997; Kielhofner, 1997; Polatajko, 1992).

However, as the quote from Sherr Klein (see case 1) indicates, the therapeutic value of every occupation is not the same for every person. The therapeutic potential of occupations, and the power and positive effects of occupation, are greatest when choice and control can be exercised, and a sense of accomplishment from performance is obtained (Laliberte Rudman, Cook, & Polatajko, 1997).

Occupation is a very personal thing; **occupations are idiosyncratic**. While all humans need occupation, the specific occupations in which a particular person engages in are idiosyncratic to that person, as is that person's experiences of those occupations. This is very evident when Sherr Klein writes, "The occupational therapist worked with humiliating seriousness. ... Everything seemed random and irrelevant (to me)" (CAOT, 1997a, 2002, p. viii). Engagement in occupations that are situated in a person's life and hold meaning for that individual are particularly potent, bringing validation to the person and helping them gain a sense of self.

> When (the patient) gets down to honest work with her hands she makes discoveries. She finds her way along new pathways. She learns something of the dignity and satisfaction of work and gets an altogether simpler and more wholesome notion of living. This in itself is good, but better still, the open mind is apt to see new visions, new hopes and faith. There is something about simple, effective work with the hands that makes (humans) ... creators in a very real sense – makes them kin with the great creative force of the world. From such a basis of dignity and simplicity anything is possible (Hall & Buck, 1915, pp. 57-58)

The idiosyncrasy of occupations points to an important caveat. Not all occupations lead to health, well-being and justice, or have therapeutic value, even if they hold meaning, organize time, and bring structure to life. Occupations can be "maladaptive," even harmful, either to the individual or society (Golledge, 1998), examples being self-abusing behaviour, vandalism, arson, or illegal drug use. Many people are engaged in risky, unhealthy or even illegal and illicit occupations, which can undermine health, well-being, and justice.

1.5 Specification of an occupational perspective: Our Canadian model

In setting the stage for enabling occupation, the Canadian Association of Occupational Therapists (1997a) introduced the Canadian Model of Occupational Performance (CMOP). With the introduction of the CMOP, the CAOT placed particular emphasis on occupational performance, an important construct of human occupation of interest to occupational therapists. The CMOP, updated from the Occupational Performance Model (OPM) in earlier guidelines (CAOT, 1991), conceptualizes occupational performance as the dynamic interaction of person, occupation, and environment. Accordingly, the CMOP was designed so that occupational performance is not actually a construct in the model; rather, the entire model is understood to portray the interaction that results in occupational performance. The *person*, depicted as a triangle at the centre of the model, is portrayed as having three performance components — cognitive, affective, and physical — with spirituality at the core. The model depicts the person embedded within the *environment* to indicate that each individual lives within a unique environmental context — cultural, institutional, physical, and social — which affords occupational possibilities. *Occupation* is depicted as the bridge that connects person and environment indicating that individuals act on the environment through occupation. Although the 1997 publication of *Enabling Occupation* indicated that occupation can be classified in numerous ways, the CMOP identified three occupational purposes: self-care, productivity, and leisure.

The CMOP achieved two important functions for the profession. First, it specified three core constructs of interest for the profession and provided a graphic representation of our occupational perspective: that human occupation occurs in context as a result of the dynamic interaction of person, occupation, and environment (see figure 1.3, part A). Second, by considering a transverse section (see figure 1.3, part B), the CMOP can

---

Figure 1.3   The CMOP-E[1]: Specifying our domain of concern

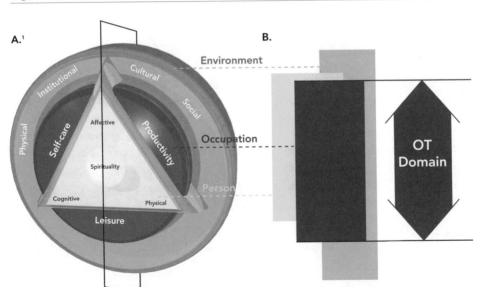

A.[1] Referred to as the CMOP in *Enabling Occupation* (1997a, 2002) and CMOP-E as of this edition
B. Trans-sectional view

Polatajko, H. J., Townsend, E. A., & Craik, J. (2007). Canadian Model of Occupational Performance and Engagement (CMOP-E). In E. A. Townsend & H. J. Polatajko, *Enabling occupation II: Advancing an occupational therapy vision of health, well-being, & justice through occupation* (p. 23). Ottawa, ON: CAOT.

---

be used to show that occupation is of central interest and delimits our concern with the person and environment. The transverse view — with occupation front and centre — presents occupation as our core domain of interest, showing that we are only concerned with what is related to human occupation and its connection with the occupational person and the occupational influences of the environment; those aspects of person or environment that are not related to occupation are beyond our scope.

Beyond performance

The *Ottawa Charter for Health Promotion* (WHO, 1986), states:

> To reach a state of complete physical, mental and social well-being, an indi-vidual or group must be able to identify and to realize aspirations, to satisfy needs, and to change or cope with the environment. Health is, therefore, seen as a **resource for everyday life**, not the objective of living (p. 1).

From the perspective of occupational therapy, to be able to realize aspirations, to sat-isfy needs, and to change or cope with the environment, a person must have occupa-tion — occupation is the stuff of everyday life. To *have* occupations is not the same as to *perform* occupations. At any given point in time, only one occupation can be performed; yet an individual or group has numerous occupations, and as occupa-tional therapists we are concerned with engagement in all of them. Further, humans frequently engage in occupations without performing them.

Consider the case of Rick Hoyt a 43 year old who has participated in 26.2 mile marathons 85 times without ever taking a step, thanks to his father, Dick (see text box 1.1). On eight occasions, Dick not only pushed his son in a wheelchair while running a marathon, but also towed him for 2.4 miles in a dinghy while swimming and pedaled 112 miles with Rick in a seat on the handlebars of his bike.

The focus of the CMOP on performance highlights only a segment of our concern with human occupation. Beyond occupational performance, occupational therapists are also interested in other modes of occupational interactions. Among these are occupational behaviour, capacity, competence, development, engagement, history, mastery, satisfaction, and participation, to name a few (see Glossary). Each of these has specific meanings and specific uses (see table 1.1). Each mode will be discussed in this text in a context-appropriate manner; the term *occupational engagement* will be given special prominence.

The construct of occupational engagement captures the broadest of perspectives on occupation. To perform is less broad, meaning to "begin and carry through to com-pletion; do; to take action in accordance with the requirements of" (Houghton Mifflin Company, 2004). The broader term *engage* encompasses all that we do to "involve oneself or become occupied; participate" (Houghton Mifflin Company, 2004). To engage is to occupy oneself or someone else. As discussed at the start of this chapter, early in our history there was strong objection raised to describing our work as occupying people because of its association with ordinary diversion or keeping busy, without the professional value of therapy. Today, occupational ther-apy concerns are congruent with the broad meaning of occupational engagement.

Rick and Dick Hoyt

This love story began in Winchester, Massachusetts, 43 years ago, when Rick was strangled by the umbilical cord during birth, leaving him brain-damaged and unable to control his limbs. "He'll be a vegetable the rest of his life," Dick says doctors told him and his wife, Judy, when Rick was 9 months old. "Put him in an institution.

But the Hoyts weren't buying it. They noticed the way Rick's eyes followed them around the room. When Rick was 11, they took him to the engineering department at Tufts University and asked if there was anything to help the boy communicate. "No way," Dick says he was told. "There's nothing going on in his brain." "Tell him a joke," Dick countered. They did. Rick laughed. Turns out a lot was going on in his brain. Rigged up with a computer that allowed him to control the cursor by touching a switch with the side of his head, Rick was finally able to communicate. First words? "Go Bruins!" And after a high-school classmate was paralyzed in an accident and the school organized a charity run for him, Rick pecked out, "Dad, I want to do that."

Yeah, right. How was Dick, a self-described "porker" who never ran more than a mile at a time, going to push his son 5 miles? Still, he tried. "Then it was me who was handicapped," Dick says. "I was sore for two weeks." That day changed Rick's life. "Dad," he typed, "When we were running, It felt like I wasn't disabled anymore!" And that sentence changed Dick's life. He became obsessed with giving Rick that feeling as often as he could. He got into such hard-belly shape that he and Rick were ready to try the 1979 Boston Marathon. "No way," Dick was told by a race official. The Hoyts weren't quite a single runner, and they weren't quite a wheelchair competitor. For a few years, Dick and Rick just joined the massive field and ran anyway, and then they found a way to get into the race officially: In 1983, they ran another marathon so fast they made the qualifying time for Boston the following year.

Then somebody said, "Hey, Dick, why not a triathlon?" How's a guy who never learned to swim and hadn't ridden a bike since he was six going to haul his 110-pound kid through a triathlon? Still, Dick tried. Now they've done 212 triathlons, including four grueling 15-hour Ironmans in Hawaii. It must be a buzzkill to be a 25-year-old stud getting passed by an old guy towing a grown man in a dinghy, don't you think?

Hey, Dick, why not see how you'd do on your own? "No way," he says. Dick does it purely for "the awesome feeling" he gets seeing Rick with a cantaloupe smile as they run, swim and ride together. This year, at ages 65 and 43, Dick and Rick finished their 24th Boston Marathon, in 5,083rd place out of more than 20,000 starters. Their best time? Two hours, 40 minutes in 1992 — only 35 minutes off the world record, which, in case you don't keep track of these things, happens to be held by a guy who was not pushing another man in a wheelchair at the time.

"No question about it," Rick types. "My dad is the father of the century."

"The thing I'd most like," Rick types, "is that my dad sit in the chair and I push him once."

— Reprinted courtesy of Sports Illustrated: Strongest Dad in the World.
June 20, 2005. Copyright 2005, Time, Inc. All rights reserved.

Examples of occupational therapists' breadth of interest in occupational engagement are in its nature (active or passive), intensity (sporadic or constant), degree of establishment (novel or long-standing and established), extent (fully engaged or barely attentive), competency of performance (novice or expert), and so on. Accordingly, to assert the broadest perspective on occupation, this book will emphasize occupational engagement.

Table 1.1   Modes of occupational interaction

Occupational ...	Definition
Capacity	That aspect or class of human action that encompasses mental and physical doing*
Competence	The actual or potential ability to engage in occupations Adequacy or sufficiency in an occupational skill, meeting all requirements of an environment*
Deprivation	The influence of an external circumstance that prevents a person from acquiring, using, or enjoying occupation over an extended period of time (Whiteford, 1997; Wilcock, 1996)
Development	The gradual change in occupational behaviour over time, resulting from the growth and maturation of the individual in interaction with the environment*
Engagement	To "involve oneself or become occupied; participate"(Houghton Mifflin Company, 2004)
Enrichment	The deliberate manipulation of environments to facilitate and support engagement in a range of occupations congruent with those that the individual might normally perform. (Molineux & Whiteford, 1999)
History	The record of how one progresses from one occupation to another, often due to a transitional event such as a marriage or divorce (Meltzer, 2001)
Identity	How an individual sees the self in terms of various occupational roles; an image of the kind of life desired (Kielhofner, Mallinson, Forsyth, & Lai, 2001)
Mastery	Competent occupational functioning (adopted from Schkade & Schultz, 1992)
Participation	Involvement in a life situation (WHO, 2001) through occupation
Pattern	The regular and predictable way of doing that occurs when human beings organize activities and occupations (Bendixon et al., 2006, p. 4)
Performance	The actual execution or carrying out of an occupation*
Potential	The capability of being or becoming occupationally engaged **
Role	The rights, obligations, and expected behaviour patterns associated with a particular set of activities or occupations, done on a regular basis, and associated with social cultural roles (adapted from Hillman & Chapparo, 1995)
Satisfaction	The state of being satisfied or content with ones occupational performance or engagement **

* From *Enabling Occupation: An Occupational Therapy Perspective* (CAOT, 1997a, 2002)
** Adapted from http://dictionary.reference.com/browse/capacity

It is interesting to consider the potential impact on occupational therapy practice if our Canadian model had from the beginning been focused on engagement rather than on performance — or if it had been named the Canadian Model of Occupational Engagement or simply the Canadian Model of Occupation. As discussed above, occupational performance is not actually captured in the CMOP. It is only implied as the result of the interacting constructs of the CMOP, and is specified in the model's name.

Our concern with human occupation is not only regarding the actual performance of an occupation, but is also with the level of importance it holds or the degree of satisfaction it brings to the individual. In fact, there is already awareness of occupational therapy interests beyond performance in the *Canadian Occupational Performance Measure* (COPM) that invites clients to self-rate importance and satisfaction, in addition to performance.

Furthermore, we are concerned with the potential and the possibility for occupational engagement that is afforded by the person-occupation-environment interaction. A profession based on a model that goes beyond performance, as our model has the potential to do, would offer a broad scope of practice and entrench our concern for occupationally supportive environments while maintaining our focus on the occupational human. Adoption of the expanded CMOP-E advances a vision of health, well-being, and justice through occupation, not limited to occupational performance. Therefore, throughout this publication the model will be renamed the Canadian Model of Occupational Performance and Engagement (CMOP-E), and our profession will be defined accordingly:

> *Occupational therapy is the art and science of enabling engagement in everyday living, through occupation; of enabling people to perform the occupations that foster health and well-being; and of enabling a just and inclusive society so that all people may participate to their potential in the daily occupations of life.*

1.6 The CMOP-E and other models of occupation

The CMOP-E is the graphic representation of the Canadian perspective on occupation, or more specifically on occupational performance. Its predecessor, the CMOP, is nationally and internationally acclaimed, enjoying wide use throughout the world, and stands among the major international models of occupation developed in the past 20 years (see table 1.2). While each of these models is unique, each has commonalities with the others and with the CMOP-E (see table 1.3 for a comparison of models).

One of the early models, first published in 1980, is the *Model of Human Occupation* (MOHO) (Kielhofner). In the 2002 version of the MOHO, Kielhofner and his colleagues (2002) identify three constructs: person, environment, and occupational performance. The MOHO asserts that what a person does in work, play, and self-care is a function of motivational factors, life patterns, performance capacity, and environmental influences (Forsyth & Kielhofner, 2003, p. 48). Unlike other occupational therapy models, the MOHO does not discuss or define occupation separate from person, environment, or occupational performance. Furthermore, in the 2002 edition of the MOHO, there is more emphasis on occupational participation than on occupa-

Table 1.2   The CMOP-E and other major models of occupational performance

Model	Occupational performance
Canadian Model of Occupational Performance and Engagement (CMOP-E) (CAOT, 1997a, 2002, Townsend & Polatajko, 2007)	• Provides a three-dimensional depiction of the relationship of the person with 3 performance components, 3 areas of occupation, and the environment with 4 elements; conceptualizes occupational performance and engagement as the dynamic interaction of person, occupation, and environment • By virtue of its name, the CMOP-E focuses on performance and engagement

The Model of Human Occupation (MOHO) (Kielhofner, 2002)	• Defines occupational participation as "engagement in work, play, or activities of daily living that are part of one's sociocultural context and that are desired and/or necessary to one's well-being" (p. 115). Engagement involves performance and subjective experience — thus occupational participation is "doing things with personal and social significance" (p. 115)
	• Occupational performance is "doing an occupational form" (citing Nelson, 1998)
	• Views occupational skill as a set of discrete purposeful actions and skills: "observable, goal-directed actions that a person uses while performing" (p. 117, citing Fisher, 1999):
	  - Motor skills: "moving self or task objects"
	  - Process skills: "logically sequencing actions over time, selecting and using appropriate tools and materials, and adapting; performance when encountering problems"
	  - Communication skills: "conveying intentions and needs and coordinating social action to act together with people"
	• Occupational participation in roles is comprised of occupational performance, which is comprised of skills

The Ecology of Human Performance (EHP) (Dunn et al., 1994; Dunn et al., 2003)	• The interaction between person and context affects human behaviour and performance • "Performance occurs as a result of the person interacting with context to engage in tasks" (Dunn et al, 2003, p. 228) • Performance range (number and types of tasks available) is determined by the interaction of the person variables and context variables
Person-Environment-Occupation (PEO) Model (Law et al., 1996)	• Outcome of the transaction of person, occupation, and environment • Defined as "the dynamic experience of a person engaged in purposeful activities and tasks within an environment" (p. 16) • Takes place within the environment • Occurs optimally when the fit among the person, occupation, and environment is maximized
Person-Environment-Occupational Performance (PEOP) Model (Baum & Christiansen, 2005)	• Occupational performance and participation sit in the middle of the model, represented by the overlap of person, occupation, environment, and performance • Occupational performance is the "central construct of participation and requires the understanding and linking of occupation and performance" (p. 246) • Satisfactory occupational performance is a "consequence of individual and group goals and characteristics and environmental characteristics that either limit or support participation" (p. 244) • Performance is defined as the "actual act of doing the occupation" (p. 245) • "The interaction of capacity, environment, and chosen activity lead to occupational performance and participation" (p. 245) • Describes occupational performance in terms of type of occupation as well as their degree of complexity

Continued ...

Occupation: The core domain of concern for occupational therapy

Table 1.2 The CMOP-E and other major models of occupational performance

Model	Occupational performance
Kawa Model (Iwama, 2006b)	• Is distinct because it is essentially metaphoric. It uses a familiar phenomenon from nature — a river — as a medium to translate subjective views of self, life, well-being, and the meanings of occupations • Regards individual or collective clients as inseparably integrated into their daily life contexts. Occupations are products of a multitransactional dynamic between client, environment, and circumstances, located in time and place. Changes to any component of a river are seen to affect all other parts of it • Depicts occupational performance metaphorically, as the quality (relative location, volume, rate, and clarity) of multiple water channels (occupations) that combine to form the client's river (life flow). Enhanced occupational performance is evidenced by increased quality of flow in specific occupations, effecting increased overall quality of life flow

tional performance, and the outcomes of participation are named occupational identity, occupational adaptation, and occupational competence.

Like the MOHO, the Ecology of Human Performance (EHP) Framework (Dunn, et al., 1994), updated in 2003 (Dunn, Brown, & Younstrom), was also among the early models. The EHP is built around four constructs: person, task, context, and performance. The authors state that although their model includes four constructs, they are specifically concerned with context: the interaction between person and environment affecting human behaviour and performance. Within the EHP model, performance cannot be understood outside of the environmental context (Dunn et al., 1994).

Three models depict the interaction of person, occupation, and environment: our own CMOP-E, the Person-Environment-Occupation (PEO) Model (Law et al, 1996; CAOT, 1997a, 2002); and the Person-Environment-Occupation-Performance (PEOP) Model (Baum & Christiansen, 2005; Christiansen & Baum, 1997). Although the three are similar, each is composed slightly differently.

The authors of the PEO Model identify six constructs: person, environment, activity, task, occupation(s), and occupational performance (Law et al., 1996). The fundamental difference between the CMOP-E and PEO Models lies in the discussion of occupation. The authors of the PEO Model view occupation as part of a hierarchical structure — occupation, task, and activity — whereas the CMOP-E discusses three purposes of occupations: self-care, productivity, and leisure. The authors of the PEOP Model (Baum & Christiansen, 2005; Christiansen & Baum, 1997) present four constructs: occupation, performance, person, and environment. Based on the PEOP Model, person and environment are bridged "through the process of personal agency or the transaction that occurs when people act with intention within environments in the performance of everyday occupations" (Baum & Christiansen, 2005, p. 251). Therefore, person and environment remain unconnected except through occupational performance and participation. This follows the graphic representation of the model whereby the person and environment only come together through occupation, performance, and occupational performance. The PEOP Model describes two important features of occupation: (a) types of occupations; and (b) level of complexity of occupation, thus bringing together the depiction of occupation within both the CMOP-E and the PEO Model. The PEOP model also lists person factors and environmental factors similar to those of the CMOP-E and PEO Model.

The Kawa Model (Iwama, 2006b) provides a metaphoric representation of human occupation. Using a river as a metaphor to depict an Eastern world way of thinking about occupational performance, the Kawa Model, focuses on a collective-oriented, interdependent view of doing. The river illustrates how one's life flow (the river water) defines, and is shaped and regulated by its context (the river's structural

Table 1.3   Comparison of key concepts across the major models of occupation

Model	Person	Occupation	Environment
Canadian Model of Occupational Performance and Engagement (CMOP-E) (CAOT, 1997a, 2002, Townsend & Polatajko, 2007)	**Performance and engagement:** • Cognitive • Affective • Physical **Essence of the person:** • Spirituality	**Areas of occupation:** • Self-care • Productivity • Leisure	**Environmental components:** • Cultural • Institutional • Physical • Social
The Model of Human Occupation (MOHO) (Kielhofner, 2002)	**Volition:** "an ongoing process" occurring "over time as people experience, interpret, anticipate, and choose occupations" (p. 16) • Personal causation: "refers to one's sense of competence and effectiveness" (p. 15) • Values: "refer to what one finds important and meaningful to do" (p. 15) • Interests "refer to what one finds enjoyable or satisfying to do" (p. 15) **Habituation:** "semi-autonomous patterning of behaviour" (p. 19) – "allows us to recognize and respond to repetitive temporal cues and time frames" (p. 19) • Habits: "acquired tendencies to respond and perform in certain consistent ways in familiar environments or situations" (p. 21) • Internalized roles: "incorporation of a socially and/or personally defined status and a related cluster of attitudes and behaviours" (p. 22) **Performance Capacity:** • Physical and mental capacities • Subjective experiences	• The model appears to view occupation separately from the environment and does not discuss it separately • **Physical:** - Natural and human made spaces and the objects within them • **Social:** - Groups of persons and the occupational forms that persons belonging to those groups perform - Occupational forms: Rule-bound sequences of action that are available to do within a social context • **Occupation:** "action that occupies a particular social and physical space" (p. 111)	

Continued ...

Table 1.3   Comparison of key concepts across the major models of occupation

Model	Person	Occupation	Environment

The Ecology of Human Performance (EHP) (Dunn et al., 1994; Dunn, Brown, & Younstrom, 2003)	• Past experiences
	• Personal values/interests
	• Ability/skill sets
	  - Sensorimotor skills
	  - Cognitive skills
	  - Psychosocial skills
		• **Tasks:**
		  - "objective sets of behaviors that are combined to allow an individual to engage in performance that accomplishes a goal" (Dunn et al., 2003)
		  - An infinite number of tasks exist around the person
		  - A person uses their skills and abilities to "look through" the context at the tasks they want to and need to do
		• **Occupation:**
		  - Specific constellation of tasks.
		• **Life roles:**
		  - "A constellation of tasks" (Dunn et al., 1994, p. 600) Tasks can be a part of more than one role
		  - The configuration of an individual's role is unique to that person
			Context (factors that operate external to the person)
			  - "a set of interrelated conditions that surrounds a person" (Dunn et al., 2003, p. 226)
			  - "a lens from which persons view their world" (Dunn et al., 1994, p. 595)
			• Temporal context (resides within the person but considered context because of the social and cultural meanings attached)
			  - chronological
			  - developmental
			  - life cycle
			  - health status
			• Environment (external to the person)
			  - physical
			  - social
			  - cultural

Person-Environment-Occupation (PEO) Model of Occupational Performance (Law et al., 1996)	"A unique being who assumes a variety of roles simultaneously" (p. 15)
	• Roles
	• Attributes and life experiences:
	  - self-concept
	  - personality style
	  - cultural background
	  - personal competencies
	  - motor performances
	  - sensory capabilities
	  - cognitive aptitude
	  - general health
	• Set of learned and innate skills
		• **Occupation:** "groups of self-directed, functional tasks and activities in which a person engages over the lifespan"
		• **Occupations:** "those clusters of activities and tasks in which the person engages in order to meet his/her intrinsic needs for self-maintenance, expression and fulfillment"
		• **Tasks:** "set of purposeful activities in which a person engages"
		• **Activities:** "the basic unit of a task"(p.16)
			• Cultural
			• Socio-economic
			• Institutional
			• Physical
			• Social (considers each domain from the perspective of the person, household, neighbourhood and community)

Continued ...

Table 1.3 Comparison of key concepts across the major models of occupation

Model	Person	Occupation	Environment

Person-Environment-Occupational Performance (PEOP) Model (Baum & Christiansen, 2005)	*(Person factors – intrinsic)*
	• Psychological
	  - Personality traits, motivational influences, and internal processes
	• Cognitive
	  - Mechanisms of language comprehension and production, pattern recognition, task organization, reasoning, attention, and memory
	• Neurobehavioural
	  - Sensory and motor systems
	• Physiological
	  - Physical health and fitness: endurance, flexibility, movement, strength
	• Spirituality
	  - Meanings that "contribute to a greater sense of personal understanding about self and one's place in the world" (p. 248)
		1) Occupations: what people want and need to do in their daily lives
		2) Hierarchy of occupation-related behaviours and supportive abilities
		• **Roles**: positions in society having expected responsibilities and privileges, typically involving the performance of many occupations
		• **Occupations (segments of goal-directed behaviour that are recognizable by others and typically include a number of related tasks performed over time ... in text):** goal-directed pursuits that typically extend over time, have meaning to the performer, and involve multiple tasks
		• **Tasks:** combinations of actions sharing a common purpose recognized by the performer
		• **Actions:** observable behaviours that are recognizable
		• **Abilities:** general traits or individuals characteristics that support occupational performance (pp. 252-253)
			(Environmental factors – extrinsic)
			• Social support
			• Social and economic systems
			• Built environment and technology
			• Natural environment
			• Culture and values

The Kawa Model (Iwama, 2006b)	• Individuals, or collectives, such as families, corporations or communities and their circumstances, are metaphorically presented as "rivers" • The person is embedded in broader context as part of the encompassing frame/milieu; these are inseparable and interrelated, so that changes in environment and/or person affect changes in the entire frame/milieu	• Conceptualized as *life flow* or *life energy*. Occupation is the expression of life, the evidence of being "alive" • Demonstrated in the model as the spaces within the structures/contexts (environment, circumstances, assets, and liabilities) of the river, through which water (life) fills/occupies and flows through • As water touches all elements in the frame, so is occupation viewed to be inseparably connected with all aspects of the broader context	• Named and conceptualized by the person as the outer context in which the person is embedded. Demonstrated in the model as the river's walls and sides, forming the substrate that shapes and influences the quality of the water (life) flow. The river walls and sides combine with other structures in the frame to determine the forms, functions, and meanings of occupations

formation, rocks, and driftwood). These contextual structures are viewed as inseparable from the river (life) since they regulate and shape its flow; therefore, life is viewed
as a part of the natural context. When life flow weakens an "individual or collective
can be described as unwell, or in a state of disharmony" (Iwama, 2006a).

1.7 The CMOP-E and the International Classification of Functioning, Disability, and Health

The CMOP-E captures the occupational perspective of our profession and positions
it as an internationally important occupational model. However, since its inception,
occupational therapy has been located and funded within the health system, which
operates primarily within a medical model. It is therefore important to understand
how our occupational model fits with the medical model and how we can frame our
practice in occupational therapy with our medical and non-medical colleagues
(Martini, Polatajko, & Wilcock, 1995; Polatajko, 1992; Stamm, Cieza, Machold,
Smolen, & Stucki, 2006; Townsend, Ryan, & Law, 1990). One avenue for exploration is the translational bridge that the occupational model provides between the
medical model and everyday life.

In 2001, the World Health Organization (WHO) published the latest in a series of
models, the *International Classification of Functioning, Disability and Health* (ICF)
(WHO, 2001). The ICF, which describes the impact of health conditions on people's
lives, illustrates the relationship between health conditions, activity, and participation
in daily life, and positions functioning and disability within a context.

The ICF model (figure 1. 4) is a graphic representation of the dynamic relationship
between a person's functioning, disability, and contextual factors. The ICF has two
parts: Part one covers functioning and disability and includes two constructs: body
functions and structures, and activity and participation. Part two covers contextual
factors, including environmental factors and personal factors.

Figure 1.4   International Classification of Functioning, Disability, and Health

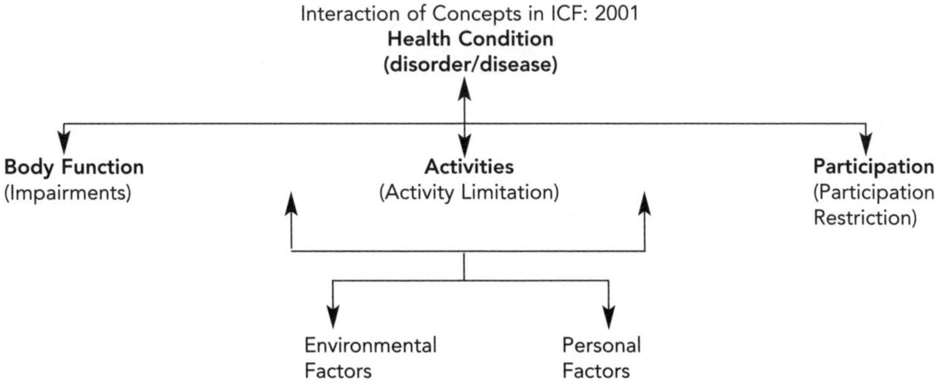

Interaction of Concepts in ICF: 2001
Health Condition
(disorder/disease)

Body Function
(Impairments)

Activities
(Activity Limitation)

Participation
(Participation Restriction)

Environmental Factors

Personal Factors

World Health Organization. (2001). *Classification of functioning, disability and health*. Geneva, Switzerland:
World Health Organization. P. 18.
COPYRIGHT © 2001 World Health Organization (WHO). Reprinted with permission of WHO. All rights reserved.

The ICF focuses on healthy human functioning which, from an occupational perspective, must include occupation. There are many similarities, and some important differences, between the ICF and the CMOP-E (see table 1.4). Occupational therapists have begun to study these similarities and differences. Of particular interest is the identified relationship between the ICF concept of body function and structure and the CMOP-E concept of person; also of interest is the relationship between the ICF concepts of activity and participation and the CMOP-E concepts of occupation and occupational performance (Desrosiers, 2005; Hemmingsson & Jonsson, 2005; Stamm et al., 2006).

The body function and structure concept in the ICF is similar to the performance components — cognitive, affective, and physical — associated with the person factor in the CMOP-E. The ICF includes a variable called *personal factors*, as part of the context. It captures components of the CMOP-E concept of person that would not otherwise be captured by body function and structure.

The ICF defines activity, along with its domains (see table 1.5) as "the execution of a task or action by an individual" (WHO, 2001, p. 17), much the same way as the TCOP defines it. In the ICF, activity is conceptually viewed as representing health functioning at the individual level, and a problem at this level is labeled activity limitation.

Table 1.4 Comparison of ICF (WHO, 2001) and CMOP-E (CAOT, 1997a; 2002, Townsend & Polatajko, 2007)

ICF	CMOP
Body functions and structures • Body functions are the physiological functions of body systems (including psychological functions) • Body structures are anatomical parts of the body such as organs, limbs, and their components	**Components of the person** • Contribute to the successful engagement in occupation • Physical, cognitive, affective functions and structures of the person

Activity and participation
• Presented as one "component" where:
  - activity is the execution of a task or action by an individual
  - participation is involvement in life situations
• Names nine dimensions: learning and applying knowledge, general tasks and demands, communication, mobility, self-care, domestic life, interpersonal interactions, major life areas, and civic life
	Occupational performance and engagement
	• The result of a dynamic relationship between persons, environment, and occupation
	• Names three main occupational groupings: self-care, productivity, and leisure
	• Occupations are composed of activities, which are composed of tasks, which are, in turn, composed of actions composed of voluntary movement or mental processes

Environmental factors • Make up the physical, social, and attitudinal environment in which people live and conduct their lives	**Environment** One of the three major variables • External contexts, including physical, cultural, institutional, and social elements
Personal factors • Are the particular background of an individual's life and living, and comprise features of the individual that are not part of the health condition or health states	**Person** • One of the three major variables • Described in terms of the component variables cognitive, affective, physical, and spiritual • Although not specifically stated in the model, the background information specified by the ICF is of interest and implied

World Health Organization, (2001). *International classification of functioning, disability and health*. Geneva, Switzerland: World Health Organization p.14

Occupation: The core domain of concern for occupational therapy

Table 1.5   Domains of activity and participation in the ICF (WHO, 2001)

Activity and participation domains

D1 Learning and applying knowledge

D2 General tasks and demands

D3 Communication

D4 Mobility

D5 Self-care

D6 Domestic life

D7 Interpersonal interactions and relationships

D8 Major life areas

D9 Community, social, and civic life

Reprinted with permission from International Classification of Functioning, Disability, and Health by WHO, 2001. Geneva, Switzerland:Author.

In the ICF, participation and its domains (see table 1.5), are defined as "involvement in a life situation" (WHO, 2001, p. 17). Participation is conceptually viewed as functioning at the societal level, and a problem is called *participation restriction.* Participation represents a dynamic interaction between personal and contextual factors. The construct of participation would appear to fit well with the construct of occupational performance captured by the CMOP-E. However, the two are not synonymous. The most important difference is that the ICF does not refer to the subjective experience of participation. For occupational therapists, the subjective meaning that the person and the culture ascribe to participation in occupation is an important factor (Hemmingsson & Jonsson, 2005). From a CMOP-E perspective, it would not be sufficient to simply observe a person's performance in participation as the ICF suggests. Occupational therapists believe that assessment of occupational performance or of participation should be person- or client-centred, using such tools as the *Canadian Occupational Performance Measure* (Law, Baptiste, et al., 2005; Law, King, & Russell, 2005).

Another concern expressed by occupational therapists writing about the ICF is the lack of distinction between activity and participation. Although the ICF model depicts activity and participation as two separate constructs, the ICF manual offers one list of domains for both activity and participation. Recent work by occupational therapy researchers is helping to distinguish these two key constructs. For example, Jette, Haley, and Kooyoomjian (2003) found that within physical functioning, level of complexity and the concept of social role helped to distinguish between activity and participation. Desrosiers (2005) cited several studies that confirmed that activities and participation should be measured separately, and she described how social roles, as valued by a person and society, are important in distinguishing participation from individual activities.

Adding to these emerging conceptual discussions, occupation itself may be the key construct that distinguishes between activity and participation. According to the ICF, activities are tasks and actions that individuals perform without meaning or a defined social role. Participation is imbedded with occupation — individual meanings and social roles are part of participation. For example, printing or writing a word or sentence is an activity performed by an individual, but when this activity takes on personal meaning and a social role, and is therefore an occupation — such as writing a book — then it is participation (Desrosiers, 2005). Indeed, one could call that occupational participation.

In summary, the ICF has a goodness of fit with the CMOP-E. Both point to the importance of the interaction of person and environment to human functioning. Both consider that the interactions contribute to functioning in context. In the case of the ICF, function is described as activity and participation, and in the case of the CMOP-E it is described as occupational performance and engagement. Activity is not specifically named in the CMOP-E, it is a subset of *occupational performance*. The distinction between the two is that the ICF uses the term participation and the CMOP-E uses the term *occupational performance*. These concepts are related, but not synonymous. Participation may be an outcome of occupational performance or a context for occupational performance, and thus may be achieved through occupation, but it is not fully occupation. Similarly, there are occupations that are not participatory, but are solitary, and still have meaning and value. Given the strength of the congruence between the ICF and the CMOP-E, it is possible, following the example of Polatajko (1992), to translate the CMOP-E into an ICF-type model to create an occupational model of health and well-being that shows the relative perspectives of occupational therapy and health (see figure 1.5). As will be discussed in chapters 7 and 8, an occupational model of health can be used to guide enablement.

Figure 1.5   Models of health and well-being

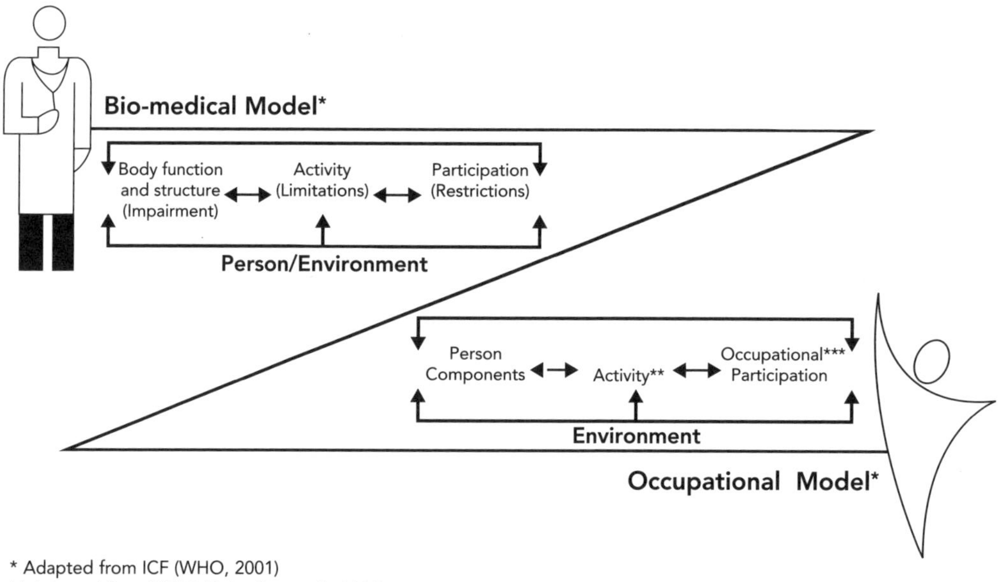

* Adapted from ICF (WHO, 2001)
** Adapted from TCOP (Polatajko et al., 2004)
*** Adapted from CMOP-E (CAOT 1997a, 2002, Townsend & Polatajko, 2007)

Occupation: The core domain of concern for occupational therapy

Chapter 2

Human occupation in context

Helene J. Polatajko
Catherine Backman
Sue Baptiste
Jane Davis
Parvin Eftekhar
Andrew Harvey
Jennifer Jarman
Terry Krupa
Nancy Lin
Wendy Pentland
Debbie Laliberte Rudman
Lynn Shaw
Bice Amoroso
Anne Connor-Schisler

CASE 2 A Burundian perspective in Canada

Eight adult Burundian refugees were torn from their homes. Literally overnight, they found themselves in Canada, which was a new and strange place. For each individual — whether young or old, male or female, married or single — the impact of environmental transformation caused changes to their everyday occupations: many daily occupations were novel and constituted new additions to the refugees' occupational repertoire, while some old occupations were abandoned, some were altered, and a few remained the same. These changes occurred because the Canadian environment imposed upon and/or offered the refugees occupational opportunities that were distinct from those of their Burundian homeland. When the Canadian environment afforded occupational opportunities, the Burundian refugees could make decisions in opposition to the Burundian culture but congruent with their personal value systems and Canadian society:

> "It is not easy for me to give up my culture; there is a thing you have to put away and there are other things that you have to pick up here in Canada. I have kept some habits from Burundi."

Fleeing Burundi in the Sub-Saharan area of Africa for continental North America, specifically Southwestern Ontario, resulted in a physical environment that imposed changes to everyday occupations. Winter snow and ice conditions mandated different forms of housing, food choices, and clothing style:

> "Weather (in Burundi) is very different and it is uncommon to wear coats. Only wear coats on wedding days."

Socioculturally, the new Canadian context emphasized the individual more than the social collective. The Burundian refugees learned Canadian values for individual human rights, women's and children's rights and policing, an emphasis on self-reliance and non-obligation to care for one's parents and siblings, freedom to choose one's life partners and to provide for one's own housing, education, and career direction after age 18. Politico-economically, the Burundian refugees found that Canadian society encouraged people to strive for their dreams and contribute to society and the world. However, they also found that foreign training and experience were not valued in Canada. The Burundian refugees had to learn to live with less money, bank loans and social assistance, occupy low paying manual jobs, and adjust their lives to the rhythm of machines, shop hours, public bus operations, and other people's schedules:

> "My career is broken ...You have to know what is out there. The more they tell you the more you want to know ... I have to keep looking.

Through the generosity of the Burundian refugees, we learn the power of the individual and the power of sociocultural structures as mediators of change.

— By Anne Connor-Schisler
(Based on Connor-Schisler, 1996)

Occupation: The core domain of concern for occupational therapy

2.1 Introduction

Occupation is a curious thing
It pervades our lives and marks our days
It defines us and is defined by us
It both shapes the world and is shaped by the world
It can be known by the tools it uses and the wake it leaves in its path
It is intangible and invisible until a person engages in it
It is a performing art
It can only be seen when a person performs it and only understood when a
person tells you its meaning

By Helene J. Polatajko

Occupation is indeed a curious thing. At one level, we know it all too well; we have engaged in it from infancy and it fills our day-to-day existence. At another level, it is extremely complex, difficult to grasp, difficult to explain, and difficult to define. Naming occupation as the core domain of concern for our profession brings with it the responsibility of knowing it at all levels (Polatajko et al., 2004). This requires us not only to make explicit the assumptions we hold about occupation, as was done in chapter 1, but also to have a comprehensive understanding of the concept and phenomenon called occupation.

In occupational therapy, an emerging literature on occupation is beginning to enhance our understanding of what is meant by occupation (CAOT, 1997a; 2002; Polatajko et al., 2004), the factors that determine engagement in occupation (Christiansen, 1999; Csikszentmihalyi & Larson, 1987; Kielhofner, 1997a), the experience of engaging in occupation for the individual (Emerson, Cook, Polatajko, & Segal, 1998; Nagle, Cook, & Polatajko, 2002), and the context that shapes occupation (Laliberte Rudman, 2005; Whiteford, 2005). Outside the profession there are also broad literatures that can contribute to our comprehension of topics important to our understanding of occupation. These subjects include systems of classification, time use patterns, work-life balance, the meaning of work, and social structure. This chapter draws together information from various sources to present the state of the art of our understanding of human occupation.

2.2 Understanding human occupation

The process of understanding a concept and phenomenon starts with description. As a first step, the observable characteristics are described; that is, the aspects that help to identify it, tell it apart, describe it recognizably, or distinguish it (Houghton Mifflin Company, 2004). In the case of *occupation*, the description of the essential characteristics is difficult; we highlight three reasons. First, occupation is not one unitary phenomenon, rather a broad class that, as defined in *Enabling Occupation* (CAOT, 1997a, 2002), is composed of all the tasks and activities in which a person engages in everyday life that are both culturally and personally meaningful. Second, occupational engagement is an event; it is a performing art. Accordingly, it is not observable until a person engages. Finally, again by definition, occupation has a meaning component, a subjective component that cannot be understood by observation alone, which is personal and unique to the individual (Hasselkus & Rosa, 1997).

Journalists are often required to describe complex events that cannot be seen until they occur and that are laden with meaning. They have created a structure that allows them to report comprehensively the specifics of a story; they ask questions about who, what, when, where, how, and why. Similarly, the CMOP-E has been created as a structure to describe critical characteristics of human occupation. The journalists' questions and the CMOP-E structure are used to describe the characteristics of human occupation.

2.3   The characteristics of human occupation

Who: The person

Occupation is a performing art; it is essentially intangible and invisible. Occupation only becomes visible through performance, either because the performance is observed or because the performance effects a visible change in the world. Because occupation is a performing art, it cannot exist without people. However, unlike other performing arts, it is not exclusive to people with special skills or talents (see figure 2.1).

All humans are occupational beings; doing is central to human life (Wilcock, 1993, 1998a, 2006). Accordingly, all people — regardless of age, ethnicity, gender, race, color, or creed — engage in occupation. Indeed, occupational engagement is so much the norm that when an individual ceases to engage in occupation, or simply changes the typical pattern of engagement, it is a good indicator that something is amiss.

Individuals accumulate their occupational repertoires and develop their occupational patterns over the course of their lives; each individual's occupational repertoire and pattern being as unique to that individual as their fingerprint. The occupations in which someone engages and the amount of time spent doing the occupation is idiosyncratic to that person and is determined by the complex interaction of internal and external factors, such as current life stage, ability, and opportunity as well as the cultural, institutional, physical, and social factors of the environment (CAOT, 1997a, 2002).

While human occupation is idiosyncratic, it is seldom done in isolation. There are many occasions when one person's engagement in occupation is intimately intertwined with that of another person or group (Rowles, 2000). This may involve persons in close proximity or at a distance, persons who support occupations or present barriers to them. It may concern occupations that are complementary, synergistic, or those that create barriers. Thus the who of occupation may not only be a single person, but pairs, groups, communities, populations, and even societies.

What: The occupation

Occupation is not a unitary phenomenon; it encompasses all the activities and tasks of everyday life for all people (see figure 2.1). Accordingly, there are a vast number of occupations in which humans may engage, almost more than can be counted,

Figure 2.1   Characteristics of human occupation

Who

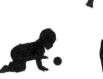 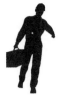

What

When

Where

   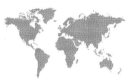

How

 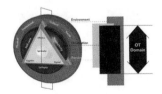

Why

- Meaning
- Fulfillment
- Social connectedness
- Contribute rest

- Relaxation
- Challenge
- Achievement
- Success
- Satisfaction

- Purpose
- Self-expression
- Sustenance
- Relief of boredom
- Joy

while at the same time more continue to be created. Numerous systems have been developed to classify the myriad of occupations, each based on the purposes and assumptions of those who design the classification. There is no right or wrong way of classifying occupations; each system serves a different analytical purpose.

Dunton's (1919) credo employed what is probably the first example of classification in occupational therapy literature. Basing his system on the type of human capacity required of an occupation, Dunton named two classes of occupations: physical and mental. Numerous others have been proposed since; perhaps the most constant among these has been that used in the CMOP-E with three classes based on the purpose of the occupation: self-care, productivity, and leisure. Neither Dunton's nor the CMOP-E's classes is optimal; yet each offers insights about occupation. Dunton's is not a mutually exclusive system; most occupations require both physical and mental abilities. The advantage is that the idea of physical and mental occupations is easily understood and frequently used in day-to-day conversations about occupation (Laliberte Rudman et al., 1997). The CMOP-E is a subjective and situation-specific system; only the individual engaged in an occupation can truly determine its purposes, which may be multiple and may shift from situation to situation. Some, like Hammell (2004a), have argued that the CMOP framework is too simplistic and fails to capture the determinants of occupation, its value, and its importance in the lives of individuals. Nonetheless, the CMOP-E framework is simple to use and allows for a fairly comprehensive categorization of occupations.

Outside occupational therapy literature, numerous other systems of classification have been developed, particularly in time use literature. The systems appearing in that literature are akin to those used in the CMOP-E as they are intended to capture all manner of occupational engagement. Ås (1982), on the one hand, defined a classification system based on obligation or constraint with the following categories: necessary (to meet survival and self-maintenance needs); contracted (paid or educational activities); committed (work or productivity-like occupation that is unpaid such as child care, home maintenance); and free time (left over and not necessarily leisure). Little (1983), on the other hand, proposed a classification of occupations that entails grouping those related to an individual's goals at any one point in time, such as raising a child or completing a university degree. He termed these *personal projects*. Christiansen (1996) recognized that we rarely perform one occupation at a time; most of us multi-task in occupations that may be primary, secondary, and tertiary.

While all systems of classification aim for a comprehensive categorization of all occupations, none are fully comprehensive. Government agencies need systems with considerable precision so that they can uncover the impact of occupations on a variety of socially important factors, including labour market behaviour, life expectancy, prevalence of disease and illness, voting behaviour, and attitudes about various social issues. Furthermore, government agencies need an occupational classification to make comparisons. Accordingly, government agencies are only interested in systems that objectively identify very specific factors related to formal work: one's manner of earning a living, one's profession or life calling. Statistics Canada, the United States Census Bureau, and parallel agencies in other countries have created occupational classification schemes that are relatively precise and objective to allow occupations to be classified uniformly from workplace to workplace, region to region, and country to country (Jarman, 2004). The International Labour Office, part of the United Nations, has developed a system of occupational classification for countries that do not have the resources to develop their own. The *International Standard Classification of Occupations* (International Labour Organisation, Bureau of Statistics, 2004) (see table 2.1 for an excerpt) has been carefully developed to allow for the considerable complexity of occupations that occur around the world. This type of classification system allows occupations to be compared meaningfully across regions and even nation-states, thereby helping to understand the social and economic processes of work-based occupations.

As indicated above, occupational classification systems are based on the purposes of those engaged in classifying. Sociocultural norms attribute a set of expectations for

---

Table 2.1   Excerpt from the *International Standard Classification of Occupations* (ISCO-88)

Major, sub-major, minor, and unit group titles

MAJOR GROUP 1
LEGISLATORS, SENIOR OFFICIALS, AND MANAGERS

11 LEGISLATORS AND SENIOR OFFICIALS

111 LEGISLATORS

1110 Legislators

112 SENIOR GOVERNMENT OFFICIALS

1120 Senior government officials

12 CORPORATE MANAGERS (This group is intended to include persons who, as directors, chief executives, or department managers, manage enterprises, or organizations, or departments requiring a total of three or more managers.)

121 DIRECTORS AND CHIEF EXECUTIVES

1210 Directors and chief executives

122 PRODUCTION AND OPERATIONS DEPARTMENT MANAGERS

1221 Production and operations department managers in agriculture, hunting, forestry, and fishing

13 GENERAL MANAGERS (This group is intended to include persons who manage enterprises, or in some cases organizations, on their own behalf, or on behalf of the proprietor, with some non-managerial help and the assistance of no more than one other manager who should also be classified in this sub-major group as, in most cases, the tasks will be broader than those of a specialized manager in a larger enterprise or organisation. Non-managerial staff should be classified according to their specific tasks.)

131 GENERAL MANAGERS

1311 General managers in agriculture, hunting, forestry/and fishing

1312 ...

the acceptable, pro-social, and legal behaviours of people — and if expectations are not met, the person's occupation may not be supported or tolerated and may even be criminalized (Christiansen & Baum, 1997). Accordingly, not all meaningful occupations are acceptable, considered pro-social, or even legal. Loitering, alcohol abuse, or littering, which demonstrate a lack of judgment or concern for others, are occupations usually regarded as antisocial. Drug use, theft, arson, or vandalism, which are in violation of a law, are regarded as criminal occupations (Cara & MacRae, 1998). Occupational engagement is important from a criminogenic perspective, not only because some occupations are criminal, but also because the lack of structured meaningful time use has been implicated in criminal re-offence (Quinsey, Coleman, Jones, & Altrows, 1997; Whiteford, 1997).

When: The temporal environment

People engage in occupation at all times of the day, week, month, year and life, (see figure 2.1). Since occupational engagement is a performing art, it occurs in time and over time, forming patterns of occupational engagement that are frequently evaluated with respect to the degree of balance that the patterns represent.

Occupational patterns

Everyday occupations are woven into habits, which affect a person's use of time and performance (Christiansen & Baum, 1997; Clark, 2000). Habits may be considered occupational patterns. This term does not have one single agreed-upon definition and is loosely used to refer to the overall ways a person or persons arrange and integrate different occupations into an entire day, week, or life plan. Occupations and their patterns are outward evidence of who we are in the world; how we organize our lives; connect with, adapt to, and have a sense of control over our environment; express who we are; develop our self identity and self-actualize. As such, they are a powerful way to describe or distinguish between individuals and groups, and to evaluate change in individual and cultural behaviours over time. Just as occupational patterns vary between individuals, fields such as sociology, anthropology, and history reveal to us that occupational patterns vary across communities, cultures, and centuries. Human occupational patterns are windows on the lifestyles of individuals, cultures and eras and — over time — are evidence of social change.

The formal examination of human occupational patterns began in the early 20th century in Europe and the United States. It stemmed from concerns about working-class lifestyles and living conditions caused by demands associated with the rise of industrialization. Since then, many countries have conducted national time use studies as part of their census data collections. Time use research is conducted by scholars in various fields, including economics, health sciences, marketing, occupational science, and social psychology. There is an International Society for the Study of Time Use with multinational and multidisciplinary participation. The majority of our information on human occupational patterns is drawn from time use research.

Time use studies are specifically designed to capture the flow of tasks and activities inherent in occupations and the contexts in which they are carried out. Typically individuals are asked to keep a record or recall their tasks and activities minute-by-minute and day-by-day. They may be asked to complete a written time diary or use specially programmed electronic devices such as a palm computer. Individuals record what they were doing, and when they started and stopped the tasks and activities, as well as contextual data such as where, when, and with whom they took place, enjoyment of the task or activity, and perceived control over it. These data are then typically reported as average time spent in many different activities or occupations within an overall classification rubric; for instance, the occupational groupings of self-care, productivity, leisure; and free time.

As an example, 2005 Canadian data (Statistics Canada, 2005c) by gender are shown in table 2.2. These data are readily collected and applied by occupational scientists to glean occupational patterns, because they classify what people typically do through an occupational lens; for instance, the three occupational categories in the

Table 2.2 Canadian patterns of occupation (Statistics Canada, 2005c)

Activity	Females (over 15 years) Hours per day	Males (over 15 years) Hours per day
Total	24.0	24.0
Total work	7.9	8.0
Paid work and education	7.7	8.8
Paid work and related activities	7.7	8.8
Paid work	7.1	8.2
Activities related to paid work	.5	.7
Commuting	.8	.9
Education and related activities	6.3	6.0
Unpaid work	4.6	3.2
Cook/wash up	1.3	.7
Housekeeping	1.8	1.5
Maintenance and repair	2.0	2.7
Other household work	1.1	1.6
Shop for goods and services	1.9	1.8
Child care	2.4	1.8
Civic/voluntary work	1.9	2.0
Personal care	10.6	10.2
Night sleep	8.2	8.0
Meals (excl restaurant)	1.2	1.2
Other personal activities	1.4	1.2
Free time	5.7	6.1
Socializing, including restaurant meals	2.8	3.0
Restaurant meals	1.5	1.6
Socializing in homes	2.3	2.5
Other socializing	2.6	2.7
TV, reading, other passive leisure	3.1	3.3
TV	2.7	3.0
Reading (newspaper, books, magazines)	1.4	1.3
Other passive leisure	1.1	1.1
Sports, movies, other entertainment events	2.8	2.6
Active leisure	2.2	2.6
Active sports	1.7	2.3
Other active leisure	2.1	2.4

Reprinted with permission from Statistics Canada. Source: Statistics Canada website: http://www40.statcan.ca/l01/cst01/famil36a.htm extracted May 24, 2007.

CMOP-E classify three major purposes that appear to underlie human occupation: self-care, productivity, and leisure (CAOT, 1997a, 2002, Townsend & Polatajko, 2007).

Human occupational patterns are the result of complex and sometimes subtle factors that interact. Factors reside both within and outside the person in her or his environment. Table 2.3 identifies some of these internal and external factors.

It is important to note that most of the publications describing human occupational patterns are based on aggregate data from large groups of people. Data are classified using an externally applied standard classification system. Yet occupation broadly defined is idiosyncratic; not everyone views their occupations in the same way (see text box 2.1). For example, what one person calls work, another may call leisure. Furthermore, we may not classify our occupations the same way each time. On weekends, cooking dinner often feels like leisure but it may feel like work during the week!

In thinking about human occupational patterns, it is important to remember that we rarely perform one occupation at a time. The concept of multitasking has been criticized due to the negative effects of increasing demands and time pressures on many people in our society. Nevertheless, humans have always multitasked: harvesting the hay and minding the children; driving to work while planning a meeting and listening to the radio. Varying levels of occupations can be differentiated as primary, secondary, tertiary, and so on. Multitasking is part of our occupational patterns.

Occupational balance

Inherent in the concept of occupational patterns is the concept of occupational balance — the idea that there is an ideal mix of occupations that one ought to have. This ideal is caught in such expressions as "all work and no play," There is, in our Canadian culture, a conventional wisdom that we need a balance between work, rest, and play.

Table 2.3 External/internal factors for occupational patterns

A. Factors internal to the individual
- Personality/character style
- Preferences/experience
- Aptitudes, abilities, knowledge
- Survival and other basic needs
- Health/chronic illness disability
- Biological rhythms
- Age, gender, socioeconomic status
- Values/attitudes/meaning we give to what we do/spirituality

B. Factors external to the individual
- Temporal-spatial environment
- Socio-economic environment and social support
- Cultural expectations and environment
- Natural and human-made physical environments
- Circumstance
- Zeitgebers (physical and social), etc.
- Resources (time, money, space)

Adapted from Harvey AS, Pentland W (2004). What do people do?. In Townsend L, Christiansen C, *Introduction to Occupation.* 1st ed, .pp. 63 - 90 . New Jersey. Prentice-Hall.

Reflections on time and occupation

How might different social groups experience and understand time and structure? While dominant Canadian perspectives view days being organized by occupational engagements, Aboriginal Canadians may think about time as spanning generations of ancestors and extending many generations into the future. This concept of time is likely to be part of their occupational understanding. Similarly, many Buddhists see time in nonlinear ways: they understand ancestors and future generations to be present, they live in the moment, and do not think in terms of future accomplishments. How might these views affect understandings of occupation, or occupational therapy practice?

While for many of us, prolonged, consistent occupational engagement can lead to the formation of habits and routines, this is not always true for everyone. For members of some social groups, life seems more random, arbitrary, and unpredictable. For example, one living in poverty is more likely to be at the whim of circumstances that totally disrupt routine. For a disadvantaged mother whose child loses a shoe and must buy a new pair, she will not be able to buy a bus pass that month, won't make it to her minimum wage job on time, and so loses her job. People living in poverty often have precarious housing situations and move frequently, disrupting their routines. How might it affect one's understanding of occupations if no matter what efforts one made, it seemed impossible to establish predictable routines? How might this affect occupational therapy?

— By Brenda Beagan

The notion of balance has been discussed in the occupational therapy literature from its inception (Christiansen, 1996). In 1922, Adolph Meyer (1922, 1977), a founding father of occupational therapy in the United States, wrote about the importance of occupational balance. In 1983 Rogers made the relationship between occupational balance and health explicit when she wrote, "Occupational therapy rests on the belief that a balance of self-care, play, work and rest is essential for healthy living" (p. 47). In occupational therapy literature, occupational balance is considered to be "subjectively defined by individuals in terms of how they choose to spend time on valued, obligatory, & discretionary activities" (Backman, 2005, p. 203), occurring when "the perceived impact of occupations on one another is harmonious, cohesive, and under control" (Christiansen, 1996, pp. 445-446). The profession generally views occupational balance as an "important aspect of the health experience" (Wilcock et al., 1997, p. 28).

Over the past two decades there has been a flood of research pertaining to life balance, with most pertaining to work-life balance. Stemming from the fields of organizational psychology, business, and management, work-life balance is typically defined as having "sufficient time to meet commitments at both home and work," to obtain "perceived balance between work and the rest of life" (Guest, 2002, p. 263). Duxbury et al.,1999) have noted slightly more than one in three Canadian employees experience a high level of work-life conflict; half experience high levels of perceived stress; and, one quarter feel "burned out" from their jobs, a prime example being nurses (Gallew & Mu, 2004). Men and women with dependent care responsibilities report substantially more work-life conflict than their counterparts without such obligations. High work-life conflict is associated with decreased wellness, greater perceived stress, depressed mood, burnout, poorer physical health, reduced job satisfaction and organizational commitment, greater use of the medical system, and increased absence from work.

Where: The physical, social, cultural, and institutional environment

Occupations are performed everywhere – at home, at school, at work, in the community, indoors, outdoors, underwater, and even in space (see figure 2.1). As case 2, the Burundian refugees, shows the environment is not only a context for occupational performance, but it also shapes occupational choice, influences health and well-being, and structures options for social inclusion or exclusion (CAOT, 1997a, 2000; Law et al., 1996; WHO, 2001). As indicated in the CMOP-E, the environment encompasses factors that greatly influence occupational performance. Interestingly, the environment and occupation have a reciprocal relationship; the environment impacts on occupation and, in turn, occupation impacts on the environment (Do Rozario, 1997; Manuel, 2003). The environment is multifaceted, including everything from the physical world to sociocultural mores. The environment is both naturally occurring and constructed. The CMOP-E conceptualizes the environment as consisting of two essential factors: physical and social. The social factor includes the social environment in general, and two specific instances of the social environment — institutions and culture. For the sake of clarity, each environmental factor is discussed separately. In reality, the different factors do not exist in isolation; each affects the other, and together they affect and are affected by human occupation. The observation of Ugandan children in their community (see text box 2.2) demonstrates this vividly.

Physical environment

The physical environment enables and limits occupational engagement, occupational choices, and methods of achieving occupational goals. People have varying skills and abilities, and their ability to engage in chosen occupations depends on an optimal fit among their personal skill set, the demands of the occupation, and the environment in which that occupation is pursued (Law et al., 1996). The physical environment encompasses natural and built factors (Hamilton, 2004): a multilevel office building with no elevator can pose a barrier to employees who have mobility impairments, as can a snow-covered sidewalk.

The natural physical world comprises all living and non-living things that occur naturally in the world. There are various ways in which the natural environment can influence the occupations of individuals, groups, and societies. The natural environment has the potential to influence what occupations people do, when people do occupations, how people do occupations, and which and how many people engage in occupations. In addition, the occupations that people do, individually, or as groups and communi-

Reflections on Ugandan children in their community

Through direct study of occupations, researchers can lend scientific support to many of the values and beliefs held by occupational therapists. In addition, we can gain knowledge about the context and meaning of occupations to facilitate client-centred practice. Observational research of Ugandan children in outdoor spaces revealed that children engaged in a broad spectrum of occupations that were clearly linked to the environment. In addition to play or games, which are often considered the primary occupation of children, children were observed to be willingly and actively involved in a broad spectrum of occupations, in particular occupations that contributed to household function.

For example, children were frequently observed transporting water, caregiving for younger infants, washing clothing and dishes, buying and selling produce, and stacking wood. Most developed nations have laws or taboos about young children being responsible for caregiving towards other children, or being involved in paid employment. However, in Uganda it appeared from observations that children are expected and encouraged to care for their other siblings. It was also common to observe children assisting with family revenue generation by selling produce or other goods and services. These observations thus lend support to the idea that occupations are culturally bound.

A further example of occupations being embedded in an environmental context was the observation that children's games tended to revolve around reclaimed objects such as old bicycle tires, discarded milk cartons, or old ropes. Children were rarely observed playing with toys specifically manufactured for them. This is likely tied to several aspects of the country's infrastructure: manufacturing plants are uncommon due to poor availability of electrical power, import of goods is limited by the country's economic status, and garbage is not collected in the same manner as in developed nations, thus making discarded objects accessible and ideal candidates for a child's imagination. This observation highlights the way in which occupations are economically bound and influenced by the availability of goods and services.

— *By Amy Sedgwick*

ties, influence the natural environment. For example, Willows (2005) has highlighted the need to study the ways in which elements of the natural environment —such as seasonal variations, the availability of fish and game, and distance between communities — influence how Aboriginal peoples in Canada procure, prepare, and distribute food. Some occupations, such as gardening, hiking, or mountain climbing, require natural environments containing certain elements and features and can contribute in unique ways to health and well-being (Hamilton, 2004; Manuel, 2003).

Bhatti (2006) drew on survey data from 244 older British people who were asked to write about the meaning of gardening across their lives. Bhatti found that gardening was associated with a variety of meanings and experiences, such as a source of identity, social connections, an outlet for demonstration, an exercise of physical capability, a connection to childhood, and a sense of being at home. Bhatti concluded that, "how older people are supported in their gardening activities in their own homes, and how well retirement homes are designed and managed can be crucial in the health and well-being of residents" (p. 391).

Gardening is an interesting example of an occupation situated in both the natural world and the constructed world. The constructed physical world refers to buildings, products, technology, tools, and equipment — the manufactured things around us (Stark & Sanford, 2005). These include homes and their furnishings, playgrounds, schools, shopping centres, office buildings and other structures in the community, and the tools, furnishings, and equipment within them. The constructed physical world is distinct from the natural environment because it has been built. It may be designed in accordance with expectations from other environmental aspects, such as sociocultural preferences, or institutional policies or law.

Take the design features of a house, for example. Design may be influenced by cultural beliefs or social desires as well as by building codes. The constructed, physical environment places demands on human occupation and also affords opportunities to participate in meaningful occupations when constructed to accommodate individual and societal occupational goals. Universal access refers to a particular approach to the design of buildings and equipment created in an attempt to ensure all users, regardless of ability, can access the built environment. Modifications to doorways, such as level grade entrances or ramps, automated doors, or levered handles in place of knobs, are examples of constructed physical environments that minimize barriers and facilitate participation in occupation. Tools and equipment may also be specifically designed to enable performance when personal skills may be insufficient; for example, a lid opener may assist with opening jars. Tools may be selected due to cultural mores; for example, chopsticks or forks are culturally determined eating utensils. Or equipment may be chosen to meet institutional requirements; for example, hard hats and steel-toed boots are mandated by law on most construction sites to minimize the risk of personal injury. In the gardening example, natural and built environments are brought together as elements of the garden; for instance, a trellis or a pathway, are constructed. Both natural and built environmental factors may facilitate occupational engagement.

Social environment

The social environment or social world is complex, multilayered, and dynamic. The nature of the social environment, and how to understand it holistically and by layers or components, has been the subject of continuous debate within sociology and other disciplines; various frameworks have been proposed to explain it. For example, one can think of the social environment in terms of micro, meso, and macro elements; in terms of various types of systems and structures; or in terms of social groups with various accesses to resources and power (Giddens, 1987; Layder, 1994). Consistent with contemporary models of occupational performance like the CMOP-E, these various ways of conceptualizing the social environment can be used to understand how occupations are shaped by the social environment and, in turn, how occupations shape the social environment (O'Brien, Dyck, Caron, & Mortenson, 2002).

Micro elements of the social environment pertain to personal and immediate aspects of social interaction in daily life, whereas macro elements refer to social structures such as the policies and regulations of organizations and institutions. Meso elements refer to social groups existing between the levels of the individual and social structures, such as families or work groups (Layder, 1994). At a micro level, an individual's occupational participation can be influenced by the people encountered in daily life and the negotiations on what, how, when, and with whom the individual will do occupations.

To illustrate, the way a new mother carries out the occupations associated with feeding her infant can be influenced by her encounters with health professionals who discuss and negotiate values and beliefs about various ways to feed infants. At a meso level, the ways in which one carries out occupations associated with being a mother can be seen as occurring in the context of groups, such as in a marital relationship, an extended family, or a mothering group. A woman may draw on family members for information and support when making decisions about how to feed or discipline a child. The presence or absence of a partner with whom to carry out parenting occupations will also influence how a mother will approach and carry out occupations.

The ways that social phenomenon like motherhood are collectively shaped and viewed at a macro level influence what comes to be taken for granted about the occupations people should engage in and how they should carry these out. Macro level influences are sometimes described as social constructions. Socially constructed discourses influence what is viewed as normal or as abnormal, non-ideal, or subversive occupations (Aronson, 1999; O'Brien et al., 2002; Rose, 1999). Discourses about parenting, for example, prevalent within a particular sociohistorical context can influence community responses to questions about the rights of parents to maternity or parental-leave practices. Discourses about parenting shape and are shaped by beliefs about parenting activities, such as breast-feeding an infant, toilet training a toddler, or disciplining an adolescent.

Cultural environment

Culture is a special feature of the social environment. Tylor (as described by Bonder, Martin, and Miracle, 2004) broadly defined culture in the late 19th century as "a complex whole which included knowledge, belief, art, morals, law, custom, and any other capabilities and habits acquired by man as a member of society" (p. 160). In the mid-20th century, anthropologists began noticing the impact of individual psychology on culture. Durkheim (as cited in Trafford, 1996) stated that culture was produced in any interaction that humans engage in. The definition moved further towards the individual level when Wallace (1961) noted that the basics of cultural traits were embedded within specific individuals; even though some individuals in society shared behaviours or had similar values, the core of culture remained in each individual.

Our understanding of the link between the individual and the collective continues to evolve today. Some see culture as a way of discussing collective identities (Kuper, 1999) whereas others see culture as the filter for all of a person's experiences (Krefting & Krefting, 1991). Fitzgerald, Mullavey-Obryne, and Clemson (1997) further explain the concept of a cultural filter as "learned and shared patterns of perceiving and adapting to the world" (p. 3). This ideational perspective of culture looks at culture's underlying influence on each individual's experiences and views. As Geertz stated, "culture is the fabric of meaning in terms of which human beings interpret their experience and guide their action" (Geertz, 1973, p. 83). This viewpoint is contrasted by the materialistic perspective of culture, where culture is not defined by abstract principles; rather it is defined by its expression in the more concrete aspects of "science, art, and technology, the sum total of achievements, inventions and discoveries"(Wagner, 1975, p. 78).

The evolving ideas on culture have given rise to different approaches or models. The most thorough and encompassing dynamic model in occupational therapy literature is the Cultural Emergent Model (Bonder et al., 2004, p. 161). This approach states that culture is a symbolic system, such as talk and action, which emerges as people interact. The model is based on each person's learning experiences through her or his life.

Culture has long been defined with respect to its underlying influence on individual views, or in terms of its artistic or scientific expression. It is, however, unfortunate that culture in today's society is often immediately replaced with the idea of race or ethnicity, as well as the prejudgments that may accompany those ideas. It is important to note that neither race nor ethnicity is synonymous with culture.

Bonder and colleagues (2004) suggest that culture has an essential impact on occupational patterns and occupational choices that are indicative of cultural beliefs. Kluckhuhn and Srodtbeck (1961) indicate that "everyday culture has a conception of human activity that conveys values that may be expressed through orientations on 'being', 'being-in-becoming', or 'doing'" (p. 165).

Even though there are many cultural influences on occupation, individual personality and personal experience are major contributing factors. Cultural patterns are constantly present during one's daily occupations. What becomes known as *appropriate* occupations are related to the community, country, gender, age, size, colour, past experiences, religious upbringing, social relationships, obligations, and responsibilities of those in a particular context. Thus, culture makes life meaningful and provides transparency in what we do. The culture and structure of our world are closely related to the meaning of occupation in our lives (Hasselkus, 2002a, p. 44).

Institutional environment

Institutional policies, funding, and legislation are a special case of macro social environments, and are the formal and informal structures that promote social order and govern society. Institutions organize society socially, economically, politically, and legally. They are complex and highly interrelated and reflect a society's values, ideals, and distribution of power and resources.

The influences of the institutional environment on human occupation are particularly profound because they are so embedded in the day-to-day experience as to become almost imperceptible. The work of people like Foucault (Danahar, Schirato, & Web, 2000), who studied prisons and medicine, and Goffman (1961), who studied psychiatric hospitals, popularized the relevance of social institutions to the purpose and function of health-related care.

The International Classification of Functioning, Disability, and Health (ICF) (WHO, 2001) recognizes that the outcomes of health conditions are related to the broader institutional context of society. The ICF identifies a detailed list of institutional factors for clinical, research, and policy development (see table 2.4). People with disabilities have long been advocating a model of disability that acknowledges that sociopolitical forces create limitations in activity and participation restrictions (Jongbloed, 2003). Despite the explicit protection of their citizenship rights by the *Canadian Charter of Rights and Freedoms* (see text box 2.3), the actual enactment of the rights of Canadians with disabilities continues to be restricted by institutional challenges.

Recently, interest has grown to understand how institutions enable or limit the occupations of people with disabilities and, ultimately, their experience of citizenship and community inclusion. The development of ideas related to occupational justice illustrate how to link occupation to individual and population health, and to the values and power relations of society (Stadnyk, Townsend & Wilcock, in press). The international work of Thibeault (2002) demonstrates how the development of occupation influences the health of communities. We know that gender is a factor that limits women with disabilities from receiving full disability benefits because Canadians still accept the idea that it is natural for women to be at home (Dyck & Jongbloed, 2000). We also know that efforts to employ more people with mental illness through the development of affirmative business are constrained by regulations regarding government disability income (Krupa, Lagarde, & Carmichael, 2003). Finally, Townsend's (1998) work on empowerment illustrates how the routine organizational structures and processes that govern occupational therapy practice can overpower the best intentions of occupational therapists in enabling occupation.

Table 2.4 Environmental factors of the International Classification of Functioning, Disability, and Health: Services, systems, and policies (WHO, 2001)

- Services, systems, and policies for the production of consumer goods
- Architecture and construction services, systems, and policies
- Open space planning services, systems, and policies
- Housing services, systems, and policies
- Utilities services, systems, and policies
- Communication services, systems, and policies
- Transportation services, systems, and policies
- Civil protection services, systems, and policies
- Legal services, systems, and policies
- Associations and organizational services, systems, and policies
- Media services, systems, and policies
- Economic services, systems, and policies
- Social security services, systems, and policies
- General social support services, systems, and policies
- Health services, systems, and policies
- Education and training services, systems, and policies
- Labour and employment services, systems, and policies
- Political services, systems, and policies
- Services, systems, and policies, other specified
- Services, systems, and policies, unspecified

Canadian Charter of Rights and Freedoms
(Government of Canada, 1982)

Equality Rights

15. (1) Every individual is equal before and under the law and has the right to the equal protection and equal benefit of the law without discrimination and, in particular, without discrimination based on race, national or ethnic origin, colour, religion, sex, age or mental or physical disability

Canadian Human Rights Act
(Government of Canada, 1977)

3. (1) For all purposes of this Act, the prohibited grounds of discrimination are race, national or ethnic origin, colour, religion, age, sex, sexual orientation, marital status, family status, disability and conviction for which a pardon has been granted.

How: Occupational development and change

Humans are occupational beings; that is, we do not become occupational over time or as a result of a particular event. Rather, we are occupational from the beginning. What does develop or change over time are the particular occupations in which an individual or group engages. The occupations of individuals are distinct and evolve with the ebb and flow of life.

Each person's unique occupational repertoire is the result of the interaction of that person, with her or his unique set of skills, talents, and interests, with the opportunities the world holds and the events life presents. Personal factors, such as an acquired disability, may disrupt a person's usual occupations and provide the impetus to develop new occupational habits (Haertl & Minato, 2006; Wallenbert & Jonsson, 2005). Similarly, environmental change can impact human performance and competence in everyday self-care, productivity, and leisure occupations. Occupations can change gradually (as in the course of development), predictably (as a result of transitions), or suddenly (as a consequence of unexpected loss). The process of change is essentially developmental.

Occupational development

The human process of accumulating an occupational repertoire and establishing occupational patterns begins at birth and continues across the lifespan. The individual's abilities, talents and interests, and the cultural, institutional, physical, and social factors of the environment will delimit and determine which occupational opportunities are available and who will engage. Accordingly, occupational development is the systematic process of change in occupational behaviours across time, resulting from the interaction of the person with the environment and the occupational possibilities, at the level of occupation, individual, and species (Davis &

Polatajko, in press). Occupational development occurs at three levels: micro, meso, and macro.

Micro occupational development: Developing occupational competence. At the micro level, occupational development occurs competence by competence, with an individual gradually moving along a continuum from novice to mastery for a specific occupation (Davis & Polatajko, 2006). Micro occupational development is an iterative process with the progression from novice to mastery repeated again and again for each new occupation (Davis & Polatajko, 2006). The trajectory and speed of competency development is relatively individual. It is dependent on the ability, capacity, growth and maturation of the individual, the demands of the competency, and the supports in place to enable the competency development. Thus competency development is specific to the individual and the specific competence to be developed. Understanding the intention of an occupation is key to developing competence (Humphry, 2002), as is having a rudimentary understanding of the occupation (Polatajko & Mandich, 2004); without knowledge of the intention or a representation of the occupation, development of competence is not possible.

Children offer an example of occupational development: in order to learn to feed themselves with a spoon, they need to understand that a spoon is intended to get food to the mouth and to have some idea about how they might use their hands, the spoon and the food to perform the occupation of feeding. Once these notions are in place, trial and error, and practice become the essential ingredients for developing competence. In the course of a lifespan, a person engages in a large variety of occupations and accumulates an occupational repertoire that is as unique to the individual as a fingerprint.

Meso occupational development: Developing an occupational repertoire. As individuals develop competence in an ever-increasing number of occupations, they build an array of occupational competencies — an occupational repertoire. The development of an occupational repertoire has multiple patterns and changes continuously throughout the lifespan, sometimes expanding, sometimes shrinking. There is no *a priori* determination of the number or specifics of occupations that constitute an individual's repertoire, either at a particular point in time or across the life course (Davis & Polatajko, 2006).

An individual's occupational repertoire develops as a result of a complicated process of interactions. Findings from a study by Wiseman, Davis and Polatajko (2005) suggest that occupational repertoires, at least in children, are established through an ongoing process of initiation, continuation, transformation and cessation, and are influenced by a complex combination of innate drive, exposure, resources, opportunities, and values.

Macro occupational development: Developing occupations. Occupational exposure and occupational opportunities play an important role in the development of an individual's occupational repertoire. The myriad of occupations available to the developing child in our society is the direct result of the continuous development of new occupations. The gradual emergence of a seemingly limitless number of occupations is referred to as macro occupational development (Davis & Polatajko, 2006). Macro occupational development occurs across time with the evolution of a species. As with development at the meso level, there is no predetermination of the number or specifics of occupations that a species will have at any given point in time or place; rather, occupations will develop continuously throughout time, sometimes expanding and sometimes shrinking in keeping with the species' needs, creativity, and ingenuity as well as the environmental supports, demands, and possibilities (Davis & Polatajko, 2006).

Occupational transitions

An occupational transition is a point in time during which there is a shift away from a particular occupation or set of occupations towards an alternative occupation or set of occupations. Such transitions can be self-initiated, occur in response to life events (for example, marriage or the onset of disability), or be part of a developmental process (for example, shifting from being a preschooler to entering school).

Occupational transitions can occur at the level of the individual, the level of the group (for example, a family shifting from a two-parent household to a single-parent household), and at the level of a society (for example, a shift in the types of jobs predominant within a region).

Occupational transitions at the level of the individual can be classified as micro, meso, or macro. A micro individual occupational transition occurs when one stops an occupation and shifts to another in the same context. Meso individual occupational transitions refer to larger transitions in occupations, such as leaving work and coming home or shifting from the occupational routine of a workday to that of a holiday. Macro individual occupational transitions occur with life transitions, such as getting married or retiring from full-time employment (Jonsson, in press).

Individuals experience macro occupational transitions throughout the lifespan. The timing and nature of these transitions are shaped within a sociocultural context. An important part of this context is the life course, which can be thought of as "a set of publicly shared meanings and expectations of the course of human lives" (Dannefer & Unlenberg, 1999, p. 319) that is created or constructed through social processes.

Research has begun to examine how an individual's beliefs, expectations, and occupational choices are shaped within this larger occupational life course. For example, the timing of occupational transitions, such as from school to work, or from non-parent to parent, have changed within North American society as social policies, labour market, and gender relations have changed (Moen, 1996). In turn, the occupational choices and behaviours of people within a particular sociohistorical context alter shared expectations and beliefs about the occupational life course. For example, changes in women's labour force participation in the Western world have contributed to changes in the timing of parenthood, and may also be impacting how men engage in child care and homemaking (Aldous, Mulligan, & Bjarnason, 1998).

It is evident that gender, culture, socioeconomic status, and other characteristics also influence the occupational life course. For example, retirement became an increasingly salient occupational transition for North American women in the last quarter of the

20th century. The timing and experience of retirement for females is different than that of males due to variations in factors such as the timing of entry into the workforce, periods of temporary exit from the workforce for child rearing, and rates of remuneration and access to private pensions (Moen, 1996; Townson, 2001).

Occupational transitions can also be examined at the population level. Statistics Canada routinely analyzes markers such as the average age of marriage and the average age at which a woman has a first child. Such analyses clearly show changes in the typical Canadian life course. Illustrations of occupational transitions are that the average age at which a Canadian woman had her first child rose from 25.7 years in 1986 to 27.1 years in 1996, and the average age of marriage for Canadian men rose from 27.4 in 1979 to 34.4 in 2001 (Statistics Canada 2001, 2002). There are also data available on typical patterns of involvement in various types of occupation over the life course. Another illustration of occupational transitions is that participation in volunteer occupations generally rises from a low in adolescence to early adulthood to a peak in the fourth and fifth decades of life, followed by a decline in later life (Selbee & Reed, 2001).

Occupational loss

Occupational loss, a special instance of occupational transition, is an imposed, unanticipated transition. Occupational loss occurs when a person or group of individuals can no longer participate in the normal routines and activities performed within their life context. Occupational loss can be characterized and understood by considering the nature and impact of the loss on the person in their lived context. Occupational loss may arise from environmental factors or events, for example, unemployment or loss of a family member. Loss may also be from personal factors, for example, there may be permanent or temporary loss of body functions due to illness or injury. Occupational loss can negatively impact health and well-being, and change what people can do, with whom they interact, the meaning of their occupations, and how daily routines and occupations are performed. The extent (duration and intensity) and consequences of occupational loss can be defined further by three levels: micro, meso, and macro.

Micro occupational losses are short-term occupational losses with a critical impact upon the routines and occupations of an individual as well as others in her or his life situations. These losses can lead to problems on personal and emotional levels, for example, injured athletes report feelings of frustration, isolation, and decreased motivation from not engaging in activities or occupations they enjoy and are passionate about. Similarly, individuals who lose their jobs — even for short periods — report negative effects on health and well-being. The loss of a job may be emotionally and socially devastating. The sudden lack of employment limits a person's capacity to contribute to society and may in turn erode a person's sense of self-worth. The loss of a workplace also includes the loss of access to social support from co-workers. In some contexts, there is a negative stigma associated with unemployment; this change from a worker-identity to an unemployed person-identity may decrease a person's self-esteem and lead to depression.

Meso occupational losses are long-term or permanent, progressive or cumulative losses that require the adaptation of occupations or the addition of new ones.

Permanent losses may occur due to a plant shutdown, an injury, a progressive disease, or a change in life circumstances, such as becoming a refugee, as shown in the Burundian refugee case, or becoming an *empty-nester* as a parent whose children have left home. Losing occupations of choice can deeply affect a person's sense of identity and self-efficacy, and can cause emotional distress, depression, and periods of sadness. Experiencing a long-term or permanent loss may also narrow or change the choices, scope, and number of everyday occupations in which a person engages. Such loss can also require people to involve others in making changes to their daily occupational patterns and routines. For instance, a person with Parkinson's Disease may need to give up driving a car and become a passenger. When this occurs, other people, such as a spouse, may need to alter occupations to assume the role of driver.

Macro occupational losses involve the immediate disruption of many or all daily occupations for groups of people and are typically triggered by a major event, such as the institution of a broad policy (see text box 2.4), political unrest or war, or large acts of nature such as a tsunami or hurricane. They can lead to the loss, change and disruption of many or all daily occupations conducted by groups of people and can give rise to physical health problems like illness and disease. Events that cause the immediate relocation of groups can lead to losses of basic necessities — such as food, clean water, and sanitary systems — as well as the cooking, bathing, and washing routines supported by these essential elements. People who are unexpectedly relocated tend to focus primarily on survival and can experience increased periods of heightened stress in trying to overcome the enormity of daily challenges such as acquiring food and resources to rebuild homes, or locating employment. These changes and tensions can also lead to behaviours like begging, stealing and violence, and can strain relationships among family members as they try to re-establish normal routines and occupations.

External circumstances that lead to losses across all occupations in the life context — such as education, work, economic, creative, community, social, civic, and family areas — may be planned or unplanned. On the one hand, a family that immigrates to another country likely anticipates major occupational losses but may plan steps to facilitate the move. On the other hand, traumatic life-changing events, such as a hurricane, are unplanned. Understanding the difference between these types of losses is imperative. When people immigrate to a new country, they retain some control over the process unless those immigrating are refugees. When people experience an environmental catastrophe or an unplanned event that leads to sudden and traumatic occupational losses, they experience a loss of control. The latter group typically lacks economic or financial supports, the power to make decisions about living arrangements, and access to information to determine the feasibility of returning home. Occupational loss that is unplanned can completely disempower individuals, families, groups, communities, organizations, and populations; this lack of control can give rise to feelings of hopelessness, helplessness, and despair.

Why: Health, well-being, and justice

Humans engage in occupation for many reasons, the most primal of which is to ensure survival of the individual and the species; that is, to obtain food and shelter,

Reflections on macro occupational disruptions

Macro-level occupational disruptions can have effects that last for generations. Residential schools operated in Canada from the 1840s to the 1950s and 1960s, although the last federally run one did not close until 1990. When Aboriginal people in Canada were forced by law to attend these schools, they were forbidden to speak their languages, wear their traditional clothing or hairstyles, communicate with their family members, practice their spiritual or cultural rituals, or engage in the daily occupations through which individuals had historically learned to be members of their Nations. In some families four, five, six, or seven generations attended residential schools. How might this have affected Aboriginal peoples occupationally, in terms of spirituality, community and family relationships, education, employment, and health practices? How might we as occupational therapists take into account both the detrimental effects of this intergenerational, macro-level occupational disruption, and the tremendous strength and resilience Aboriginal peoples have shown as survivors of such collective trauma?

— By Brenda Beagan

and to procreate. However, the human need for occupation continues even when the need for food, shelter, and procreation has been satisfied. The importance of occupation to health, well-being, and justice is becoming more evident as research elucidates the impact of engaging in meaningful occupation (Aubin, Hachey, & Mercier, 1999, 2002; Eklund, 2004; Goldberg, Britnell, & Goldberg, 2002) and the impact of social structures on occupational inclusion, equity, and justice (Wilcock & Townsend, 2009).

To completely understand the complexities of occupation and its effect on humans, we must first understand the experience of engagement from the perspective of the individual, as stated by Yerxa et al. (as cited in Hasselkus & Rosa, 1997):

> *To fully understand occupation, it is necessary to comprehend the experience of engagement …The same occupation may have a myriad of different meanings depending upon the goal of the individual, the environmental context, or mood … Eating may be done for survival, for social interaction as an important cultural ritual, as a symbol of a child's growing independence, or as a spiritual form of communion (pp. 9-10).*

Meaning is thought to be an important factor in understanding the relationship between occupational engagement, and health and well-being, and is likely related to experiences of injustice or justice in everyday life. However, no single theory that describes the characteristics of meaningful occupation currently exists. Some occupational scientists position meaningfulness in occupation within a framework of spirituality. Indeed, *Enabling Occupation* (CAOT, 1997a, 2002) states that spirituality is a source of meaning; "it resides in persons, is shaped by the environment, and gives meaning to occupations" (p.33). Spirituality in this context is not necessarily seen to have a religious base, although it may for some people, and is regarded as the essence that makes us distinctive and unique. Some theorists postulate that spirituality is an innate force that drives us to seek meaning and happiness through doing (Kang, 2003).

Meaning is also a central driving force for occupational engagement. Kielhofner's (2002) description of the Model of Human Occupation (MOHO) alludes to the importance of meaning as a determining factor of occupational engagement. It is postulated that humans have an inherent set of values that govern the occupations that are important and set a standard to measure performance. In addition, past experiences of engaging in occupation may result in feelings of competence, confidence and security regarding physical and mental abilities. An assumption underlying the MOHO is that by engaging in occupation, humans learn values and skills and develop interests, a sense of self-confidence, and competence. Feelings of satisfaction and pleasure may be factors that determine meaningful occupational engagement and motivate individuals to engage in occupation (Emerson et al., 1998; Mee & Sumsion, 2001). Research confirms that when individuals engage in meaningful occupations that promote feelings of self-worth and confidence, they are further motivated to engage in other occupations that are meaningful and result in feelings of satisfaction and pleasure (Mee & Sumsion, 2001; Rebeiro, 1999).

Not only is meaning considered a driving force to occupational engagement, it is also an outcome of occupational engagement. The Value, Meaning, and Occupations (ValMO) Model directly addresses the relationship between meaning and occupation by framing occupational engagement in terms of meaning (Persson, Erlandsson, Eklund, & Iwarsson, 2001). The ValMO states that meaning is created or discovered through engagement in everyday occupations and that occupations consist of the task(s) that the individual chooses to complete because they have some value to that individual. Value, an important component of meaning, is unique to each individual, can change throughout a person's life course, and is determined partly by cultural factors. Therefore, meaning occurs through engaging in occupations that have value to the individual. According to the ValMO, the environment plays an important part in determining an occupation's value: as occupation occurs in the context of the environment, the interaction between the two is imperative.

Christiansen (1999) proposed that one's identity is the source from which meaning is derived. Christiansen argued that the relationship between well-being, life satisfaction, and occupational engagement can be understood by examining identity. He proposed that identity is created and reaffirmed through occupational engagement, and is further shaped by our interactions with others and their reactions to our actions. Therefore, identity forms a context by which we view and interpret the world around us.

Whiteford (1997, 2000, 2004) found that unplanned and long-term losses of occupation deprived people of the sense of meaning required to thrive. Loss of meaning in occupational deprivation and occupational alienation are forms of occupational injustice, which in turn undermine health, well-being, and equitable participation in society (Stadnyk et al., in press). Therefore, inclusion and justice form a context in which to understand the essential nature of occupation.

Although definitions of meaning differ, it seems that meaningful occupation is a major factor of health, well-being, and justice. The literature consistently supports the view that meaning is determined by a complex interaction of societal, cultural, and personal factors and that it occurs within the context of occupation.

Deriving meaning

Meaning is a central focus in philosophical studies as well as in linguistics. The way in which the word is used in common speech is as intriguing as the roots of the word. Meaning is a significant piece of our thinking, our cognitive state, and our reality. Meaning is what we create for ourselves in our mind that explains experiences and, in turn, motivates and spurs us on to create new experiences.

Individuals seek to understand reality in many different ways. For some, the knowledge and beliefs inherent within a faith or tradition are invaluable in providing a framework and set of guidelines for creating a meaningful existence on earth. For others, the knowledge and empowerment that comes from close relationships with family, friends, and others is what affirms an individual's existence and creates a sense of self and awareness in place. Still others find their passion and commitment, the meaning of their reality, in working for the greater good of humankind. The interpretations through actions and decisions of our search for meaning are innumerable.

Our sense of meaning and purpose is essentially communicated to others and to those in our world through what we say, how we say it, and what we do. How we dress, the choices we make in spending our leisure time, and the manner in which we make our living are all vehicles that express our own personal meaning. The profound link between meaning and occupation is inextricably interwoven into what we believe, who we are, and the self that we portray to our external environment through occupation.

Occupation: The core domain of concern for occupational therapy

Chapter 3

Occupational science: Imperatives for occupational therapy

Helene J. Polatajko (Editor)
Daniel Molke
Sue Baptiste
Susan Doble
Josiane Caron Santha
Bonnie Kirsh
Brenda Beagan
Zofia Kumas-Tan
Michael Iwama
Debbie Laliberte Rudman
Rachel Thibeault
Robin Stadnyk

CASE 3.1 Emma in waiting

"Give me the card! Give me the card!" Bob grabs the card from Emma's arthritic hand and puts it down in the game of solitaire, in the wrong spot. With very limited range of motion at the shoulder, Emma cannot reach and correct the situation. And she wouldn't oppose Bob anyway: given his relatively advanced dementia, he is prone to sudden, frightening tantrums. As usual, Emma simply moves back to her bedroom, sits in its only chair, and stares out the window. In the early stages of Alzheimer's disease, Emma still enjoys fairly good cognitive function and feels more disabled by her increasing rheumatoid arthritis. In the special home where she has been placed — the only one available in her area so she could stay close to her family — most activities are designed for more physically independent residents with severe cognitive deficits. She can't play shuffleboard or throw beanbags, and she is bored beyond measure with the reminiscing group where the majority of people can't even remember their children's names. And watching residents dip their hands in the butter or lick the serving utensils has killed any appetite that had existed. With each day that passes, she ventures outside her bedroom less and less; instead she sits idly and cries. Her anxiety and blood pressure have continued to rise, as her weight and alertness have continued to drop. The attending caregiver looks in and asks, "Why don't you join us, Emma? What are you waiting for?" "For the day to end," replies Emma.

— By Rachel Thibeault

3.1 Introduction

Naming occupation as the core domain of concern for our profession brings with it the responsibility of knowing it at all levels (Polatajko et al., 2004). This requires us not only to make explicit our assumptions about occupation, as was done in chapter 1, but also to undertake careful study of occupation, to become *occupationologists*. In the late 1980s, Yerxa and her colleagues at the University of Southern California, initiated a new field of inquiry dedicated to the formal study of occupation. The intention was to create a science that would provide the foundational knowledge necessary for effective occupational therapy practice and to develop a professional identity focused on occupation.

Occupational science is the study of the occupational nature of people and how they adapt to the challenges and experiences of their environments through the use of occupations. Occupational science provides a way of thinking and a knowledge base in which the fundamentals from many theories are integrated to provide an understanding of the occupational human.

Since its inception, occupational science has been building our occupational knowledge base. It has also begun providing us with perspectives and data on a variety of topics that have important practice implications. This chapter will present an overview of selected areas of occupational study and the practice imperatives they

Occupation: The core domain of concern for occupational therapy

are pointing towards. This is an edited chapter with each distinct topic written by a recognized expert.

The areas presented in this chapter have special relevance for the understanding of the occupational human in context. Together, they provide an insightful picture of the relationship between the self and one's occupations as well as the roles played by the cultural, institutional, physical, and social environments in influencing that relationship.

The presentation of the selected topics starts with a discussion of the spiritual dimension of the self as it relates to occupation and is followed by a description of the relationship between occupational engagement and well-being. First, however, the chapter provides a description of the origins of occupational science as it emerged in the context of occupational therapy. The chapter introduces the importance of choice and presents an exploration of how it is influenced by social context. To further understand context, the concepts of culture and geography are presented. The chapter concludes with a discussion of occupational deprivation and a call for occupational justice for all. The question posed for readers is: How might occupational science knowledge, as presented in the summaries that follow, help occupational therapists work with individual clients like Emma (see case 3.1), or organizational clients like the nursing home?

3.2 Occupational science and occupational therapy from the perspective of Daniel Molke

Occupational science reflects not just the realization of a set of ideas that emerged at one place and time, but also the fulfillment of a need identified repeatedly throughout occupational therapy's history internationally and in Canada. Moreover, Wilcock (2001a, 2002, 2006) has identified sciences of occupation prior to the 20th century. She underlines the enduring importance of developing occupational science for understanding human nature, the human condition, and the structural factors that influence occupation.

Crisis in occupational therapy

Throughout much of its history, in order to obtain support and gain legitimacy, occupational therapy has relied heavily on the ideas and evidence generated by others. We use knowledge from various professions, disciplines, and administrations that may not have shared or even understood occupational therapy's concern with the importance of human occupation (Molineaux, 2001; Wilcock, 1991; Yerxa, 1992). Yerxa (1991a) argued that occupational therapists' reliance on others to define our concerns sacrifices control of our knowledge, vocabulary, and practice. We allow others to mold occupational therapy without developing our central constructs.

For example, from the 1930s to 1970s, we focused on specialized equipment and the treatment of performance components (CAOT, 1997a, 2002). In the 1970s and

1980s, leaders in the field felt that occupational therapy was in danger as a profession in part because there was no clearly articulated research foundation (Molke, Laliberte Rudman, & Polatajko, 2004). To take control of occupational therapy knowledge development, Yerxa (1981, 1987) called for two distinct avenues of research and knowledge development: practice-based research and basic research. Basic research was to pursue greater understanding of occupation as the profession's core domain.

The birth of a new academic discipline

In the late 1980s, the first doctoral program in occupational science was founded at the University of Southern California. The intention was that this new academic discipline would focus on "the study of the human as an occupational being including the need for and the capacity to engage in and orchestrate daily occupations in the environment over the life span" (Yerxa et al., 1989, p. 6). Occupational science was described as a basic science that would develop a broad and complex understanding of occupation without concern for immediate application to occupational therapy practice. Yerxa et al. (1989) argued that, occupational science should be multidisciplinary and concentrate on understanding occupation in relation to varying ability levels. They hoped that a basic science of occupation would generate knowledge as a foundation for developing occupational therapy practice.

International growth of occupational science

Since its establishment in the late 1980s, occupational science has grown and developed internationally and in Canada (Molke & Laliberte Rudman, 2003). For example, between the years 1990 and 2000, the number of countries, academics, and publication sources involved in disseminating occupational science literature grew substantially (Molke et al., 2004). Figure 3.1 provides a visual timeline of some of the important growth that has occurred in occupational science internationally and, more specifically, in Canada since its establishment.

Debate and controversy

The increased interest and participation in the development of occupational science gave rise to disagreement and debate regarding its intended focus and relationship to occupational therapy (Lunt, 1997). Debates focused primarily on questions about the appropriate type of scientific inquiries for occupational science and occupational therapy as well as the degree to which the two should be seen as distinct entities with differing focuses of concern.

Occupational science was created as a basic discipline to study the multifaceted nature of occupation without a concern for how knowledge would be used in practice. Some have espoused a focus on developing a science that would be intimately linked to the concerns of occupational therapy and the development of practice knowledge (Kielhofner, June 2002; Zemke & Clark, 1996). Others have argued that occupational science has distinct concerns from those of occupational therapy; they

Figure 3.1 International/Canadian growth of occupational science from 1989 to 2006

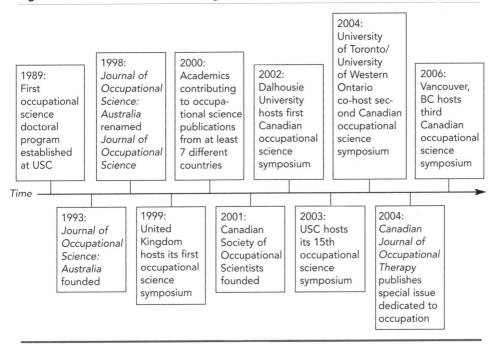

suggest that if occupational therapy leads the way, much of occupational science's potential may be lost (e.g., Mounter & Ilott, 2000; Wilcock, 2001b). In fact, development of a body of knowledge about occupation requires a radical shift to ensure the survival of occupational science (Molke et al., 2004).

The continuing pursuit of differing positions

Some might feel discouraged by the lack of consensus regarding the proper focus of occupational science's knowledge development. Kuhn (1996) indicated that the emergence of new forms of science results in intense debate among academics who develop and defend various positions. DiCenso (1990) pointed to the need for "interchange of divergent standpoints":

> *"Truth occurs by a continuing openness to otherness and to transformation. Its pursuit requires the free and critical interchange of divergent standpoints rather than the imposition of fixed standards" (DiCenso, 1990, p. 151).*

Farnworth and Whiteford (2002) argue that debate and dialogue is not only positive, but also essential for growth and development. One thing has become clear: as occupational science evolves and is exposed to a variety of perspectives, occupational therapists are faced with decisions about how best to apply knowledge developed by occupational science and other academic disciplines.

3.3 Occupation and spirituality from the perspective of Sue Baptiste

Spirituality is not finally a matter of technical expertise but of shared humanity at its deepest level.

(Kroeker, 1997, p. 66)

For many decades, the occupational therapy community in Canada has recognized the special place that the concept of "spirit" and personal meaning play in individuals' unique abilities to deal with unexpected events and to move forward in a new life direction after experiencing trauma, adversity, and hardship. In Canada's first set of three national occupational therapy guidelines, *Guidelines for client-centred practice of occupational therapy* (CAOT, 1991; DNHW & CAOT, 1983, 1986, 1987), spirituality was included as one of four components of the individual in the Occupational Performance Model (OPM). In the next iteration of guidelines, that is to say in *Enabling Occupation* (CAOT, 1997a, 2002), spirituality was placed in the centre of the Canadian Model of Occupational Performance (CMOP). Spirituality was defined as the very essence of who we are as human beings. In translating ideas about spirituality into practice, occupational therapists engage in partnerships with clients in a manner that respects their uniqueness, values their interpretation, and facilitates the optimization of skills to reach an integrated future.

Ideas about spirituality may, at first glance, appear high flown and ethereal, especially since there is still little clarity of definitions or applications to practice. Many questions arise with this concept. What does spirituality really mean? How can we assess it and how do we know that we are working with someone around or about spirituality? How can we implement spirituality in busy practice environments? How can occupational therapists' attention to spirituality compete if funding agencies, administrators, colleagues, and clients place a high value on evaluating measurable outcomes? How do we evaluate what we do surrounding spirituality?

Since the early 1990s, occupational therapists in Canada and around the world have undertaken a great deal of exploration into this complex and compelling concept (Belcham, 2004; Hasselkus, 2002b; Howard & Howard, 1997; Kang, 2003). A special issue of the *Canadian Journal of Occupational Therapy* (1997) explored spirituality from the perspectives of occupational therapists and colleagues in other disciplines.

McColl, in her Muriel Driver Lecture (2000), provided a rich and thoughtful exploration of spirituality from a non sectarian, faith-based foundation that offered much to those who were seeking some enhanced understanding. She outlined five specific areas of familiar occupational therapy practice within which spirituality emerges as clearly recognizable: in the use of narrative, ritual, appreciation of nature, creativity, and work. In 2003, McColl's edited book on spirituality provided an even broader canvas for occupational therapists and others to explicate their views on the integration of true partnership through human connectedness, using occupation as the core of that relationship.

Various authors have explored their own views, experiences, and insights on spirituality. Unruh, Versnel, and Heintzman (2001) completed an "Outcomes that Matter" project for the Canadian Occupational Therapy Foundation exploring the evidence around definitions of spirituality and possible ways of measuring spiritual outcomes. They uncovered multiple approaches that centre on the dichotomy of religiosity and spirituality. Debates about spirituality exist broadly across the literature on related concepts: spiritual crises, distress, need, wholeness, and well-being.

There is no clear and incontrovertible definition of spirituality. The absence of a single definition is not helpful to the occupational therapist struggling for understanding, the educator striving for clarity of thought, the researcher searching for measures to support the exploration of a question, or the busy practitioner hungry for something upon which to pin the rationale for a practice direction. However, this is the nature of spirituality itself. Each one of us would define it in our own way, and perhaps that is how it should be. This is an elusive element of human existence and interaction that seems to defy concrete explanation. Perhaps we should resist attempts to define spirituality. While we currently remain uncertain about how to weave the notion of spirituality into occupational therapy practice, we can seek understanding about personal meaning and uniqueness. We can learn more about what being human means as we explore occupations with our clients.

3.4 Occupational well-being from the perspective of Susan Doble and Josiane Caron Santha

Occupational therapy is grounded on the premise that individuals' health and well-being are supported by participation in culturally and personally meaningful occupations (CAOT, 1997a, 2002; Kielhofner, 1997; Wilcock, 2006; Yerxa, 1998). However, our understanding of occupation, as it relates to health and well-being is poorly developed. Efforts to enable individuals to perform valued occupations with less effort, greater efficiency, greater safety, or greater independence — or interdependence — may contribute to individuals' satisfaction with their performance of specific occupations. However, we propose that health and well-being are enhanced when people experience *occupational well-being*. Occupational well-being is an experience in which people derive feelings of satisfaction and meaning from the ways in which they have orchestrated their occupational lives (Caron Santha & Doble, 2006; Doble, Caron Santha, Theben, Knott, & Lall-Phillips, 2006).

Several assumptions ground the theoretical understanding of occupational well-being. First, at any one point in time, an individual's occupational life is comprised of a unique constellation of occupations. For example, Jill[1] works full-time as an elementary schoolteacher, goes to concerts and the theatre with friends, and volunteers to lead hikes through her local trail association. Christina is a full-time parent of two elementary schoolchildren, takes her children to swimming lessons, plays cards weekly with friends, and makes arrangements for her and her husband to get together with friends.

---

[1] A pseudonym, as with all names used.

Second, occupational well-being is enhanced when the unique constellation of occupations that comprise individuals' occupational lives enables them to meet their needs. These needs are assumed to be universal and include the needs to (a) derive feelings of mastery and achievement, (b) contribute to the well-being of others and/or community, (c) experience a sense of belonging and connection with others, (d) experience pleasure and fun, and (e) relax and restore energy levels (Hammell, 2004b; Laliberte Rudman, Yu, Scott, & Pajouhandeh, 2000; Pierce, 2001; Piskur, Kinebanian, & Josephsson, 2002; Rebeiro, Day, Semeniuk, O'Brien, & Wilson, 2001; Wilcock, 2006).

Third, occupational well-being is a subjective experience (Weinblatt & Avrech-Bar, 2001) and thus reflects an individuals' own perceptions. For example, Jill and Christina will make a personal judgment about whether the occupations in which they engage have enabled them to meet their needs. That said, individuals are more likely to experience well-being if they engage in occupations that they perceive (a) are consistent with their values and preferences, (b) support their abilities to competently perform valued roles, (c) support their occupational identities, and (d) support their plans and goals (Christiansen, 1999; Wilcock, 2006).

Fourth, even when individuals engage in the same tasks or sets of tasks, different needs may be met. The occupation of playing basketball, for example, is not the same for all. John prefers a pick-up game with a group of close friends on the outdoor court of the neighbourhood school. He plays basketball to meet his needs for belonging and to maintain a connection with others, whereas Dave plays in a competitive basketball league so he can challenge his physical skills and his ability to play strategically. Basketball provides Dave with an opportunity to meet his needs for achievement and mastery.

Fifth, several needs may be met through one occupation. A father, Kevin, and his 5-year old son, Brett, illustrate how people experience pleasure and fun through occupation as well as feelings of mastery and achievement. Kevin and Brett experience the enjoyment of occupational well-being while meeting their need to express their love for a family member by baking and decorating a cake to surprise Brett's mother on her birthday.

Sixth, an individual may experience an occupation in different ways at different points in time (CAOT, 1997a, 2002; Primeau, 1996). When preparing dinner for her family, a mother, Mariel, sometimes feels relaxed and takes the opportunity to try out new recipes. On other evenings, the same occupation of preparing dinner becomes a test of her skills and emotional control as she tries to get something ready before family members rush off to evening events.

Finally, opportunities for individuals to participate in culturally and personally meaningful occupations vary between individuals and over time (Becker, 1997). The orchestration of individuals' occupational lives is an ongoing and ever-changing process affected by both internal and external factors. As a result, individuals' occupational well-being will vary over time. On the one hand, one woman's opportunities to engage in and derive satisfaction from meaningful occupations may be affected by symptoms of multiple sclerosis. On the other hand, Peter is challenged to meet his own occupational needs because he spends most of his time caring for his frail mother. Huang Lee, a recent immigrant to Canada, has limited occupational opportunities because she does not speak English.

Ongoing and future steps for action

It is critical to empirically test the assumptions that ground the construct of occupational well-being. The first step in that process has been to develop a questionnaire to measure it (Caron Santha & Doble, 2006; Doble, Cameron et al., 2002; Doble et al., 2006). Development of the Occupational Well-being Questionnaire (Doble et al., 2002; Doble et al., 2006) will enable researchers to (a) examine the relationship between occupational well-being and health, (b) identify the level of occupational well-being experienced by different individuals and groups of individuals, (c) determine how social and environmental factors (for example, employment, access to health care and other services) affect individuals' occupational well-being, and (d) determine the effectiveness of interventions designed to support individuals as they discover, explore, and redesign their occupational lives.

3.5 Occupational choice and control from the perspective of Bonnie Kirsh

The constructs of occupational choice and control include the concept that occupational engagement is selective and variable across individuals, groups, communities and cultures; it emanates from a set of preferences, needs and values. Embedded in these concepts is the assumption that the right and power to exert preferences in occupational engagement exists. Perceptions of choice and control are socially and culturally constructed and some research has pointed to variations in conceptualizations of empowerment across cultures (Brunt, Lindsey, & Hopkinson, 1997; Mok, 2001).

Occupational choice and control have emerged as constructs of interest to occupational therapists from a significant literature on empowerment, rooted in the field of community psychology, adult education, and community development. The community psychology literature has emphasized the importance of individual determination over one's life as well as democratic participation in the life of one's community (Rappaport, 1987). Riger (1993) pointed out that mastery and control need consideration along with connectedness in human life; both are integral to human well-being and for well-functioning communities. Therefore, efforts might be directed at understanding and increasing individual control to link individuals with their larger social and political environments (Perkins & Zimmerman, 1995). Choice and control are not only individual constructs but also organizational, political, social and economic ones. It is important for groups, neighborhoods, communities, and institutions to make decisions and exert control over their status and destiny.

Occupational choice and control are imperatives for occupational therapy practice, as they pave the way for client-centredness and satisfying, successful outcomes. The opportunity to weigh options, make choices and exert decision-making capacity has been associated with the development of a positive working alliance (Kirsh & Tate, 2006) as part of client-centred practice. Research conducted with consumers of mental health services points to a direct relationship between perceived control and overall life satisfaction (Rogers, Chamberlin, Ellison, & Crean, 1997; Rosenfield, 1992; Segal, Silverman, & Temkin, 1995). Creating opportunities for choice and control ensures that clients are doing the things they wish to do in the ways, time frames and places that they wish to do them.

Choice and control are also important determinants of positive outcomes on a programmatic level. Programs that are flexible, offer a range of services, and provide opportunities for client choice and control are witnessing outcomes that demonstrate important changes in clients' lives (Kirsh, Cockburn, & Gewurtz, 2005). Provision of full information on the goals, operations and expectations of programs and services enables clients to make choices regarding occupational engagement. Enabling choice and control contributes to perceptions of client-centered practice (Sumsion, 2005).

Conversely, lack of choice and control produces negative outcomes. The absence of choice and control results in perceived paternalism, conflict and limited disclosure within the therapeutic relationship (Hendrickson-Gracie, Staley, & Neufeld-Morton, 1996). Lack of control has detrimental effects on health. High-demand workplaces that offer few opportunities for control produce increased depression, lower vitality, psychological strain, and sickness absences amongst workers (Karasek & Theorell, 1990; Niedhammer, Goldberg, & Leclerc, 1998; Stansfeld, Fuhrer, Head, Shipley, & Work, 1999).

Choice and control are severely restricted by stigma and occupational injustices. Conditions such as racism, poverty, homophobia, ageism, illness, or disability and policies that reinforce exclusion from mainstream occupational engagement are, unfortunately, still a reality in today's society. Such conditions limit the choice and degree of control that people can exert in their occupational lives. The mobilization of power through advocacy, community development, and peer support is gradually breaking down barriers that limit choice and control. Occupational therapy practice and research have the potential to delineate, understand, and remove barriers to optimize conditions in which choice and control can be exerted.

3.6 Social context and occupational choice from the perspective of Brenda Beagan and Zofia Kumas-Tan

Each of us makes individual choices several times a day, rarely aware of the extent to which our social group influences these choices. There are many different kinds of social groups, including those defined by race, ethnicity, age, gender, sexual orientation, ability or disability, and social class. Social groups influence our values, beliefs, and experiences. Obviously, not every member of a social group is the same, yet there are discernible commonalities that influence occupational choice, meaning, and participation within these groups.

Occupation: The core domain of concern for occupational therapy

While occupational choice is ultimately individual, our social group provides us with a framework of unwritten rules that tell us what is okay, depending on who we are, in social terms. It is not that we cannot break those rules, but rather that our social context promotes some choices and hinders others. For example, while it is increasingly acceptable for women to perform occupations that were once seen as men's work, men who engage in women's work may face ridicule and doubts about their masculinity and heterosexuality (Evans, 2004). At home, women still do the vast majority of child care, food-related occupations, and housework — although men's contributions have increased slightly in recent decades. While many women may actually enjoy *men's work* occupations, there is also social pressure to engage in them regardless of whether they experience pleasure; at the same time there is pressure on men *not* to enjoy or engage in *women's work* occupations (Wada & Beagan, 2006).

Similarly, while the meanings of occupations are always highly individual, historical and collective experiences shape occupational meanings differently for different social groups. For example, generations of Aboriginal peoples were forced to attend residential schools until as late as the 1980s. Understandably, the meaning of schooling for Aboriginal people today is likely to differ from that of other Canadian citizens.

Social class also influences the collective meanings of occupations (Humphry, 1995). People living in poverty — especially over generations — develop cultural routines and habits that arise directly from the realities of their lives. For example, insecure, unstable jobs may lead to placing heightened priority on family-related occupations, as family constitutes an irreplaceable source of security (Kiefer, 2000). Over time, when you rarely see members of your social group engaging in particular occupations, those occupations may take on a meaning of *belonging* to others, to people unlike yourself. Some leisure occupations, for example, become seen as middle, or upper-class — for example, ballet, theatre, skiing — while others become seen as belonging to the working class — for example, bowling, bingo, playing cards (Beagan, 2007).

Occupational participation is also affected by our social group, in terms of how we experience the occupation as well as why we participate. For example, schools tend to operate on the basis of middle-class values, leaving students from working-class families feeling like outsiders (Olson, 1995). Individuals with working-class backgrounds are then more likely to disengage (drop out of school) or to engage in occupations that are intended to show resistance — for example, truancy, substance use. When a simple shopping trip means you are likely to be followed, ignored by staff, or treated as unworthy to be in the store — as is the experience of many African Canadians (Beagan, Etowa, Acton, & Egbeyemi, April 2006), straightforward occupational participation becomes an experience charged with feelings of guardedness and vigilance against racism. Even the experience of child care can be vastly different when the mother is a woman with a disability; pervasive social assumptions that people with disabilities are always recipients of care cast constant doubt on their ability *to provide* adequate care to others (Grue & Laerum, 2002).

We engage in occupations in part to express or mask our social identities. For example, a young woman from an impoverished family background might use self-care occupations to pass as, or pretend to be, middle class (Beagan, 2007). Similarly, a young gay man may throw himself into hockey and football, attempting to pass as heterosexual. In contrast, particular occupations may be avoided as too disclosing of a stigmatized identity since, "The idea of playing a certain instrument in the [school] band is abandoned when doing so would contribute to the rumor that one is gay" (Kivel & Kleiber, 2000, p. 227).

Occupational engagement is also a way to convey social identities or forge belonging. A young lesbian joins the softball team to challenge gender expectations, to display her sexual orientation, and to attempt to connect with other lesbians. A young woman attends aerobics classes, reads fashion magazines, and learns to apply make-up to convey femininity. Boys and men with disabilities, who are often seen as un-masculine, may engage in sports as a way to convey their masculinity, health, fitness, and capability (Taub, Blinde, & Greer, 1999). Participation and non participation in specific occupations help to construct the social environment that, in turn, dictates the appropriateness of particular occupations. Participation in differing occupations produces social identity, just as social identity influences individuals' participation in occupations.

3.7 Culture and occupation from the perspective of Michael Iwama

Culture is a specific example of the social context of the occupational human. Culture has been defined in numerous ways according to varying social contexts of time and place (Arnold, 1879; Geertz, 1973; Mill, 1863; Williams, 1958). Culture can represent everything from the lifestyles of people in high society, versus those of ordinary citizens, to physically embodied distinctions and patterns of dress and food preparation attributed to one's race, or place of origin (Iwama, 2005). Historically, culture has been connected with the cultivated lifestyles and preferences of the social elite (Bourdieu, 1984). This understanding endures to this day, when we connect culture with the fine and performing arts, and to forms and symbols of everyday life as seen in language, fashion, and food preparation. In social scientific contexts, there have also been many definitions and debates over how culture ought to be explained and analyzed (Smith, 2005). Culture has evolved into a pervasive construct used in all aspects of daily life in the industrialized world, yet it remains problematic from the viewpoint of universal definition and meaning. There is, however, an evolving common understanding that is well captured in Hays' (1994) conceptualization that defines culture as shared meanings. Hays includes shared meanings in features such as the "beliefs and values of social groups, language, forms of knowledge and common sense, as well as material products, interactional practices, rituals and ways of life established by these" (p. 65). In the postmodern era, culture is discussed as a process by which groups of people share (Bates & Plog, 1990), create, and ascribe meanings to occupations.

The treatment of culture within the occupational literature has historically mirrored prevailing academic discourses of the day. In the 1980s and early 1990s, our literature regarded culture as distinct features located in the client (Kinebanian, 1992; McCormack, 1987). We admonished occupational therapists to be sensitive to the unique cultural patterns and features of their clients. Little attention was paid to the cultural features embedded in the occupational therapists themselves, nor in occupational therapy itself, its knowledge base, theory, or practice norms. Isabel Dyck (1998) captured the current consensus in the social sciences in defining culture as "a shared system of meanings that involve ideas, concepts and knowledge and include the beliefs, values and norms that shape standards and rules of behaviour as people go about their everyday lives" (p. 68). Iwama (2005) added that culture is as much a system of shared meanings as it is a dynamic process by which "meanings are ascribed to commonly experienced phenomena and objects" (p. 8.)

By assuming this broad perspective of culture, the construct of occupation can be appreciated from a variety of levels and dimensions (Iwama, 2005). One particularly useful approach is to organize cultural views of occupation by layers of complexities, as is done in Connor-Schisler's (1996) *micro, meso, and macro* analytical framework. By employing this three-level framework, a constellation of factors that influence the meaning, choice, and enactment of occupation by individuals can be better understood. When we understand how individuals choose, organize, and enact occupations, we can appreciate how the context of groups and communities support certain occupations and influence their meanings. We can also understand how larger institutions, such as modern medicine or the welfare state, political systems, and economic conditions can influence access to meanings and the performance of occupations.

Micro perspectives: Culture and occupation at the individual level

Perhaps the most familiar comprehensions of occupation have been taken at the fundamental micro, individual level of experience. Consideration focuses on the form, function, and meanings (Yerxa et al., 1989) of occupations by the client who is regarded as an occupational being. The impetus of occupation is seen to come from within the individual, supported by an essential system of values and beliefs. Culture is viewed as individual embodiment and becomes the explanation for the unique patterns and meanings formed through the client's action on the world.

Meso perspectives: Culture and occupation at the collective level

Most people understand that what an individual regards as worth doing encompasses much more than a solitary or individual phenomenon. The importance we attach to what we do is found in the interface between self and context and is affected by an interplay of social dynamic experiences and shared meanings. From this vantage point, the motivation and reason to engage in an occupation is thought to be influenced by a common set of values, beliefs, and situated conditions shared by a greater collective wherein one abides and to which one belongs. Occupations tied to the greater needs of a social group, be it a family or community, are examples of this cultural regard for the form, function, and meaning of occupation. An elderly client's need to maintain dependence in basic activities of daily living, to enable the caring roles of younger family members in certain Asian societies, is an example of a meso perspective of culture and occupation. The emerging interest in matters of context (Whiteford & Wright St-Clair, 2005) as a means to understand occupation is testament to this way of looking at the meaning of occupation from a cultural perspective.

Macro perspectives: Culture and occupation at the societal level

The macro level retains the same interests as the micro and meso levels concerning factors that affect the form, function and meaning of occupations, and the client as an occupational being. However, analyses focus more on systems and the broader context of conditions that influence culture at the meso and micro levels.

What does a socio-economic model have to do with individual occupations? How do gender norms in one's own society affect one's choice of occupations and desire to participate in them? What does the occupational therapist do in cases where meaningful occupations are accessible to some but not to others? These are some examples of questions that draw attention to macrostructures and their influences on human occupation.

3.8 Human geography and occupation from the perspective of Debbie Laliberte Rudman

Human geography seeks to understand material (physical) and immaterial (symbolic, social) aspects of space in relation to human doing and being. Concepts and research from the discipline of geography, related to the interaction of humans and space, point to the intricate interconnections between space and occupation, including their interactions over time in the lives of individuals, communities, and societies.

Rowles' (2000) geographically informed concept of *being in place* is an example of a concept that can inform our understanding of occupation and its enablement. Rowles, a geographer, proposed the concept after a qualitative examination of the occupations of older people living in an isolated rural community. Rowles' research demonstrates how the use of home, neighbourhood, and broader community spaces, through engagement in routine occupations, contributes to developing a sense of being in place. He found that the result of being in place is a sense of *autobiographical insideness* that sustains a coherent sense of self, despite changes occurring with the ebb and flow of life. Engaging in occupations within the individual and shared spaces of one's life reinforces identity and a sense of successful adaptation. Disruptions, such as disability or the relocation of significant others, can alter occupations and the use of space, thereby necessitating ongoing adaptation to attain an altered sense of being in place.

When occupational therapists work with seniors who aim to remain within their familiar places, such as homes, neighbourhoods, and communities, it may help to work towards being in place to shift the focus away from "obsessively striving for independence" (Rowles, 2000, p. 64S) and assessing risk. There is increasing sensitivity in society to the complex reasons why some older adults steadfastly seek to remain in their homes despite their inabilities to do so safely. Working towards being in place amongst community members would enable seniors to engage in familiar spaces and occupations. Alternately, working to enable seniors to carry familiar occupations and elements of space into new places would enable them to minimize disruption to their sense of self when they move.

A second example of human geography and occupation is Manuel's (2003) analysis, from an environmental planning perspective, of the impact of the removal of a pond from a suburban neighbourhood. She argues that change in place changes occupational opportunities. Access to diverse types of spaces, including natural ones, can support healthy emotional, cognitive, and physical development through diverse occupational opportunities. Manuel raises questions about the promotion of modern "landscapes of deprivation" (p. 37) in suburban and urban areas, which may contribute to decreased occupational opportunities. She also suggests that occupational therapists should advocate for the creation of spaces that facilitate engagement in a diversity of occupations. Manuel notes that differences in regional spaces can lead to varying access to occupation. For example, the location of post-secondary institutions in urban spaces may contribute to lower rates of post-secondary enrolment of youth from rural and remote communities.

A third example highlights the relationships between spaces where various types of occupations are located, such as home or work. Hanson and Pratt (1988), working from an economic geographic perspective, argued almost 20 years ago that it is essential to look beyond the workplace space to understand employment patterns and choices. Similarly, it is essential to look beyond the home space to understand housing decisions. The authors illustrated the interconnection between home and work spaces with data regarding the fact that women's workplaces tend to be closer to home than men's. Decisions regarding work spaces are also often connected to support services available in one's residential or home space.

3.9 Occupational alienation, apartheid and deprivation from the perspective of Rachel Thibeault

There is no meaning to life except the meaning man gives to his life by the unfolding of his powers.

(Fromm, 1962, p. 45)

As summarized eloquently by Erich Fromm, the need for meaningful occupation is rooted so deeply in human nature that when no venue exists to give shape to this need, with full or residual powers, life either drains away or explodes into anger and chaos (Camus, 1942; Fromm, 1962; Lang-Étienne, 1983; Lang-Étienne, 1986).

Among other impacts, meaningful occupation plays a pivotal role in fostering growth and development (Miller, 1992; Wilcock, 1998), providing psychological stability and well-being (Lang-Étienne, 1983, 1986; Mosey, 1986), sustaining health and social networks (Townsend, 1993; Wright-St. Clair, 2003) and harmonizing relations within civil society (Dürckheim, 1974; Marx, 1992). Conversely, blocking access to meaningful occupation can trigger a cascade of negative events, from the individual to the societal level.

CASE 3.2 Hussein and the cab

Hussein sighs behind the cash register: Now that the local grocery store has extended its business hours, customers are few and far between in the corner store he owns with his cousin. For him, the days are long and boring and his mind often drifts back to the prestigious engineering positions he held in his native Iran. Ten years ago, while still in his early forties, Hussein chose to leave his country so that his young sons wouldn't be eventually drafted into compulsory military service. The political instability of the region worried him and the prospect of war was very real. But ever since his arrival in Canada, he has been unable to get his initial training officially recognized, in full or in part, a fate shared by his dentist wife. So they make ends meet, with jobs they haven't chosen and for which they have few affinities. Hussein speaks of poor sleep, anxiety, back pain, lack of appetite, and general malaise. Another customer asks him if he would consider trying something different. Hussein shakes his head: "Too much energy, not enough hope." He has lost weight recently and his smile is not quite as bright as it used to be. Despite the risks and the difficulties, Hussein thinks that maybe he should move back home. But he can't talk much right now: Like every night, it's time for him to take his evening shift driving a cab.

— By Rachel Thibeault

Occupational alienation and apartheid

One injustice in everyday life has been called *occupational alienation*, a lack of control over one's life and an experience of meaninglessness or purposeless (Townsend & Wilcock, 2004a, 2004b). Occupational alienation results when external forces modulate occupational choices in such a way that they no longer fit the individual's potential or aspirations. Kohn (1976) was among the first to demonstrate how elements of occupational structure could lead to alienation. Such elements may be found in rising technological demands, work overload, lack of adequate ergonomic features or social interactions, and loss of meaning in life (Bryant, Clark, & McKay, 2004; Townsend & Wilcock, 2004a, 2004b). At the personal level, occupational alienation may exact a toll in the form of stress and feelings of inadequacy or futility that in turn may induce insomnia, addictive behaviours, depression (Greenberg,

Occupation: The core domain of concern for occupational therapy

Grunberg, & Moore, 2003; Utsugi, Saijo, Yoshioka, Horikawa, Sato, Yingyan, et al., 2005) and a significant increase in work-related injuries (Grunberg, Moore, Anderson-Connolly, & Greenberg, 1999). To be cast in the wrong occupational role deeply affects social relationships. For Hussein (case 3.2) the shift in professional status has meant a loss of identity, friendships, and a sense of belonging. Although he likes his customers and the delivery crews, he does not feel towards them the same kinship he used to experience with his engineering colleagues. In the end, a poor, alienating fit between the task and the individual culminates in high social costs: absenteeism and dissatisfaction. Their resulting destructive behaviours all undermine positive forces and contribute to the destabilizing of society (Fromm, 1962).

Akin to the concept of occupational alienation is *occupational apartheid*. The term occupational apartheid should be used with caution since, in itself, apartheid refers to the willful exclusion of a group. It should therefore be limited to those contexts where access to meaningful occupation is denied not out of fear or ignorance, but out of an organized political or social desire to deliberately exclude access. Before using the term — because it implies an active intent to exclude — one must ensure that no unfair assumptions are being projected on governments, agencies, or communities. A thorough and fair analysis of the motives underlying ostracism, which may range from the ignorant to the malicious, must be carried out prior to suggesting that governments and other agencies support apartheid.

In the case of people with disabilities, a charge of occupational apartheid would be a damaging strategy especially when most bureaucrats have only been minimally exposed to issues relating to people with disabilities. An inadequate use of the term occupational apartheid may lead to polarization that can seriously jeopardize constructive dialogue and impair efforts towards equity and justice for people with disabilities. An appropriate use of the term would be a powerful use of language to signal the impact of deliberate exclusion on the occupational lives of those involved.

Occupational deprivation

If extreme or prolonged, blocking access to meaningful occupation can result in *occupational deprivation*. The term occupational deprivation refers to ongoing restrictions arising from environmental, not personal, influences. Restrictions may be cultural, institutional, physical, political, or social (Townsend & Wilcock, 2004a, 2004b). Despite the wide range of potential sources, all forms of restricted occupational expression can lead to occupational deprivation. At the individual level, occupational deprivation can translate into stunted growth and ill health. As Emma's case at the beginning of this chapter illustrates, she has lost most of the control over her own life, and meaning in life is now imposed on her from the outside. Passivity is replacing interest, gradually eroding her sense of self. At the social level, her current living situation lacks opportunities for occupations that could connect her to family and friends or to higher-functioning residents with whom she could establish relationships. Occupational deprivation forces Emma into a social void that further draws her into discomfort and accelerates the degenerative process in body function, thereby undermining health and well-being through unjust deprivation of meaningful occupation.

At the societal level, groups that are denied access to meaningful, sustainable occupations can become marginalized and potentially disruptive. Emma (see case 3.1) represents the groups of seniors who end up removed from society, in an occupational no-man's land sanctioned by current social practices. Marginalization is even more apparent with captive populations or oppressed minorities (Provident & Joyce-Gaguzis, 2005; Thibeault, 2002; Whiteford, 1997). Life in refugee camps or prisons speaks to the destructive power of occupational deprivation: lack of occupation leads to lack of purpose, which can trigger depression, suicide, or violence (Frankl, 1962; Fromm, 1962; Seligman, 2002).

In the extreme, occupational deprivation may result in profound social fragmentation leading in turn to unrest and political instability, threatening the very foundation of civil society. When faced with near total occupational deprivation in the demobilizing camps of Sierra Leone, many rebel soldiers opted to wage war, as they needed something meaningful to do. And in the fall of 2005, despite its substantial welfare benefits, France paid the high price of violent riots as a result of relegating immigrant populations to situations of unemployment and/or meaningless work (Morice, 2006). Félix Leclerc (1972), a Quebec poet and singer, summarized it best: "There is no better way to kill man than to pay him to do nothing."

3.10 Occupational justice and injustice from the perspective of Robin Stadnyk

The devastating effects that can result from inadequate access to meaningful occupation should move occupational therapists to defend the Husseins (case 3.2) and the Emmas (case 3.1) of the world. Townsend (1993) captured this notion of a call to action in analyzing that social justice is occupational therapy's implicit social vision. She joined with Wilcock to propose the concept of *occupational justice* as both an embedded value and an implicit outcome of occupational therapy (Townsend & Wilcock, 2004a, 2004b; Wilcock & Townsend, 2000, 2009). Our profession's focus on occupation means that we are concerned that people have access to opportunities and resources to participate in culturally defined, health-building occupations. Occupational justice is a concept that can be used to guide consideration of diverse occupational needs, strengths, and potential of individuals and groups, while taking into account occupational enablement, empowerment, rights, and fairness (Stadnyk et al., in press).

In an occupational justice framework, access to occupations of personal meaning and societal value is seen as a right, based on one's citizenship. Townsend and Wilcock (2004b) outlined four occupational rights: (a) to experience occupation as meaningful and enriching; (b) to develop through participation in occupations for health and social inclusion; (c) to exert individual or population autonomy through choice in occupations; and (d) to benefit from fair privileges for diverse participation in occupations. These rights must be interpreted in a cultural context. For example, dominant Western cultural groups focus on choice and meaningfulness of occupations to individuals, while other cultures might instead focus on occupations that allow people to fit in or to contribute to their families, communities, or social groups.

Occupation: The core domain of concern for occupational therapy

Occupational justice, particularly in a Western context, is founded on three beliefs:

1. In an occupationally just world, people have a voice on how occupations in which they participate are organized. Justice relates to the power that individuals and groups have with respect to social structures that affect occupational opportunities for individuals and groups (Galheigo, 2005; Kronenberg & Pollard, 2005; Townsend & Wilcock, 2004a, 2004b; Townsend & Whiteford, 2005). Occupational therapists must understand these structures and work to enable occupational empowerment.

2. Honouring differences is important (Townsend & Wilcock, 2004a). People have different occupational needs, abilities interests, social situations, and resources. Young (1990) states that justice "… requires not the melting away of differences, but institutions that promote reproduction of and respect for group differences without oppression" (p. 47).

3. The occupational therapist can be an agent of change (Kronenberg & Pollard, 2005; Townsend & Whiteford, 2005; Townsend & Wilcock, 2004b). Occupational therapists have the skills to recognize and reflect on situations causing occupational injustices, and to work to change them.

Figure 3.2   A framework of occupational justice: occupational determinants, instruments, contexts, and outcomes

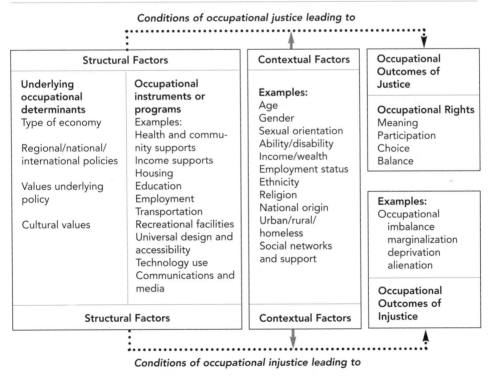

Conditions of occupational justice leading to

Structural Factors		Contextual Factors	Occupational Outcomes of Justice

Underlying occupational determinants
Type of economy
 	
Regional/national/ international policies
 	
Values underlying policy
 	
Cultural values
	Occupational instruments or programs
	Examples:
	Health and community supports
	Income supports
	Housing
	Education
	Employment
	Transportation
	Recreational facilities
	Universal design and accessibility
	Technology use
	Communications and media
		Examples:
		Age
		Gender
		Sexual orientation
		Ability/disability
		Income/wealth
		Employment status
		Ethnicity
		Religion
		National origin
		Urban/rural/ homeless
		Social networks and support
			Occupational Rights
			Meaning
			Participation
			Choice
			Balance
			
			Examples:
			Occupational
			  imbalance
			  marginalization
			  deprivation
			  alienation
			
			Occupational Outcomes of Injustice

Structural Factors		**Contextual Factors**	

Conditions of occupational injustice leading to

Stadnyk, R. L. (2007). A framework of occupational justice: Occupational determinants, instruments, contexts and outcomes. In E. A. Townsend and H. J. Polatajko, Enabling occupation II: Advancing an occupational therapy vision for health, well-being & justice through occupation, p. 81. Ottawa, ON: CAOT Publications ACE. Adapted from Townsend, E. A. & Wilcock, A. A., In C. Chistiansen, & E. A. Townsend (2004). *Introduction to occupation: The art and science of living* (p. 251). Upper Saddle River, NJ: Prentice Hall. Adapted with permission from Pearson Education.

Structural factors, in interaction with personal contexts, can create conditions of occupational justice or injustice (see figure 3.2). Underlying occupational determinants (Townsend & Wilcock, 2004a), such as the type of economy, national and international policies, policy values and cultural values, influence what occupations are valued, how they are rewarded, and who may participate in them. Occupational determinants are often experienced as funding priorities that inhibit or enhance occupational forms, which in turn will affect how work, parenting, play, recreation and sports, and supportive care are organized and fostered. Occupational determinants are operationalized in occupational forms (Townsend and Wilcock, 2004a). Occupational determinants and forms are experienced differently by different people which may be intentional, for example, in the case of programs targeted to people with low incomes, or unintentional, such as when accessibility to opportunities differs on the basis of age, sex, or other factors (Fast, Eales, & Keating, 2001; Kronenberg. & Pollard, 2005; Nussbaum, 2003, 2004; Stadnyk, 2005; Young, 1990). Contextual factors are individual group, or community characteristics that mediate the effect of occupational determinants and forms.

In the Canadian occupational justice framework, outcomes of occupational justice are conceptualized as having one's occupational rights met. Occupational injustices may result in outcomes such as occupational imbalance, occupational deprivation, occupational marginalization, and occupational alienation (Townsend & Wilcock, 2004b).

Occupational therapists address outcomes of occupational injustice by enabling change at various levels. At the level of the individual experiencing occupational injustice, an occupational therapist might enable a client's participation in occupations that are more aligned with choice and meaningfulness to self or society, or that allow for more balance. In interaction with occupational forms, enablement might occur through lobbying programs to be more inclusive, or to reduce discrimination. At the level of occupational determinants, an occupational therapist might be involved in advocating for change to regional, provincial, or federal policies. Occupational therapists can be partners and supporters of lobbying efforts by client or citizen groups.

Occupation: The core domain of concern for occupational therapy

SECTION II

Enablement: The core competency of occupational therapy

Introduction

Plato ranked reasoning as the highest form of human endeavour. We can reason carefully scrutinizing our body of professional knowledge for its thin, its flimsy, its fuzzy claims. We can scrutinize our body of professional knowledge for the clear, the substantial, the well formulated methods of practice. Both good and bad must be viewed critically, not necessarily negatively (Driver, 1968, pp. 59-60).

Occupational therapists are all too familiar with the question, *What do occupational therapists actually do?* Muriel Driver, a Canadian occupational therapy pioneer who is honoured nationally through an annual CAOT lectureship in her name, noted that occupational therapists "lag not so much in stating our role and function, but in enunciating clearly and positively the exact details of our methodology" (Driver, 1968, p. 59). Section II embraces Muriel Driver's challenge to articulate the often taken-for-granted "exact details of our methodology" (Driver, 1968, p. 59).

The centerpiece of Section II is a new Canadian Model of Client-Centred Enablement (CMCE). The CMCE is a visual metaphor for enablement and displays occupational therapy competency as a spectrum of enablement skills for client-centred, occupation-based practice. Chapter 4 presents the evolving definition and language of enablement, aligned with client-centred practice, with clients who may be individuals, families, groups, communities, organizations, and populations. The CMCE portrays practice based on enablement foundations, client-professional relationships, enablement skills, and critical reflection on influences that result in ineffective or effective enablement. Chapter 5 illustrates the CMCE in asset-based, client-centred enablement with individuals, families, and groups, using appreciative narrative inquiry, transformative learning and coaching approaches as examples. Chapter 6 highlights occupational therapists' longstanding, yet lesser-known interests in enabling systems-level, social change through community development, organizational development, and population health. It is noteworthy that the 10 key enablement skills in the CMCE are congruent with the seven core competency roles in the new *Profile of Occupational Therapy Practice in Canada* (CAOT, 2007).

Vision

To embrace enabling as the core competency of occupational therapy.

Purpose

To raise critical awareness about how occupational therapists practice.

Objectives

- To reflect on evolving definitions and reasoning about client-centred, enabling (verb) or enablement (noun) in occupational therapy
- To emphasize the breadth of occupational therapy with individual, family, group, community, organization, and population clients
- To introduce the Canadian Model of Client-Centered Enablement (CMCE), with:
    - enablement foundations
    - client-professional relationships
    - key and related enablement skills
    - an enablement continuum
- To illustrate use of the CMCE framework in:
    - appreciative narrative inquiry
    - transformative learning
    - coaching
    - community development
    - organizational change
    - population health

Practice implications

Section II introduces a new framework for embracing enablement as the core competency of occupational therapy. It alerts readers from outside occupational therapy to recognize the invisible complexity of a profession committed to enablement with others rather than doing things to or for them. This section promotes an appreciation of the power relations of enablement, and facilitates the adoption of enablement as a world view for participatory, collaborative, power-sharing ways of working and living. You are encouraged to adopt enablement as the language and methodology of client-centred practice focused on occupation — be you a clinician, educator, researcher, administrator, manager, consultant or other type of practitioner, or a reader who is not an occupational therapist. Immerse yourself in a language framework and model to respond to the question, What do occupational therapists actually do? The response offered here is that occupational therapists do enablement — our core competence is in client-centred *enablement* through occupation.

Chapter 4

Enabling: Occupational therapy's core competency

Elizabeth A. Townsend
Brenda Beagan
Zofia Kumas-Tan
Joan Versnel
Michael Iwama
Jennifer Landry
Debra Stewart
Jocelyn Brown

CASE 4 Joshua, Beth, and Joanne: Enablement possibilities

Joanne, a sole-charge community occupational therapist in a small rural hospital, opens Joshua's file at her desk. Joshua and his mom, Beth, will soon arrive for their weekly appointment. Joshua is 20 months old and has been diagnosed with Rubinstein Taybi Syndrome, a rare genetic disorder that can result in multiple medical, physical, and developmental disabilities.

Joshua lives in a loving home with his parents and two older siblings, David, age 9, and Brittany, age 4. Joanne has been working with Joshua and his family since he was discharged home from a children's hospital where he spent the first 6 months of his life. Beth will be bringing Joanne the latest home program designed by the occupational therapist at the children's hospital. Beth and Joanne will discuss how to incorporate the program into Joshua's daily routine. The request from the children's hospital asks Joanne to follow up with recommendations for speech language development because there are no speech therapy services available locally.

The micro-level goals of Joshua's occupational therapy program have been continually revised with the children's hospital and Joanne to accommodate Joshua's fragile health status and his slow but steady progress. Joanne is coaching Beth in promoting Joshua's independent sitting and hand function to enable him to play with his toys for occupational and social development, a specialized skill and an important step to improve the health and well-being of both Joshua and Beth, who is extremely worried about Joshua's future. The 10-year vision is that Joshua will start to participate in local daycare, recreation, and school programs with the help of Beth and attendants. Together, Beth and Joanne coordinate Joshua's team. Joanne will meet Joshua's new respite worker, who will attend the next appointment with Beth and Joshua. Joanne will involve Beth in an upcoming meeting with local health and community service providers, and the director of a daycare centre experienced with children with special needs. Joanne is collaborating to improve the inclusion of children with disabilities by sitting on the provincial board for special needs transportation planning.

In the hall Joanne hears voices. As Beth enters with Joshua in her arms she is beaming. "We've got great news! Joshua clapped his hands for the first time today!"

— By Patricia Moores and Brenda Head

4.1 Introduction

Enable or *enabling* (verb) or *enablement* (noun)[1] are words that describe what occupational therapists actually do. Occupational therapy enablement is focused on

---

[1] The authors use the noun enablement and the verbs enable or enabling depending on syntax.

Enablement: The core competency of occupational therapy

occupation, the primary domain of concern of occupational therapists. Thus enablement is the other core construct, with occupation, on which occupational therapy rests. Why do occupational therapists enable occupation? Critical analysis reveals a historic, implicit, social vision of enabling individual and social change to advance occupational justice (Townsend & Wilcock, 2004a, 2004b; Townsend, 1993; Wilcock, 2006). The imperative of articulating what occupational therapists do will be clearly recognized by Joanne and Beth. Explanation of occupational therapy competency will be needed when they seek policy and financial support to continue occupational therapy to help Joshua.

Definitions of enabling are evolving from multiple sources. In 1997, the practice of enabling occupation was defined as *"enabling people to choose, organize, and perform those occupations they find useful and meaningful in their environment"* (CAOT, 1997a). Chapter 1 of this book introduces a new definition of occupational therapy:

> *Occupational therapy is the art and science of enabling engagement in everyday living, through occupation; of enabling people to perform the occupations that foster health and well-being; and of enabling a just and inclusive society so that all people may participate to their potential in the daily occupations of life.*

Why adopt enablement language?

In proposing that occupational therapists describe our core competence as enablement, one might ask: Why are occupational therapists talking about enablement? Why not explain what we do with examples? We could say: occupational therapists educate employers to provide workplace accommodations for people with mental disorders; or occupational therapists use special techniques to facilitate children with motor dysfunction to develop the skills they require to participate in school; or occupational therapists provide adaptive technology for those living at home with a physical disability. Joanne, like other occupational therapists, may not be accustomed to referring to enablement when talking about the profession's core competence. We trust that many readers will rejoice in talking and writing about enablement to describe the dynamism and complexity that underlies what occupational therapists actually do. Some may find the language of enablement uncomfortable. Still others may feel that this language works well in theory, but they would not use it in practice because they think that no one will understand. The real question is: Does it matter?

Not surprisingly, our answer is yes, it matters that we develop the language of enablement because language can spark learning, insight, self-reflection, understanding, and critical reflection (Chompsky, 1968; Foucault, 1972; Townsend, 1998). Language is a tool to communicate and document ethical and moral values as well as professional competence; examples of using professional language are in textbooks, ethical codes, scope-of-practice statements, and accountability documentation (see chapter 12). Language is the basis of professional literacy; hence, enablement language extends occupational therapists' literacy to communicate to others the values, beliefs, assumptions, and ideas underlying what may appear to be a simple or technical profession. To illustrate, Joanne will want to educate Beth, the mother, and the provincial government contact persons on the special needs transportation committee how occupational therapy enablement might help Joshua to live as full a life as possible in his family and community. The language and concept of enablement will empower Joanne to communicate and document how she enables Beth to facilitate Joshua's occupational development, and how she collaborates with Beth and others to enable policy, funding, and legislative change to develop accessible transportation options for children, like Joshua, to be included in the local school.

In documenting and communicating what occupational therapists do, we want to use the language of enablement with awareness that language is embedded in cultural meanings. Hays (1994) described culture as shared meanings that include "beliefs and values of social groups, language, forms of knowledge and common sense, as well as material products, interactional practices, rituals and ways of life established by these" (p. 65). Culture is a dynamic process by which "meanings are ascribed to commonly experienced phenomena and objects" (Iwama, 2006a, p. 149). Because of cultural diversity in Canada and worldwide, the varied meanings, forms, and functions embedded in clients' and occupational therapists' lives will require diverse approaches to enablement and the language used to describe it (Whiteford, 1995). English-speaking occupational therapists might use and explain the language of enablement in connection with the language of occupation. We are reminded that the language of enablement, as with the language of occupation, will need cultural and linguistic exploration in particular contexts. Awareness of culture, therefore, will enrich Joanne's understanding of the cultural nature of her language and of her competency in enablement.

As the language of enablement becomes known in and beyond occupational therapy, we want to consider how to use this language with attention to diversity (Beagan & Kumas-Tan, 2006). A preliminary, national occupational therapy statement on diversity reminds us that: "the profession is stimulating discussion to identify which definition or definitions of diversity most effectively move the profession forward" (ACOTRO et al., 2006, p. 1). Enablement language, used with awareness of culture and diversity, is presented to advance both the vision and practice of occupational therapy in Canada, empowering the profession's members to understand and tell others what we actually do.

Enablement reasoning — an emerging social theory of change through occupational enablement

Knowing that language is a powerful tool to empower the profession, and that attention to culture and diversity is important, one might still ask: Why is enablement named as the core competency? *Enablement reasoning*[2] to explain occupational therapists' core competency is summarized in table 4.1.

The enablement reasoning in table 4.1 displays enablement as a phenomenon of interest, a construct for research, a methodology and an emerging social theory of

---

[2] Occupational therapists were introduced to the term *clinical reasoning* through research on clinical forms of occupational therapy in medical settings. Professional reasoning for reflective practice is employed here as a broader term that encompasses occupational reasoning and enablement reasoning. *Enablement reasoning* draws on narrative, conditional, empirical, or other reasoning. (See Glossary).

Table 4.1   Enablement reasoning: Imperative of enablement as core competency

- Enablement is the appropriate methodology to engage people in occupations and extends beyond applying treatments to people who remain passive

- Enablement and client-centred practice are aligned, each explaining and delimiting the other

- Enablement methods make space to hear the voices, interests, and perspectives of others, and to share power with them as they promote health, well-being, inclusion, and justice through occupation

- Enablement methods structure and encourage citizenship with entitlement, opportunities, and resources for participation by all in a just and inclusive society, including those who are healthy, occupationally compromised, or marginalized; for example, those who are elderly, living with chronic disease, injury, illness, disability or social disadvantage

- Enablement prompts engagement in both individual and social change in occupations; these are interconnected with different entry points to effect change in occupations

- Enablement in occupational therapy draws on a spectrum of complex skills that are selected, interwoven, and dynamically shaped as enablement unfolds with different clients in different contexts

- Enablement captures occupational therapy's historic social vision in 19th-century occupation work with people with mental illness and indigent people to enable change in their individual lives and social conditions

- Enablement uses age-old methods of learning through doing is a powerful way for people to influence their own lives and societies

- Enablement challenges occupational therapists to be critically reflective and to take into account multiple perspectives, competing interests, power inequities, and diversity

- Enablement is the professional identity and trademark of occupational therapists who engage others through meaningful occupation to pursue goals for health, well-being, and justice through occupation

change through occupational enablement. Enablement, focused on occupation, goes beyond systems theory, which was cited in Canada's first three guidelines books in the 1980s on client-centred practice (CAOT, 1991). Systems theory provided insight on the environment and on relationships between actors, objects, and processes. It suggested that occupational therapists might enable change by changing systems. An analogy using systems theory might be to reason that enabling change in the train route and schedule (environment) would enable change in individuals' travel patterns (persons), and the daily routines (occupations) of those who take trains.

Enablement, focused on occupation, also goes beyond symbolic interaction and transactional social theories, as cited in *Enabling Occupation: An Occupational Therapy Perspective* (CAOT, 1997a; 2002): to examine the fit in the interaction of persons, occupations, and environments. An analogy for enablement based on transactional theory might be to reason that enabling change in the train route and schedule (environment) might produce a better fit for commuters (persons) to get to work (occupations) on time.

What distinguishes enablement reasoning as a social theory of change focused on occupation engagement, is the inclusion of a critical[3] social perspective to understand power and power relations. Occupational therapy interests are in enabling

---

[3] The term *critical* refers to a critique of social structures, not to criticism of people.

client empowerment and, with clients, in reaching toward visions of possibility for occupational dreams and futures. Enablement may draw on systems, symbolic inter-action, and transactional theories. With a critical social perspective, however, we can extend our understanding of enablement with awareness of the social construction of power and power relationships (Fay, 1987; Giddens, 1991; Habermas, 1995), which are at the heart of client-centred enablement. Effective enablement practices will display awareness of taken-for-granted power relations that are embedded in the regulatory, governance, and practice structures and organization of institutional functions like health care, education, or housing (Smith, 1987, 2005).

Occupational therapy has possibly always included an implicit, critical social perspective, given our history and aims to enable change in the environment as this influences occupational engagement (Friedland, & Davids-Brumer, 2007; Law, 1991; Wilcock, 2006). Furthermore, our profession's interests are congruent with a critical perspective given our history of concern to enable change with those who are socially disadvantaged or marginalized because of disability, chronic illness, poverty, and real or potential exclusion; our socially oriented aims in enablement target health, well-being, inclusion, and justice. Moreover our social perspective informs everyday practice as we mediate power sharing, collaboration, and empowerment with clients ranging from individuals to organizations and populations. This profession is already committed to reflective practice as championed by Schön (1983, 1987) and applied to occupational therapy (Kinsella, 2001; Mattingly, 1998; Mattingly & Flemming, 1994) to better understand enablement for both individual and social change.

Consideration of language as a tool for professional literacy and empowerment, and consideration of enablement reasoning lay the groundwork for this chapter. The chapter explores definitions from within and outside the profession as guidance for embracing a new definition and model of enablement. The new Canadian Model of Client-Centred Enablement (CMCE) celebrates our competency in a spectrum of enablement skills. The chapter ends with critical reflection on an enablement continuum to highlight factors that determine the effectiveness of occupational therapy enablement.

4.2 Defining enablement

Enablement is not unique to occupational therapy. It occurs in many fields, such as adult education, health, law, organizational management, planning, sociology, social work, and psychology. Sociocultural diversity requires diverse forms of enablement. Moreover, let us be mindful that there are ineffective and negative, as well as effective and positive, forms of enablement. Best practice in occupational therapy seeks to offer effective, client-centred, occupation-based enablement for health, well-being, and justice. Contrasting this is ineffective, unhealthy enablement, described particularly in the field of addictions as enabling substance abuse (Beattie, 1992). In the field of disability studies, enablement is viewed as potentially disabling and oppressive when norms for ability are narrowly defined (Morris, 1991, 1992).

Starting with simple dictionary definitions, enable or enablement is typically defined as creating possibilities and building power and capacity to be or do something. As in the *Oxford Dictionary* (1989), definitions are concise but too simplistic to capture the complexities of occupational therapy enablement:

> *enable: a) give power to; strengthen; make adequate or competent b) make able, give the means, to be or to do something to provide with ability or means to do something ... to make possible ... to give legal power, capacity or sanction (Barber, 2004).*

An internationally influential source, the landmark *Ottawa Charter for Health Promotion* (WHO, 1986) named enable as one of three key strategies, with advocate and mediate. In the *Ottawa Charter* (see text box 4.1), *advocate* refers to actions to create favorable conditions for health; *mediate* highlights the need for coordination. *Enable* focuses on equity and justice in opportunities, and resources to enable all

---

Text box 4.1

Defining advocate, enable, mediate

Advocate

Good health is a major resource for social, economic, and personal development and an important dimension of quality of life. Political, economic, social, cultural, environmental, behavioural, and biological factors can all favour health or be harmful to it. Health promotion action aims at making these conditions favourable through advocacy for health.

Enable

Health promotion focuses on achieving equity in health. Health promotion action aims at reducing differences in current health status and ensuring equal opportunities and resources to enable all people to achieve their fullest health potential. This includes a secure foundation in a supportive environment, access to information, life skills and opportunities for making healthy choices. People cannot achieve their fullest health potential unless they are able to take control of those things which determine their health. This must apply equally to women and men.

Mediate

The prerequisites and prospects for health cannot be ensured by the health sector alone. More importantly, health promotion demands coordinated action by all concerned: governments, health and other social and economic sectors, non-governmental and voluntary organizations, local authorities, industry and the media. People in all walks of life are involved as individuals, families, and communities. Professional, social groups and health personnel have a major responsibility to mediate between differing interests in society for the pursuit of health.

people to achieve their fullest health potential through a supportive environment, access to information, and opportunities for making healthy choices. Structural (environmental) forms of enablement are interconnected with personal attributes and performance, such as "life skills," so that people are able to have agency over those things which determine their health. The *Ottawa Charter* defines enable with attention to diversity, specifically gender, noting that "This must apply equally to women and men" (WHO, 1986, see text box 4.1).

The 1986 *Ottawa Charter for Health Promotion* captures the idealism of enabling in the context of health promotion (WHO, 1986). From an occupational therapy perspective, an important missing element from the *Charter* and other idealistic definitions is the connection between vision and real life; that is to say, a connection to what people actually do every day to promote health, well-being, inclusion, and justice through their everyday occupations.

Also from an occupational therapy perspective, the *Ottawa Charter for Health Promotion* pays explicit attention to social conditions — to what occupational therapists call the environment. Not mentioned is the challenge to hold onto the dual, interrelated approaches of enabling individual and social change. Absent is a link between enabling change in the environment (policies, sociocultural habits, built and natural context, governance, economics) and enabling change in persons (sense of meaning, physical and mental performance, thinking, making decisions, expressing feelings).

Occupational therapy reflection on the term enable, in the context of health promotion, may raise awareness around diversity in enablement. The *Ottawa Charter for Health Promotion*'s definition of enable (text box 4.1) calls for decreasing differences and ensuring equal opportunities and resources. Since occupations, people, and environments differ, occupational therapists would ideally define enable/enablement to celebrate, not reduce differences, so that all people could reach their fullest health potential.

An occupational therapy definition of enablement needs to recognize the profession's historical concern for differences and challenges associated with disability and other disadvantages. To this end, the *Canadian Charter of Rights and Freedoms* (Government of Canada, 1982) may be a useful reference in defining enablement, given that Section 15(1) of the *Charter* refers to "equality before and under the law, and equal protection and benefit under the law" (text box 2.3).

Section 15(2) continues on affirmative action programs that could include occupational therapy enablement programs or activities with disadvantaged individuals or groups:

> *Subsection (1) does not preclude any law, program or activity that has as its object the amelioration of conditions of disadvantaged individuals or groups including those that are disadvantaged because of race, national or ethnic origin, colour, religion, sex, age or mental or physical disability.*

Section 15(2) may be used to highlight the importance of enabling social, as well as individual, change in the "amelioration of conditions of disadvantaged individuals or groups." This section offers support to occupational therapists in making our concerns to enable a just and inclusive society more explicit. The *Charter* may help occupational therapists integrate both individualistic and social perspectives. It is important to note that the *Charter* cites social conditions of disadvantage as an important, national matter of social rights and justice.

4.3 Defining enablement with diverse clients

There is a heavy emphasis in occupational therapy literature, education, and practice on practice with individuals. This is natural in light of Canadian values regarding individualism (see text box 4.2).

Text box 4.2

Reflections on individualism

When referring to Canadian values regarding individualism, it is important to consider how these are embedded within larger Western ways of knowing or thinking and to acknowledge that such ways of thinking about the individual are not universal. Sökefeld (1999) and Geertz (1973) describe the Western conception of the person as emphasizing autonomy, wholeness, uniqueness, separateness from others and the environment, and capable of defining and pursuing her/his own goals. As Geertz (1973) said, this way of thinking about individuals may be "a rather peculiar idea within the context of the world's cultures" (p. 126).

In acknowledging the cultural diversity of clients with whom occupational therapists interact within Canada and internationally, there is a need for awareness of and sensitivity to the varying cultural ways of thinking about persons. Occupational therapists might consider how enablement may occur with individual, family, group, organization, and population clients who do not interpret the world in terms of themselves or view themselves as individuals who are separate from others and their environment.

Iwama (2005) pointed out that within Japanese culture there is no strong sense of a centralized self who independently acts upon a separate environment, but rather a focus on how self, others, and nature are inseparable. Sökefeld (1999) argued that, from a South Asian perspective, individuals are viewed as elements of larger social units, rather than as separate parts. Watson (2006) described an Afro-centric worldview as collectivist in which people are valued in terms of what they do within their community or collective, rather than in terms of individualistic characteristics and goals.

How might occupational therapists recognize how individualism and/or collectivism are influencing practice? How might such fundamental values be respected and given voice in practice? What are the implications of individualism for occupational therapy?

— *By Debbie Laliberte Rudman*

Reflections on individualism

In light of practice concerns for both individual and social change, the occupational therapy definition of enablement needs to be broad to encompass many categories of clients. The pyramid in figure 4.1 and descriptors in table 4.2 name six categories of clients, drawn from occupational therapy literature. The definition of an occupational therapy client is, therefore, broad.

> *Clients may be individuals, families, groups, communities, organizations, or populations who participate in occupational therapy services by direct referral or contract, or by other service and funding arrangements with a team, group, or agency which includes occupational therapy.*

The six categories in figure 4.1 evolved from the four categories in the 1997 definition (CAOT, 1997a). Without intending to delimit the addition of other client categories, the 2007 categorization adds families, communities and populations, and subsumes agencies as a form of organization. The term *family* is used broadly to recognize that there are many types of families. The message in defining clients broadly is that occupational therapy enablement extends beyond working with individuals or persons: practice may focus on the environment (Iwarsson & Slaug, 2001; Law, 1991; Whiteford, 2005) with community, organization, or population clients.

The figure 4.1 pyramid layers the six categories numerically from base to peak. Figure 4.1 and table 4.2 descriptors are not meant to communicate a moral judgment about priority, preference, or value for some categories over others. Instead, the pyramid image shows that occupational therapists work with far more individuals (at the base of the pyramid) than populations (at the peak). Some occupational therapists may wish to use additional client categories such as agencies, institutions, special interest groups, or corporations.

In the first national guidelines (DNHW & CAOT, 1983), Canadian occupational therapists chose to refer to the people or organizations with whom we work as clients. Although *client* is a business term, the reasoning was that Canadian

---

Figure 4.1   Occupational therapy clients

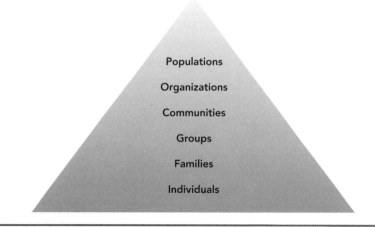

Enablement: The core competency of occupational therapy

Table 4.2   Client descriptors

Client Types	Descriptor
Individuals	A single human considered apart from a society or community: the rights of the individual. A human regarded as a unique personality: always treated her clients as individuals. A person distinguished from others by a special quality (Dictionary.com, n.d.-c).
Families	A family consists of a domestic group of people (or a number of domestic groups), typically affiliated by birth or marriage, or by analogous or comparable relationships — including domestic partnership, cohabitation, adoption, surname, among others (Wikepedia, n.d.-a).
Groups	A group is usually defined as a collection of humans [or animals], who share certain characteristics, interact with one another, accept expectations and obligations as members of the group, and share a common identity. Using this definition, society can appear as a large group. (Wikepedia, n.d.-b).
Communities	Social, religious, occupational, or other groups sharing common characteristics or interests and perceived or perceiving itself as distinct in some respect from the larger society within which it exists: the business community; the community of scholars (Dictionary.com, n.d.-a).
Organizations	A group of people united in a relationship and having some interest, activity, or purpose in common: association, club, confederation, congress, federation, fellowship, fraternity, guild, league, order, society, sorority, union (Answers.com, n.d.). Organizations may also be governmental, corporate or other business systems to manage functions such as health care.
Populations	A group of individuals of the same species occupying a particular geographic area. Populations may be relatively small and closed, as on an island or in a valley, or they may be more diffuse and without a clear boundary between them and a neighboring population of the same species (Dictionary.com, n.d-d). In health care, populations and population health research may use medical diagnosis, such as the Canadian population of adults with multiple sclerosis.

occupational therapy clients are typically active participants in therapy and their lives. Instead of using the term clients, occupational therapists may want to use occupational terminology relevant to a particular practice context. Examples of occupational terms to replace clients are: workers; residents in housing; players in recreation or sports; patients in medical settings; family members; students in educational settings; participants in research; target audiences in policy work; or representatives and members of agencies, communities, organizations, or populations.

Reflections on diversity point to the complexity, such as in a family situation, of determining: Who is the client? Unlike in a business context, the individual of concern is not likely the payer. Client diversity may also be in characteristics, such as ethnicity, race, or social class as highlighted in text box 4.3.

Reflections on clients and diversity

In defining client categories, occupational therapists might raise these questions about client diversity: Would the definition of enablement differ if Beth, the mother, was the client, or if Joshua's whole family was the client? What if the daycare was a client? Or what if Joanne held a contract with the provincial government, an organizational client, to make recommendations on special needs transportation?

Some questions worth critical reflection include: How might enablement differ if Joshua and Beth live in an Aboriginal community in Canada's North? How might it make a difference if Joanne, the therapist, is also Aboriginal? How might client participation, visions of possibility, change processes, and power relations for collaboration differ if all three are white and live in a major Canadian city? How might enablement change if the family lives in poverty or is very well off?

— By Brenda Beagan

4.4 Defining enablement in alignment with client-centred practice

A further consideration in defining enablement is the alignment of this concept with the concept of client-centred practice. Since definitions of client-centred practice and enablement differ, their alignment in occupational therapy has not been clear. Canada's first national practice guidelines, developed in 1983 (DNHW & CAOT, 1983), described occupational therapy as client-centred, based on the work of a clinical psychologist, Carl Rogers (1939, 1951, 1969). Client-centred practice was not explicitly defined in these or subsequent national occupational therapy guidelines until the publication of *Enabling Occupation: An Occupational Therapy Perspective* (CAOT, 1997a). Instead, the idea of collaborating with people — rather than doing things to or for them — was implicitly infused in guidelines for assessment and the process of practice (DNHW & CAOT, 1983). Guidelines for the implementation of client-centred practice (DNHW & CAOT, 1986) and recommendations for a client-centred outcome measure of occupational performance (DNHW & CAOT, 1987) emphasized that client-centred practice meant focusing on client goals and projected outcomes. Neither the 1991 combined publication of the 1983, 1986 and 1987 guidelines (CAOT, 1991) nor the 1993 guidelines for client-centred mental health practice (CAOT, 1993) actually defined client-centred practice.

Fourteen years after the publication of the first occupational therapy guidelines for client-centred practice, the terms client-centred practice and enablement were both included in the stated purpose of *Enabling Occupation: An Occupational Therapy Perspective* (CAOT, 1997a, 2002). The purpose was to offer readers a "perspective which makes occupation, occupational performance, and enablement the focus of client-centred practice" (p. 3). Client-centred practice was, henceforth, aligned with enablement and defined in 1997 as:

... collaborative approaches aimed at enabling occupation with clients who may be individuals, groups, agencies, governments, corporations or others. Occupational therapists demonstrate respect for clients, involve clients in decision making, advocate with and for clients in meeting clients' needs, and otherwise recognize clients' experience and knowledge (CAOT, 1997a, 2002, pp. 49, 180).[4]

Occupational therapy *enabling [enablement]* was further defined as:

... processes of facilitating, guiding, coaching, educating, prompting, listening, reflecting, encouraging, or otherwise collaborating with people so that individuals, groups, agencies, or organizations have the means and opportunity to participate in shaping their own lives; enabling is the basis of occupational therapy's client-centred practice and a foundation for client empowerment and justice; enabling is the most appropriate form of helping when the goal is occupational performance (CAOT, 1997a; 2002, p. 50, 180).

These definitions not only align client-centred practice and enablement, they put enablement at the core of client-centred practice. In occupational therapy, client-centred practice delimits the definition of enablement; conversely enablement delimits the definition of client-centred practice.

The 1997 publication included guiding principles for client-centred practice (see CAOT, 1997a, 2002, table 10 and pp. 51-54). It also highlighted issues of choice, risk and responsibility (see pp. 54-56).

The emergence of definitions and guiding principles in 1997 seems to have sparked occupational therapy research on client-centred practice without always specifying the connection to enablement. A search for the terms *client-centred* and *occupational therapy* in the *Cumulative Index of Nursing and Allied Health Literature* identified 228 peer-reviewed papers published between 1997 and 2006.

There is an increasing array of research on the concepts, power relations, justice, and tensions in client-centred practice (Sumsion & Smyth, 2000; Kirsh, Trentham, & Cole, 2006; Townsend, Langille, & Ripley, 2003; Townsend & Wilcock, 2004a; Wilkins, Pollock, Rochon, & Law, 2001). Research with minority groups has highlighted the need for occupational therapists to attend to diversity as a central component of client-centred practice (Kirsh et al., 2006). Law et al. (1998) and Sumsion (1999) recognized the need for textbooks on occupational therapy's client-centred practice, and published on the topic.

Challenges in client-centred practice — and similarly in enablement — have been identified at the levels of the client, the therapist, and the health care system (Sumsion & Smyth, 2000; Wilkins et al., 2001). At the client level, challenges relate to clients' culture, level of education, problem-solving skills, desire to be an active decision maker, and age (Black, 2005; Restall, Ripat, & Stern, 2003; Sumsion & Smyth, 2000; Sumsion, 2005; Wilkins et al., 2001). At the therapist level, challenges in trusting client judgement, sharing power, recognizing client expertise, finding

---

[4] The CAOT (1997a, 2002), Glossary definitions of client-centred practice and enabling (p. 180) differ slightly from the definitions in the text (p. 49, 50).

time to be client-centred, and lack of resources may be barriers to client-centred practice (Duggan, 2005; Restall et al., 2003; Sumsion, 2000). At the systems level, challenges to client-centred practice are in management philosophies, resource rationalization, policy restrictions, regulations, governance structures, expectations, accountability, and restrictions on implementing an occupational model in the bio-medical context of health services (Black, 2005; Restall et al., 2003; Sumsion & Smyth, 2000; Townsend et al., 2003; Townsend, 2003; Wilkins et al., 2001). Studies of client-centred practice in occupational therapy and other fields show that good intentions are often invisibly and routinely subordinated to management concerns for safety, efficiency, and cost-minimization, which are not centred on the client at all (Campbell, Copeland, & Tate, 1998; Townsend, 2003).

On the positive side, studies suggest that client-centred practice leads to better health outcomes (Black, 2005; Sumsion, 2005). This finding parallels research in nursing and medicine on the implementation of patient-centred models of care (Stewart, et al., 1995). Positive strategies to enhance client-centred practice have been proposed; by Duggan (2005), Restall et al. (2003), and Sumsion (2005). Their research showed that occupational therapists embrace client-centred practice when there is a facilitator who will prompt insights to deal with the challenges of being truly client-centred. The use of client-centred tools for occupational therapy assessment (Pollock, 1993; Swee Hong, Pearce, & Withers, 2000) and the measurement of occupational performance (Pollock, 1990) are known methods for shifting practice toward client-centredness. The *Canadian Occupational Performance Measure* (COPM) (Law, Baptiste et al., 2005; McColl et al., 2006) is a good example of occupational therapists embracing client-centred practice when they have a recognized assessment/ evaluation tool. The *COPM* has a strong international recognition as a Canadian outcome measure based on concepts of client-centred practice.

4.5 Enablement foundations

Before describing the Canadian Model of Client-Centred Enablement, consider six foundations (see figure 4.2) of occupational therapy enablement: choice, risk, responsi-bility; client participation; change; justice; visions of possibility; and power sharing. Enablement foundations are the interests, values, beliefs, ideas, concepts, critical per-spectives, and concerns that shape enablement reasoning and priorities.

Choice, risk, and responsibility

The importance of mediating client and professional choice, risk, and responsibility in client-centred enablement was raised in 1997 (CAOT, 1997b). Emphasized was the ethical commitment to respect client views, experience, interests, and safety. Also emphasized were the rights of clients to live with risk and to make choices that may differ from the suggestions of professionals. Here, we continue to remind occu-pational therapists that goal setting, choice, and decision making with clients require close attention to matters of choice, risk, and responsibility for professional and legal responsibilities. Occupational therapists are strongly encouraged to collaborate in all processes with clients, and to openly make arrangements for client choice,

Figure 4.2   Occupational therapy enablement foundations

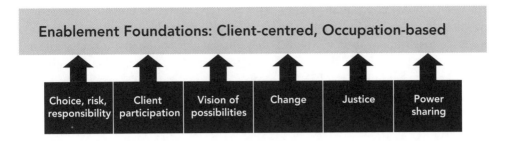

Townsend, E. A., Polatajko, H. J., & Craik, J. (2007). Enablement foundations. In E. A. Townsend and H. J. Polatajko, *Enabling occupation II: Advancing an occupational therapy vision for health, well-being, & justice through occupation*. p. 101 Ottawa, ON: CAOT Publications ACE.

risk, and responsibility. The aim in occupational therapy is to enable safe engagement in just-right risk-taking.

Client participation

Building on the focus on occupation and client-centred practice, client participation is a central feature of enablement. Participation is an active concept characterized by involvement and engagement, and is driven in part by biological needs to act, find meaning, and connect with others through doing (Wilcock, 2006). Participation in everyday occupations is shaped by a host of factors, including interests, perspectives, needs, expectations, desires, motivations, social conditions, resources, dreams, hopes, and visions of possibility. Participation exerts individual human agency and reflexivity to participate through individualistic or collectivist engagement in occupations.

As discussed in section I, the concept of participation has received worldwide attention through publication of the ICF (WHO, 2001), which defines participation as "involvement in life situations" (p. 17). Current research is mapping ICF categories of participation onto outcome measures used by occupational therapists, while also developing and testing new measures of participation (Desrosiers, et al., 2004; King et al., 2004). Since the ICF concept of participation is meant to recognize citizenship and rights, the National Organization on Disability (NOD) in the United States has adopted the notion of citizenship in its definition of participation as the "degree of connection that citizens with disabilities have to physical and social surroundings" (National Organization on Disability, 2000, p. 1). Hence, client participation in occupational therapy may be guided by the concept of occupational citizenship; that is to say optimal engagement as a fully integrated citizen in a just and inclusive society with entitlement to participate and to promote health and well-being for all.

The implication for occupational therapy enablement is to include clients as citizens who are entitled to participate in making decisions about occupational therapy, other services, and their lives. Occupational therapists understand that the personal and environmental factors influencing participation, as noted in the ICF, can support or limit enablement. In some contexts clients may not wish to participate in making choices and decisions in a professional context (see text box 4.4).

Hammell (2004a) points to the potential for the ICF to be a disabling tool for occupational therapists, not an enabling one, if our profession adopts participation and loses the focus on occupation. The ICF may also be a disabling tool if occupational therapists use it as a professional framework without client participation. For client-centred enablement using the ICF, clients would be invited to take an active role to identify and make implementation plans to enable greater participation in occupations.

Text box 4.4

Reflections on client participation

Some clients — due to age, gender, culture, social class, education level, or even personality — will not want to be part of the occupational therapy decision-making process. They will not want to express their interests, perspective, or priorities. How do we as occupational therapists respect these people's social or cultural expectations for non-participation, while not falling into the expert-therapist/passive-patient model?

— By Brenda Beagan

Visions of possibility

As clients participate through occupation, they may generate and express visions of possibility to resolve occupational challenges (Townsend & Landry, 2005). Their visions of possibility and those of occupational therapists will be grounded in particular values, beliefs, and ideals about the diverse potential of persons to engage in life — in mind, body, and spirit — beyond usual expectations. Occupational therapists' visions of possibility appear to be charged by professional beliefs, knowledge and experiences to pursue an ideal, inclusive, and just society (Townsend, 1993).

With support from occupational therapists, clients' visions of possibility may energize them to imagine a life that may not be expected of them and that they may not have expected. Adults who have been injured on the job may not imagine the possibility of returning to work until they and the occupational therapist begin to explore workplace accommodations; young offenders in detention may be unable to envision a new life until they and the occupational therapist develop a program to build their skills and confidence for living and working on their release in a new community. Visions of possibility may prompt people to perform occupations or to participate more fully as citizens beyond what they had previously imagined. Visions of possibility may also spark a readiness to participate and an openness to make new choices, take risks, and even accept previously unimagined responsibilities. In essence, visions of possibility to participate in everyday occupations challenge us to find or create opportunities to include people regardless of their ability, age, social status, or other characteristics. Occupational therapists' visions of possibility are being informed by emerging research on hope (Borel, Lija, Sviden, & Sadlo, 2001; Woodside, 1976).

Critical perspectives on disability, diversity, oppression, and inequity (Beagan & Kumas-Tan, 2006) raise important questions about structural norms that restrict visions of possibility and hope. Visions of possibility may be a counterpoint to reflections on the status quo. The implication is that visions of possibility challenge *what is* and consider *what might be* or even *what could be*. A belief in possible futures rejects the notion that change is impossible. A fundamental question of occupational therapy is whether or not to comply with the status quo and allow people and the profession to fit in with established social norms or expectations. Occupational therapists are encouraged to generate the courage and supports to enable individual and social change, thereby advancing opportunities for client empowerment and participation in society.

As a foundation for enablement, it seems that occupational therapists aim to inspire confidence, hope, respect, readiness, and resilience with tough-minded and tireless optimism. A hallmark of occupational therapy is to radiate genuine interest and empathy, expectations of success, and a belief in the potential for personal and social transformation, as the checklist in table 4.3 suggests.

Table 4.3 Sparking visions of possibility: Discussion points

- Inspire confidence, hope, and resilience through relationship
- Exert a tough-minded and tireless optimism
- Trust others
- Radiate an expectation of success
- Express genuine interest, acknowledgement of concerns, and deep empathy
- Courageously express possibilities for transformation and empowerment

— By Jo Clark

Change

Change means simply to take a different position, course, or direction (Merriam-Webster, 2003). Change may also be a process of transition or transformation to a new, altered, or different state (Answers.com). In reading about enablement foundations to this point, one might imagine an occupational therapist, charged with tireless optimism and visions beyond what others expect, inviting clients to be active participants in their transition or transformation to a new and altered state. The invitation would be, in fact, for clients to take part in effecting the changes they not only need to make but also dream to achieve toward their goals for health, well-being, and justice.

Between 1983 and 1991 (CAOT, 1991) occupational therapists were guided to develop, maintain or restore occupational performance, or to prevent problems in occupational performance. With attention to the research advances and constructs beyond performance, which were highlighted in section I, change might be directed to enable clients to (a) develop through occupational transitions across the life-course, (b) maintain occupational engagement, health, and well-being, (c) restore occupational potential and performance, or (d) prevent occupational losses and deprivation, occupational alienation, or other forms of occupational injustice.

To illustrate the relationship among enablement foundations, change processes would draw on visions of possibility and the belief that humans are active agents whose participation can effect individual and social change. Occupational therapy practice with individual, family, or group clients might focus on enabling change in occupational performance and beyond. With communities, organizations, or populations, desired change might be in collective issues, such as the occupational deprivation of community members when an industry closes. Concerns for change in organizations may be to reduce the marginalization in the workplace of persons with disabilities as a population. In client-centred enablement, occupational therapists would respect diverse perspectives and competing interests on whether changes are needed or not. Underlying concepts in enabling change are to uphold fairness, to ensure choice, and to balance risk and responsibility. When occupational therapists enable change, we ideally invite clients to imagine change or the prevention of change based on their own visions of possibility.

Change associated with occupational therapy enablement may be superficial and barely detectable, for example when seniors are enabled to cook their own meals or garden in long-term care facilities. Or, change may be radical enough to threaten some while liberating others, as when persons with disabilities secure the part-time positions that non-disabled persons covet. Radical changes may reshape the social structures that determine possibilities and limits for inclusive participation. Change may also cause clients and occupational therapists to transform their perspectives on life and re-envision their identities as individuals, family members, group representatives, and representatives of communities, organizations or populations. Enablement of change may be directed toward occupational transitions across the lifespan, such as the transition to retirement (Jonsson, in press). Occupational therapy interests in change are sometimes based on minor, physical adaptations to an individual's environment; for example, changes in a school, workplace, or kitchen for living in a wheelchair. Sometimes occupational therapists pursue major policy changes to make the educational, employment, housing, transportation, or other environmental context more inclusive or equitable. Change, then, is highly infused with questions about power: Who has the power to effect change? How will change affect the exercise of power, especially in situations where there are competing interests? What happens when the client, family, or community have different visions of possibility? What forms of power will prevail, and who may benefit and who may lose power if the changes desired by clients are achieved?

Knowledge and skill in change processes are necessary to effectively support clients to exert agency and to enable social inclusion (Kegan, 1994). While there are many models of change for particular circumstances (see chapters 5 and 6), occupational therapists may find it useful to generate and discuss their own questions. Sample questions for discussion might be: What forms of occupational engagement might draw individuals into contemplating change? How does change work in groups when they are engaged in shared occupations? What is the role of occupational therapists in enabling social change if our trademark is to engage people in occupations? What partners are appropriate when occupational therapists engage clients in changing disabling policies or physical environments?

Justice — diversity and equity

Many occupational therapists deeply value the opportunity to help people to help themselves, and to make a real, practical difference in people's lives (Kumas-Tan & Beagan, 2003). In our profession, values around helping are subsumed within the concept of enablement. Yet even as we use occupational therapy skills, techniques, and assistive technology to enable others, it is important to ask: "What else do we enable through our work with clients? Are all enabling efforts consistent with our values?"

Occupational therapists work with many populations to enable occupational transitions and wellness, and to enable the discovery of occupational potential with those who are occupationally disadvantaged. Consideration of persons with disabilities illustrates how justice is an enablement foundation (Morris, 1992). Persons with disabilities face prevalent beliefs that they are not good enough as they are — that they need to change somehow, to become more "normal." As Morris (1991) states:

> One of the most oppressive features of the prejudice which disabled people experience is the assumption that we want to be other than we are; that is, we want to be normal (p. 105).

Of course, some people insist that all they want is to be normal again. Yet what values do we act upon if we accept the view that being normal means being able-bodied? We may enable occupation, but do we also enable the belief that having a disability is abnormal, wrong, or shameful? Ironically, it is the belief that disability needs to be changed that many people with disabilities have found most disabling (Morris, 1991).

A related question to ask ourselves is: What do we enable when we work toward the goal of independence, and to what extent do we promote the beliefs that people should not have to help one another, that people should be able to care for themselves? Efforts to increase the independence of people with disabilities may be of more benefit to able-bodied people, freeing them from helping others or adapting the able-bodied world (French, 1991). At the same time, the benefits of giving and receiving help are denied to everyone when independence is expected and demanded.

> Disabled people have been conditioned to manage and overcome their disability, to be independent, to be normal ... These pressures make accepting help difficult – nowhere in the socialization of disabled people have they been encouraged to do so. Yet giving and receiving help can greatly enrich human experience (French, 1991, p. 47).

What then do we enable when promoting independence? We may enable the belief that independence is better than dependence. We may entrench the belief that people with disabilities should not ask for help, because asking for help means failure. Short-term individual benefits may have long-term collective costs.

Facing such questions honestly and grappling with possible answers allow us to reflect on what we are enabling — and what we *want* to enable — through our work with clients. We suggest that, from a justice perspective, enabling means
- recognizing the injustices systematically experienced by groups of people, including people with disabilities;

- expressing positive regard for people just as they are (regardless of ability, age, or dependency on others for help);
- expressing and acting on the belief that people should have a place in society — in their families, in their schools, in their places of work, in their community spaces — and that they have the right to participate in their society, just as they are;
- questioning ourselves and others — clients, family members, colleagues — when we imply that people are not "good" enough as they are, that people need to change in some way to be "better" (more mobile, more independent, etc.).

At times, we *will* help people to change, to find a way to fit in, to adapt to society's expectations. But when we do this, we need to make sure that our efforts are based on clients' conscious, well-informed decisions, rather than on unspoken assumptions that people should do things a certain way. At other times, we can support clients to do things differently, to stand out with pride, to show that people don't need to do things "normally" or independently to be valuable, contributing members of society.

In attending to justice, we may begin by thinking holistically about people's environments and occupations. However, our train of thought may first grasp issues of impairment, especially in biomedical contexts. In an impairment-focused context, we are likely to think about impairment as the root of a client's occupational performance issues — the one problem that leads to all the other problems. In health services teams, we tend to make our work as occupational therapists fit with that of others by emphasizing what we do to address physical and cognitive impairments, referring to body functions as defined in the ICF (WHO, 2001). We enable remediation of impairments or enable compensation for impairments. Such practices have impacts on justice.

Critical reflection on justice, diversity, and equity will help us to take a step back to remember that not all problems arise from an impairment or deficit. Sometimes the root of the problem lies in social norms that set up expectations for how people should and should not be, what they should and should not do, and how they should or should not do something. A few key points remind us about social norms:
- We internalize social norms as we become socialized into a society, and we create systems, institutions, and laws that reflect these social norms — these social norms become embodied and institutionalized;
- We are generally not aware of social norms and their pervasiveness in our everyday lives — they are a taken-for-granted aspect of our everyday world;
- We all enact and thereby reinforce social norms every day through our daily habits and routines, words and silences, actions and inactions;
- Some social norms are positive and constructive, helping us to live in harmony; for example, people should not discriminate against one another;
- Other social norms are divisive and destructive, pitting us against each other — they set up ideas about better and worse and imply that some people are better than others, simply because of what they look like, how much help they need, how much they earn, who they love, what they believe in. (for example, people should have a certain appearance; it is better to look "normal" like an able-bodied person; it is better to have youthful looks; it is better to look slim).

Enablement: The core competency of occupational therapy

For people from non-dominant social groups, social norms are particularly limiting or constraining because they generally idealize a society's dominant groups. Norms set up dominant groups as good, normal, and natural, while they cast those from non-dominant groups as not so good, abnormal, and unnatural. Examples of non-dominant groups in Canada are people with disabilities, women, elderly people, people who are gay, lesbian or bisexual, people from ethnic minority groups, and people from minority faith groups. Given the history of occupational therapy's concern for non-dominant groups, the issue of social norms is an important piece to understand justice, diversity, and equity as an enablement foundation.

When we think of social norms, we may enable clients to identify issues that do not necessarily arise from impairments. We may truly focus on occupations and the environment, on the highest outcome levels of participation according to the ICF (WHO, 2001). With attention to social norms, we are more likely to see choices for enablement congruent with justice and to consider an array of options for clients to:

- go along with and try to meet the social norms imposed on them (working around the problem, coping with the problem);
- name, question, and challenge the social norms that are limiting and constraining them (facing and dismantling the problem, working towards social change).

Enabling based on a recognition of diversity and inequity means (a) noticing how people's everyday lives, including our own, are shaped by social norms and (b) naming the situations that people with disabilities encounter because of their ability, ethnicity, race, sexual orientation, faith, gender, or age. When we recognize that social norms produce injustice for some groups, we also recognize that there are likely possibilities and solutions to work toward justice. The enablement foundation of justice is closely related to the other enablement foundations. Not surprisingly, issues of justice, diversity, and equity require close attention to client participation, visions of possibility, and power-sharing in enabling change.

Power-sharing

One of the most enduring foundations of occupational therapy is a commitment to client-centred collaboration. Fulfillment of this commitment requires a high level of conscious and explicit emphasis on power-sharing. The clients whom occupational therapists wish to enable need to know that they are entitled to share power, and they need structured opportunities and resources to share power in making choices and decisions about their occupations and occupational therapy. Ideally, occupational therapists invite clients to exert their power to express what they want, need, or are expected to do to participate in the occupations of their choice that are meaningful to them.

In the ideal, collaborative, power-sharing structure, personal power is expected and guaranteed; intra- and inter-personal power coexist (Schaeffer, 2002). Individuals develop and express gifts, talents, and abilities in mutual respect. Successful, collaborative power-sharing involves genuine interest, acknowledgement, empathy, altruism, trust, and creative communication. Through curiosity and inquiry, the genuine listener expresses authentic interest in each, unique client and probes for deeper understanding. The self-dialogue of an occupational therapist shifts from "I bet" to "I wonder" and from "What will I tell this client?" to "What will we learn from each other?"

Exploration, curiosity, and inquiry are the precursors to synergy, a phenomenon of collaboration. In synergy, the combined effect or interaction of two or more agents is greater than the sum of their individual efforts (Linden, 2003). The opposite of synergy is antagonism, which undermines efforts. What self-test will turn antagonism and domination into a synergistic sharing of power in which everyone gains? With dynamic engagement of hearts, hands, and minds — all parties leading as peers — the collaborative occupational therapist enables through relationship skills, affiliation, and communication that emanates trust.

The idealism of power-sharing is problematic given that occupational therapy is a profession. By definition, professions are structured and managed hierarchically based on the status and privilege accorded to expert knowledge and skills (Freidson, 1970, 1986, 1994, 2001). Collaboration is actually counter to the idea and expectations of a professional expert. Yet collaboration is the central concept of modern initiatives that centre upon clients, patients, and families. There is a profound difference between being a professional expert in collaborative, client-centred enablement and being a professional expert who operates by using power in a top-down relationship with the client. The central difference is that collaborative, shared power and expertise operate horizontally, not hierarchically (Schaeffer, 2002).

Occupational therapy is a profession situated within the medical hierarchy of health professions. Yet occupational therapists are reluctant dominators of clients, given the profession's good intentions for client-centred enablement (Townsend et al., 2003). Occupational therapy is located at a crossroads where contradictory power structures meet — at a point where the hierarchical structure of professions and health services confronts the horizontal, collaborative, power-sharing ideal associated with enabling client participation through occupation. In essence, occupational therapy operates across the grain (Townsend et al., 2003), at an invisible junction where hierarchical and horizontal practices potentially converge or conflict. The profession wants to both increase its status within the medical hierarchy and also to develop collaborative partnerships with non-dominant groups and marginalized populations. The challenges and potential strengths of this contradictory position continue to shape occupational therapy. Optimistically, one can point to the tremendous potential at such a crossroads to champion collaborative initiatives within the hierarchy and to empower clients through client-centred enablement.

Awareness of power-sharing is needed to manage degrees of collaboration and domination that are acceptable to the profession, clients, colleagues, funding sources, and managers. Clients may want to drive practice in a direction that the practitioner may feel is not in the client's best interests (Gage & Polatajko, 1995; Townsend & Landry, 2005). Some clients may not be able or wish to make choices or decisions, preferring instead to rely on professional expertise.

Occupational therapists who wish to explore the theoretical foundations of power-sharing in this profession are directed particularly to literature on social theories of power. Critical reflection, with attention to social structure, raises awareness of possibilities and limits for the transformation of our power as professionals and the power of our clients. Critical reflections on power sharing associated with parenting or sexism are noted in text box 4.5.

Enablement: The core competency of occupational therapy

Reflections on power-sharing

How can an occupational therapist negotiate potential conflicts between collaborative power sharing and the aim of enhancing justice when challenging a situation that is detrimental to occupation or well-being? For example, when a client's approach to parenting, which is rooted in her or his cultural background, appears to be detrimental to a child? Or when individuals manifest sexism or discrimination, in the name of cultural diversity, perhaps not allowing women or girls to engage in particular occupations or insisting that a disabled family member is of less value than others?

— By Brenda Beagan

4.6 The Canadian Model of Client-Centered Enablement (CMCE)

Building on definitions of enablement and enablement foundations, this chapter embraces enablement as the core competency of occupational therapy by introducing the Canadian Model of Client-Centred Enablement (CMCE) (see figure 4.3). Table 4.4, a 10-point checklist, summarizes the representation of enablement in the CMCE. The CMCE is a visual metaphor for client-centred enablement based on the following premises:

Enabling and enablement, focused on occupation, describe what occupational therapists actually do. Enablement is occupational therapists' core competency.

Client-centred enablement is based on enablement foundations and employs enablement skills in a collaborative relationship with clients, who may be individuals, families, groups, communities, organizations, populations, to advance a vision of health, well-being, and justice through occupation.

A central feature of the CMCE is the two asymmetrical, curved lines. They represent the dynamism, changeability, variability, risk-taking, and power differences present in the client-professional relationship. The asymmetrical curve suggests the possibility of diverse forms of collaboration. The evolving nature of client-professional collaborations means that they will not be symmetrical, straightforward, static, standardized, predictable, or prescriptive.

Client-professional relationship

The purpose of the client-professional relationship is for enabling individual and social change, through occupation, in occupational engagement and the social structures that influence engagement in everyday life. The intersecting points of the two lines signal the presence of boundaries of the relationship. Two contact points frame the start and end of each enablement encounter; they are the action points to enter/initiate and conclude/exit practice, as portrayed in the *Canadian Practice Process Framework* in chapters 9 and 10. The two action points may frame a single encounter in time, such as an hourly meeting, or they may frame a referral or contract over days, weeks,

Figure 4.3   Canadian Model of Client-Centred Enablement (CMCE)

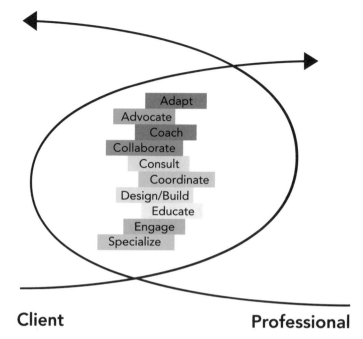

Adapt
Advocate
Coach
Collaborate
Consult
Coordinate
Design/Build
Educate
Engage
Specialize

Client   **Professional**

Townsend, E. A., Polatajko, H. J., Craik, J., & Davis, J. (2007). Canadian Model of Client-Centred Enablement. In E. A. Townsend and H. J. Polatajko, *Enabling occupation II: Advancing an occupational therapy vision for health, well-being, & justice through occupation.* p. 110 Ottawa, ON: CAOT Publications ACE.

months, or years. The CMCE portrays the lower point as the start; the upper point is the end of the contact when both client and occupational therapist proceed, as the arrows indicate, in their different directions. Some may prefer to rotate the diagram 90 or 180 degrees to read the CMCE sideways or from top to bottom.

Table 4.4   Canadian Model of Client-Centred Enablement (CMCE) highlights

Occupational therapy enablement is ...

- What occupational therapists do — core competence
- Based on values-based, conceptual enablement foundations
- Distinguished by a client-centred approach on occupation
- Framed by start- and end-points, which are defined by referrals and contracts
- Participatory and collaborative in a client-professional relationship
- Goal-directed, based on client and professional agreement on aims for individual and/or social change
- Value-based, evolving with diverse clients from individuals to populations, in diverse contexts, and non-standardized
- Practised by integrating a spectrum of 10 key and related enablement skills
- Energized by visions of possibility for health, wellness, inclusion, and justice in everyday life
- Critically reflective and attentive to structural power inequities, diversity and issues of choice, risk and responsibility

Enablement: The core competency of occupational therapy

The boundaries of enablement will vary with the referral or contract, service conditions, the physical environment, and the sociocultural, economic, political, and institutional context. As well, boundaries may support, extend, or confine the scope of practice in particular contexts. Each practice is bounded by values and concepts embedded in the policies, laws, or funding arrangements that govern enablement possibilities. Other examples of documents that govern practice include descriptions of professional scopes of practice, terms of reference for team roles and functions, funding guidelines and budgets, educational texts and articles, and public relations information.

Boundaries for the client-professional relationship are also produced by the regulation of professionals who have ethical, legal, and financial responsibilities to provide expertise and quality services. Clients make choices, take risks, and have responsibilities to respond and communicate what will work best for them. Some may express their choices through creative forms, rather than through verbal expression. Occupational therapists are responsible to guide clients to make choices to advance their goals. Regulations may encourage professionals to limit risk (and opportunity). This is especially true in some biomedical contexts where patients tend to comply with professional recommendations, even when their own experiential and scientific knowledge would caution them against doing so.

The power sharing foundation of client-centred enablement requires the professional claim of expertise and competence to be handled carefully. Professionals are usually expected to be top-down experts. Professional experts may actually disempower some clients. Client knowledge and skills may be unrecognized, and are never paid for. Client choice is not free, given the potential loss of professional services, insurance claims, or other consequences if they appear to be noncompliant or ungrateful. The commercial nature of the client-professional relationship in privately funded services will shape control around choices, risks, and responsibilities. In privately funded services, clients may express a sense of entitlement to the services for which they are paying directly. In publicly funded services, clients may be encouraged to express their preferences, but possibilities are likely limited by budgets.

4.7 Enablement skills

Occupational therapy enablement skills are based on enablement foundations, which employ complex principles and processes (Townsend & Landry, 2005). Occupational therapy enablement is, thus, beyond the ordinary enablement that occurs in everyday life by parents, friends, and others (see table 7.1). The chapter has, to this point, defined occupational therapy enablement with reference to clients, client-centred practice, enablement foundations, and the client-professional relationship. Here, we offer a refined definition of enablement with recognition of the spectrum of enablement skills portrayed in the CMCE.

> *Enabling (verb) and enablement (noun), focused on occupation, is the core competency of occupational therapy, drawing on an interwoven spectrum of key and related enablement skills which are value-based, collaborative, attentive to power inequities and diversity, and charged with visions of possibility for individual and/or social change.*

The CMCE illustrates occupational therapy enablement skills as bands of variable length and colour, like a rainbow. The 10 coloured bands represent the 10 key enablement skills which are profiled from an extensive list of related occupational therapy enablement skills (see tables 4.5 and 4.6). These 10 skills are considered key because they appear to capture the essence of occupational therapy on initial, informal field tests of the list for this book. Given the variability of clients and contexts for enablement, the order of key enablement skills is not prioritized. Rather, the ten key enablement skills are in alphabetical order as a memory trigger. They are summarized in table 4.5.

Before offering definitions for the 10 key enablement skills (see below), it is important to show briefly how these skills are enunciated in a different yet compatible, national, occupational therapy framework. To encourage congruence in defining occupational therapy competency, we have mapped the 10 key enablement skills to the seven competency roles of the updated *Profile of Occupational Therapy Practice in Canada* (CAOT, 2007) (see text box 4.6 and table 4.7).

Eight principles guide the application of enablement skills across the spectrum. First, it would be unusual for an occupational therapist to employ only one enablement skill. Rather, key and related enablement skills are interwoven and overlapping. For instance, an occupational therapist would not want to design and build assistive technology without also collaborating with the client to determine a satisfactory design based on client occupational demands and environmental conditions. To be effective, enablement would be to coach the client to incorporate the technology in everyday habits, and to educate the client or others on safety or other issues.

Second, enablement skills evolve and unfold to respond to clients in context. For instance, a request for a simple physical adaptation of an eating device for a single client in a nursing home may evolve into a consultation contract to coordinate and educate the staff in the nursing home. The contract may be to adapt or redesign the environment so that all residents may participate more fully not only in eating on their own, but also in leisure and community occupations. A nursing home manager may offer the contract both to promote health, well-being, and social inclusion for residents and to minimize the costs of caregiving and injuries for staff and residents.

Third, occupational therapists seek collaboration that is mutual and reciprocal, although different for each party. Clients are partners in enablement and, thus, contribute their own enablement skills. When occupational therapists propose home adaptations with clients, clients require skills to adapt both their emotional attachment to their accustomed home arrangement, and to adapt their routines and use of household equipment. Occupational therapists who collaborate with teams to develop mental health initiatives include mental health service consumers who require skills to communicate with the team and manage their own symptoms.

Fourth, occupational therapists develop a personalized spectrum of key enablement skills with different emphases given their particular interests, talents, and experience. Furthermore, enablement skills in one setting may not work in another setting. Clients and professionals will learn and develop their skills in each particular client-professional context. The enablement competence of individual occupational thera-

Enablement: The core competency of occupational therapy

Table 4.5   Key occupational therapy enablement skills: The spectrum at a glance

10 Key Skills	Occupational therapy enablement at a glance
Adapt	With clients, make suitable to or fit for a specific use or situation (Answers.com), to respond to occupational challenges (Schkade & Schultz, 1992) with all clients from individuals to populations given that "individuals continuously adapt their occupations" (Meltzer, 2001, p. 17)
Advocate	With clients, raise critical perspectives, prompt new forms of power sharing, lobby or make new options known to key decision makers; to speak, plead, or argue in favor of (Houghton-Mifflin Company, 2004)
Coach	With clients, develop and sustain "... an ongoing partnership designed to help clients produce fulfilling results in their personal and professional lives, improve their performance and enhance their quality of life" (International Coach Federation, 2006)
Collaborate	Power-sharing (Schaeffer, 2002) to work *with* clients on occupational issues, versus doing things to or for them in a joint intellectual effort or toward a common end (Answers.com); sharing talents and abilities in mutual respect with genuine interest, acknowledgement of others, empathy, altruism, trust and creative communication to achieve results that are greater than the sum of individual efforts (Linden, 2003), with awareness that professions operate hierarchically in a top-down manner based on the priority given to professional expertise over client experience (Freidson, 2001)
Consult	With clients, exchange views and confer (Answers.com) throughout the practice process with a wide range of clients; in management, education or research, confer with team members, community support personnel, social agencies, government personnel, business representatives, non-governmental organizations, consumer groups, special interest groups, and more
Coordinate	With clients, integrate, synthesize, and document information, link people with resources, manage teams with students and support personnel, facilitate interaction between government "silos" and otherwise harmonize and orchestrate initiatives by a broad range of stakeholders in a common action or effort (Houghton-Mifflin Company, 2004); develop an accord, combine and adapt in order to attain a particular effect (Answers.com)
Design/ Build	With clients, design and/or build products, such as assistive technology or orthotics (McKee & Morgan, 1998); design to adapt the built and/or emotional environment (Clark et al., 2001), and design and implement programs and services (Rebeiro et al., 2001) by formulating a plan or strategy (Answers.com) and in some situations actually building the technology, program, or service
Educate	With clients, employ philosophies and practices of adult and childhood education, notably experiential and behaviourial education that emphasize *learning through doing* (Dewey, 1900; Dewey & Bentley, 1949)
Engage	Involve clients in *doing*, in *participating*, that is to say, in action beyond talk by involving others and oneself to become occupied (Answers.com)
Specialize	With clients, use specific techniques in particular situations, examples being therapeutic touch and positioning, the use of neurodevelopmental techniques to enable children to participate in occupations, or psychosocial rehabilitation techniques to engage adults in their own empowerment

pists will evolve with education, experience, and opportunities within a single encounter, across diverse encounters, and throughout a professional life. Some encounters will — for a variety of reasons — come close to modeling effective enablement, while others will not.

Table 4.6   A spectrum of occupational therapy: Key and related enablement skills

Key skills	Related enablement skills
	Note: Alphabetical, single citation, highly inter-related, dynamic, evolving
Adapt	Accommodate, Adjust, 'Analyze and break down' occupations into do-able components, Configure and re-configure, Conform, Cope, Observe, Tailor
Advocate	Challenge, Champion, Develop (guidelines, policy, positions, regulations, reports), Generate critical perspectives, Politically strategize, Prompt power sharing and empowerment, Enlighten, Lobby, Make Visible, Mobilize, Promote, Raise consciousness
Coach	Encourage, Guide, Challenge, Expand choices, Hold accountable, See the big picture, Listen, Mentor, Motivate, Pose powerful questions, Reflect, Reframe, Support
Collaborate	Communicate, Cooperate, Encourage, Facilitate, Form alliances, Mediate, Negotiate, Partner, Resolve competing interests, Tap motivation
Consult	Advise, Brainstorm options, Confer, Counsel, Integrate, Recommend, Suggest, Synthesize and summarize
Coordinate	Arrange, Bring together, Case coordinate/manage, Develop and manage budgets, Document, Integrate, Identify, Interweave or weave together, Allocate human, financial, space and material resources, Lead, Link, Manage, Network, Orchestrate, Organize, Supervise, Synthesize
Design/ Build	Conceive, Construct, Create, Develop, Devise, Fabricate, Formulate, Envision, Evaluate, Manufacture, Plan, Prescribe, Propose, Re-Design, Re-Build, Strategize, Visualize
Educate	Demonstrate, Enlighten, Instruct, Inform, Facilitate learning through doing, Notify, Present just-right-challenge, Prompt learning of skills, Prompt rote and repetitive learning, Prompt transformative learning, Simulate, Teach, Train, Tutor
Engage	Build trust, Challenge normal expectations, Develop readiness and confidence, Do with/in parallel, Draw into performance in tests or use of technology, Engage in "doing," Identify occupational issues and potential, Involve, Occupy, Optimize potential, Socially mobilize, Spark visions of possibility and hope, Stimulate creative expression through occupation, Prompt optimal participation, Tap potential
Specialize	Facilitate body function, Apply hands on techniques (e.g., support physically, scaffold, etc.), Apply specialized frameworks (e.g., asset-based practice, cognitive approaches, driver rehabilitation, ergonomics, group therapy, psychosocial rehabilitation, sensory integration etc.)

Generic Skills that underpin enablement

Process Skills: Analyze, Assess, Critique, Empathize, Evaluate, Examine, Implement, Intervene, Investigate, Plan, Reflect
Professional Skills: Comply with ethical and moral codes, Comply with professional regulatory requirements, Document practice
Scholarship Skills: Use evidence, Evaluate programs and services, Generate and disseminate knowledge, Transfer knowledge

Fifth, enablement skills may be invisible to others, taken for granted, and under-valued unless they are clearly enunciated. Invisible enablement may actually be an indicator of success. In the best enablement, client empowerment may grow with minimal awareness of professional guidance behind the scenes. Such invisible

Enablement: The core competency of occupational therapy

Mapping Canadian enablement skills and competency roles

Enabling Occupation (2007) outlines knowledge, attitudes, skills, exemplars, and conditions for best practice. In contrast, the *Profile of Occupational Therapy Practice in Canada* (2007) was a project to develop a competency framework for occupational therapy education and practice.

Five roles in the *Profile* are directly comparable to the 10 enablement skills: *change agent, collaborator, communicator, practice manager,* and *expert in enabling* (focused on occupation). The core role of expert in *Enabling Occupation* is comparable with naming enablement as occupational therapy's core competence, with the profession's core domain being occupation. Enablement skills identify what occupational therapists actually do in a competency role. For example, a communicator role may draw on skills to adapt, coach, collaborate, consult, educate, and specialize; a change agent role may be to adapt, advocate, coach, collaborate, coordinate, design/build, and educate; a practice manager role may encompass skills to collaborate, consult, design, engage, and specialize.

Two roles in the *Profile* are foundations for all enablement skills: *scholarly practitioner* and *professional.* The competency role of scholarly practitioner guides all practice to seek the best possible evidence for professional reasoning. The role of professional locates enablement skills within ethical, regulatory, and continuing professional development requirements. The professional role incorporates the supervision of students and support personnel, and participation with other individuals and teams in reciprocal peer coaching, learning teams, and collaborative work arrangements.

A national, professional advisory group's choice of the core competency role of "expert" in this edition of enabling occupation is curious. In part, the naming of an "expert" competency role was driven by the methodology to name a core competency role (expert). It is also possible that the choice was an attempt to present occupational therapy as a profession that requires expertise, as do all professions. The challenge is to consider how clients participate in collaborative power sharing when the profession identifies a core competency role of expert.

Congruence in the naming of enablement skills in the 2007 edition of *Enabling Occupation* and competency roles in the *Profile* (CAOT, 2007) developed in part through a growing awareness of competency in occupational therapy. It also came about through communication between those involved in the parallel projects of updating both publications.

— *By Elizabeth Townsend & Nancy McKay, CAOT Profile Project*

success can be problematic for the profession if clients, funding agents, and the public are unaware of the enablement. Funders and the public need explicit examples to understand how the complexity of occupational therapy enablement skills extends well beyond what family, volunteers, and others do to help people.

Table 4.7   Enablement skills and competency roles (CAOT, 2007)[*]

Enablement Spectrum: 10 Key Enablement Skills	CAOT Competency Profile: Seven Competency Roles*	
Adapt	Change Agent	
Advocate	Change Agent	*Practice Scholar* and *Professional* roles
Coach	Communicator	underlie full Enablement Spectrum
Collaborate	Collaborator	
Consult	Expert in Enabling Occupation	
Coordinate	Practice Manager	
Design/Build	Change Agent	
Educate	Change Agent	
Engage	Expert in Enabling Occupation	
Specialize	Expert in Enabling Occupation	

[*] The *Profile of Occupational Therapy Practice in Canada* (2007) identifies seven competency roles: change agent, collaborator, communicator, expert in enabling, practice manager, practice scholar, and professional.

Sixth, enablement skills are guided by scholarship and evidence, including client and professional judgement. Occupational therapists are responsible to develop enablement skills based on the best available evidence, including client experience and skills (see chapter 11).

Seventh, the occupational therapy enablement skill to *educate* encompasses the education of student occupational therapists and occupational therapy support personnel. Students, as well as support personnel, formally educated or trained on the job, are very important to the occupational therapy workforce. Education to develop their enablement skills will directly impact the competency of the occupational therapist.

Eighth, the extent to which occupational therapists use enablement skills is evident when looking across the eight action points in the Canadian Practice Process Framework (CPPF) (see chapters 9 and 10): enter/initiate services, set the stage, assess/evaluate, enable agreement on objectives and plans, implement plans, monitor/modify, evaluate outcomes, and exit/conclude. The message is that enablement skills are employed throughout the process of practice. Enablement reasoning guides decisions to proceed along the full pathway in the CPPF, or to take alternate and abbreviated pathways.

The following summaries of 10 key enablement skills are intended to be introductory, not comprehensive. The brief outlines are intended to stimulate interest to describe and critically reflect on occupational therapy's core competency in client-centred enablement.

Adapt

Adapt is a classic key enablement skill in occupational therapy, which means to make suitable to or fit for a specific use or situation (Answers.com). In the *Profile of Occupational Therapy Practice in Canada* (CAOT, 2007), this skill is part of the occupational therapy competency role of *change agent*. Occupational adaptation is typically a response to occupational challenges (Schkade & Schultz, 1992) with all clients, from individuals to populations, given that "individuals continuously adapt their occupations" (Meltzer, 2001, p. 17). Adapt means to make suitable to or fit for a specific use or situation.

Given that "individuals continuously adapt their occupations" (Meltzer, 2001, p. 17), occupational therapy enablement will contribute by adjusting or tailoring occupations, based on occupational analysis of the physical, mental, cognitive, social, economic, and other environmental demands and requirements of an occupation. In one example, Gillen (2000) describes occupational therapy enablement with a 31-year-old man with ataxia. The occupational therapist adapted the man's occupations and elicited his adaptive skills to improve his performance in activities of daily living, using motor control theory as a basis for decision making. The challenge was to "identify control parameters that are most important for the client" (Gillen, 2000, p. 89).

Adapt is the key enablement skill related to the long-standing idea in occupational therapy of breaking down tasks for just-right-challenges — that is to say challenges that stretch clients to reach goals without being overwhelmed. Occupational analysis, (see figure 1.1, TCOP on task, activity and occupation), requires competency to analyze and adapt the parts, steps, processes, or components of an occupation. The competency to use that information is to consider and implement various forms of adaptation to accomplish an occupation. The adaptation process will draw on skills to reconfigure an occupation or to observe and tailor an occupation to the requirements of persons or environments.

Enablement skills to adapt common occupations can be applied at a population level. In looking at the use of transportation systems, Carlsson (2004) used a travel chain perspective to explore usability problems experienced by travelers with physical, functional limitations when using an urban public transport system in Sweden. The travel chain perspective broadens the understanding of travel to include all of the steps involved in getting from door to door. Here, analysis provided rich information about the barriers, supports, and processes required to use transportation systems successfully. The research showed that it is possible to consider population-based strategies to adapt travel processes or chains in enabling the occupation of travel.

Related enablement skills are to synthesize occupational analyses and propose recommendations for adaptations. Skills to facilitate adaptation draw on communication, collaboration, and coordination skills to mediate multiple interests; for instance, to listen to the vested interests of those in health and community services. Adaptation is often aligned with the related skills to conform and cope with what is, which is to work within existing systems. Extensive adaptations, however, may stretch and transcend existing systems to transform them.

Advocate

Advocate is a key enablement skill, given occupational therapy interests in health, well-being, inclusion, and justice for all in everyday occupations. To advocate is to speak, plead, or argue in favour of (Answers.com), and to act with or for people to raise critical perspectives, prompt new forms of power sharing, lobby, and/or make new options known to key decision makers. In the *Profile of Occupational Therapy*

Practice in Canada (CAOT, 2007), advocacy contributes to the occupational therapy competency role of *change agent*.

Advocacy is an active skill that includes raising awareness of issues that others may not have recognized, challenging others to think differently. Through advocacy, occupational therapists may champion a cause; for instance, to have ramps and hoists installed in school buses that carry children with disabilities. In advocating, an occupational therapist would champion respect for multiple perspectives in decision making and in mobilizing others to pursue their goals. Occupational therapists may advocate by proposing changes in policies or by challenging people with disabilities to try something they couldn't have imagined was possible. One example suggests that clients perceive advocacy as being blended with other skills. A qualitative study by Darragh, Sample, and Krieger (2001) examined the practitioner qualities and traits that 51 clients who had experienced a brain injury perceived as important to the therapeutic relationship. When participants reflected on the practitioners who worked with them, they consistently referred to roles that the providers played to mentor them and advocate with them.

Policy analysis and development are advocacy skills. Writing or revising policy, guide-lines, regulations, or legislation are powerful forms of advocacy to embed particular ideas and strategies in governance. Barbara and Whiteford (2005), who distinguish the difference between legislation (laws) and policy (statement of intent or clear rules for action), suggest that occupational therapists are more involved in policy than the litera-ture would suggest. Occupational therapists advocate for policy changes to enable individual, family, or group clients to engage in occupations, or to enable community, organization, and population clients to restructure occupational opportunities and the resources needed to improve the inclusion of marginalized citizens.

Interrelated skills with advocacy may be to coordinate and manage the voicing of differences, or to design program proposals that incorporate visions of possibilities. From case 4, Joanne and Beth may advocate with local authorities by referring to global initiatives, such as the 1991 United Nations Convention of the Rights of the Child, and the 1998 WHO policy on *Health For All in the Twenty-First Century*. Advocacy involves raising critical perspectives, prompting new forms of power shar-ing, lobbying or making new options known to key decision makers. For example, occupational therapists advocate as we mobilize action or promote employment sup-port programs where none had previously existed — generally raising our own and others' consciousness to oppression, marginalization, disempowerment, and the privileges of some over others.

Related enablement skills are to form alliances, partnerships, and collective lobby groups with others. Advocacy skills are key to enabling individual and social change. An occupational therapist may advocate with individual children or adults to express their interests, or advocacy may be with parents, support groups, govern-ments or international bodies to develop the services required to sustain a person with a disability and their family.

Coach

Coach was named as a key enablement skill, using the International Coach Federation's definition (2006) as "… an ongoing partnership designed to help clients produce fulfilling results in their personal and professional lives, improve their performance and enhance their quality of life" (see also chapter 5). In the *Profile of Occupational Therapy Practice in Canada* (CAOT, 2007), coaching is related to the competency roles of *communicator* and *collaborator*.

Coaching is an emerging field with literature dating to the 1960s (Grant, 2003; Stober & Grant, 2006). The skill of occupational therapy coaching is to develop a client-centred partnership in conversation about occupation. Engagement in occupation may also occur within a coaching encounter, for instance, a coach might listen to and encourage someone to start an exercise program as a solution to break out of negative occupational routines associated with substance abuse. Occupational therapists' trademark in coaching may be to link this with occupational engagement. Time may be allocated to invite a client to sit down at a computer to learn where to search on-line for addresses and times of programs in the neighbourhood. The occupational therapist may coach occupational performance through encouragement and direct handling. Where funding supports community-based initiatives, an occupational therapist might accompany the person on the first visit to their selected program, then, use that real life occupational experience for follow-up coaching in the simulated environment of an office.

Coaching is an asset-based, appreciative approach highly congruent with enabling lasting, occupational change. Used typically with individuals, coaching may involve families or others whom an individual wishes to include. The emphasis is to coach people to take responsibility for self-direction in naming priorities and goals, which are most meaningful to them. Coaching involves collaboratively identifying challenges, setting goals, and working towards the goals set. The coach may offer feedback on occupational performance in order to support and enhance occupational development.

Coaching draws on related enablement skills, such as in engaging others in occupations, and listening to client voices, meanings, and mental models. Coaching draws on skills to engage people in self-assessment of their strengths, resources, challenges, and desired goals. A central aim is to encourage clients to reflect and discover their own motivations in their desired occupations. A coach guides, mentors, and instructs others on ways to reframe their thinking and priorities for greater congruence between their sense of self and their actions. Reframing and mentoring skills are required to guide the discovery of just-right challenges in transitions or transformations in everyday life.

Collaborate

Collaborate is arguably the key enablement skill for power-sharing in client-centred practice (Schaeffer, 2002). To collaborate is to work together, especially in a joint intellectual effort or toward a common end (Answers.com). A collaborator works with clients, versus doing things to or for them. The power-sharing in collaboration is characterized by the sharing of talents and abilities in mutual respect, genuine interest, and acknowledgement of others. Collaboration is based on empathy, altruism, trust, and creative communication. In collaborative interactions, the results are greater than the sum of individual efforts (Linden, 2003). In the *Profile of Occupational Therapy Practice in Canada* (CAOT, 2007), collaborate is directly mirrored in the competency role of *collaborator*.

The idealism of collaborative power-sharing is problematic given that occupational therapy is a profession, which by definition operates hierarchically in a top-down manner based on the priority given to professional expertise over client experience (Freidson, 1970, 1986, 1994, 2001). The central difference is that collaborative, shared power and expertise operate horizontally, not hierarchically (Schaeffer, 2002).

In enabling individual change, the skill to collaborate distinguishes enablement as a way of working with clients, versus doing things to or for them. Collaboration requires skills to listen, communicate, express respect and confidence in others, cooperate with others, encourage persistence to seek solutions, and facilitate processes for expressing diverse perspectives.

In enabling social change, collaboration is aligned with shared authority and democratic principles of shared decision making. At the community, organization, and population levels, occupational therapists might design and evaluate programs in various collaborating partnerships. For example, student occupational therapists worked collaboratively with a "Friendly to Seniors"[6] committee in Toronto to develop a program logic model and pilot an evaluation process for the initiative. In developing and implementing the evaluation, the students participated collaboratively with the organizing committee with awareness of the power dynamics. The students enabled the committee to compile process and outcome data related to their initiative, something required for continued and new funding for this population-based initiative (Chenoy et al., 2003).

Collaboration has many related enablement skills. A collaborator will seek out multiple perspectives to encourage the formation of alliances. Collaboration may involve the mediation or negotiation of resolutions that take different perspectives and experiences into account. Occupational therapists may tap motivation or enable the resolution of differences in forming collaborative initiatives. Collaboration may draw on active negotiation to find common ground. Toth-Cohen (2000) examined occupational therapists' perceptions of their roles as educators for persons with dementia. While the occupational therapist's role of educator is important, results from this study also stressed the importance of the role of collaborator with families.

Consult

Consult is a key enablement skill to exchange views and confer (Answers.com). In occupational therapy, consultation is extensive and pervasive throughout the practice process with clients or in management, education, or research. Consulting in some

---

[6] "Friendly to Seniors" is a senior-led program that aims to improve seniors' quality of life and reduce ageism by providing education and recommendations to businesses and organizations about aging, and changing design and attitudes within organizations that serve seniors.

Enablement: The core competency of occupational therapy

settings, such as school-based practice, may replace direct service with similarly effective results (Three-Suchy et al., cited in Reid, Chiu, Sinclair, Wehrmann, & Naseer, 2006). The range of consultation contacts may include clients (from individuals to organizations), team members, community support personnel, social agencies, government personnel, business representatives, non-governmental organizations, consumer groups, special interest groups, such as the Multiple Sclerosis Society, and more. In the *Profile of Occupational Therapy Practice in Canada* (CAOT, 2007), consulting is part of the competency role of *expert in enabling occupation*.

Consulting with individuals, families and groups may start by listening to their different perspectives, encouraging and coaching them to respect differences, and advising them about options to adapt or to advocate for change. An occupational therapist consults with individuals, families, professional and other team members to brainstorm options. Consulting with communities, organizations, or populations may likely occur through a formal consulting contract. An occupational therapy consultant may incorporate many key and related skills to gather information, reflect on different perspectives, and design proposals for alternative choices. An occupational therapy consultant with any category of client uses skills to integrate, synthesize, and summarize multiple forms of data. Recommendations and suggestions may reframe problems, issues, challenges, and opportunities as a way of coaching clients to take a new course of action.

Consulting has always been a key occupational therapy enablement skill. However, with changing funding structures, occupational therapists increasingly use formal consultation skills, for instance, in working in early childhood education (Dudgeon & Greenberg, 1998). Sometimes consultation approaches are not the choice of occupational therapists who prefer to follow through with direct services. Yet service administrators may favour consultation as a method to increase occupational therapists' caseloads (Dreiling & Bundy, 2003). The positive potential of consulting and guiding support personnel to implement programs may need to be considered against the loss of funding for occupational therapists to actually implement the programs that consulting occupational therapists design. In one study, there were no statistically significant differences in the outcomes of direct, indirect, and consultative models in working with preschoolers with motor delays (Dunn, 1988; Kemmis & Dunn, 1996; Mezirow & Marsick, 1978).

Related enablement skills are in brainstorming options; conferring or holding counsel as a basis for advising others. Consulting may involve making recommendations and suggestions based on an integration and synthesis of information, and professional reasoning.

Coordinate

Coordinate is a key enablement skill to harmonize in a common action or effort, to bring into accord, or to combine and adapt in order to attain a particular effect (Answers.com). Coordination skills are a powerful and under-recognized hallmark of occupational therapy. In the *Profile of Occupational Therapy Practice in Canada* (CAOT, 2007), coordinate is aligned with the leadership competency role to *manage practice*.

Coordination draws on occupational therapists' strong integration skills in which therapists synthesize, analyze, and act on the broad range of information on occupations, and the personal and environmental influences. The coordination of assessment/evaluation information mirrors the coordination of people, services, and organizations. Occupational therapists link people with resources, foster networking, and orchestrate teams to focus on enabling occupation. As coordinators, occupational therapists interweave multiple perspectives, plans, tasks, and documentation with clients, families, teams, and others involved. Occupational therapy coordination makes the client experience as seamless as possible and ideally avoids team members and clients working at cross purposes, always with the client as the centre point.

Given the broad scope of occupation-based enablement, occupational therapists are ideal to orchestrate the complexity of case coordination. Occupational therapists refine coordination skills through experience in coordinating programs, services, and systems. With a broad, integrated understanding of person and environment factors that influence everyday occupations, occupational therapy coordination may be the force that enables teams and systems to cooperate and realize results.

Occupational therapists coordinate students, support personnel, and others whose work is highly interconnected with occupational therapy and the team. Coordination may be through a formal expectation for team coordination with a range of professionals, clients, and their supporters.

Coordination may include the power to decide what to document, how documentation will be done, who will access documentation and how documents will be used. Client coordination is typically aligned with documentation to record the process of practice with clients. Documentation skills may also be used for identifying, allocating, and evaluating the use of human, financial, space, and material resources to meet goals.

By coordinating services with clients across health and other sectors, such as housing and employment, occupational therapists break down the proverbial silos of separate institutional functions. Client-centred enablement, with individuals or organizations, often links and coordinates systems that tend to operate in isolation. A classic coordination skill in occupational therapy would be for Joanne (case 4) to bring together transportation, housing, education, health, and community services to support Beth, Joshua and other families touched by disability challenges in their community. Such systems-level coordination illustrates the social coordination of occupations, which Larson and Zemke (2003) describe from observing client occupations:

> ... the architecture of our daily lives is not only a product of our own making but a complex interweaving of our own life with others' lives ... social coordination of occupations is complex, requiring consideration of individuals' routines, competing desires and expectations for mutual daily activities, as well as taking into account the many social conventions such as work hours, social calendars and daily schedules that create an underlying, often taken for granted, order around which occupations and co-occupations are structured (p. 80).

Enablement skills related to coordination are the skills to listen to diverse voices and to reframe differences in seeking common ground for collaboration. Coordination may be to educate those involved, and to facilitate, mediate, or actively negotiate networking, links, and resolutions. Also related are skills to integrate, synthesize, organize, lead, and supervise.

Design/build

Design/build is an age-old, key occupational therapy enablement skill that encompasses the design and/or building of products, such as assistive technology or orthotics (McKee & Morgan, 1998), design to adapt the built and/or emotional environment (Clark et al., 2001), and the design and implementation of programs and services (Rebeiro et al., 2001). Design means to formulate a plan for, to devise, or to form a strategy (Answers.com). Design is paired with build to indicate that occupational therapists implement designs. In the *Profile of Occupational Therapy Practice in Canada* (CAOT, 2007), design/build contributes to the competency role of *change agent*.

Occupational therapists are known for conceiving, creating, designing, redesigning, rebuilding, and in some cases fabricating, constructing, or manufacturing products and environmental adaptations. Skills to design/build programs range from creating individualized client equipment and programs to designing/building service programs or policies. The occupational therapy repertoire to design/build products is possibly best known in the areas of assistive technology, splints, and orthotics (McKee & Morgan, 1998; McKee & Nyugen, 2007; McKee & Rivard, 2004). Design/build may include environmental adaptations to promote mental health (Kirsh et al., 2005) or to make buildings more physically accessible. Life style design includes the design of programs and environments (Clark et al., 2001). Architectural modifications may be designed and the construction of them monitored to promote quality of life in institutional settings and to encourage ergonomic positioning at home or in the workplace (Ringaert, 2003). Design/build skills are very prominent in developing safe environments, for instance in falls prevention programs (CAOT, 2003a). Ringaert (2003) suggests that occupational therapists can promote universal design from a community or population perspective by consulting with design teams on specific building projects, providing education applicable to universal design to architects and contractors, serving on accessibility committees, and conducting research with a universal design team. With a focus on occupation, Manuel (2003), a municipal planner, saw opportunities to design and build communities that retain and protect wild spaces to promote nature-based occupations.

Design/build skills include planning the schedules, locations, and resources required to meet goals. In this area of design/build, skills are connected with enablement skills to design a coaching strategy, to adapt environments, to advocate for social change, to collaborate with stakeholders, to coordinate multiple efforts across sectors, to educate communities about universal and inclusive design, and to engage clients in the design and building of environments that enable them to live in health, well-being, and justice.

Educate

Educate is a key enablement skill and one of the historic knowledge foundations of occupational therapy (Schwartz, 1992). Our educational foundations are well aligned with the philosophy and practice of adult and childhood education, notably experiential and behaviourial education, which were championed in the early 20th century (Dewey, 1900; Dewey & Bentley, 1949; Schwartz, 1992). In the *Profile of Occupational Therapy Practice in Canada* (CAOT, 2007), educate contributes to the competency role of *change agent*.

Occupational therapists use occupations for *learning through doing* throughout the process of practice. In occupational therapy, education skills are to stimulate growth through engagement, with active participation in the occupations of everyday life. By teaching people, communities, and organizations to actively participate and collaborate in shaping everyday life, occupational therapists put the ancient Chinese proverb into a modern context (Hopkins & Smith, 1988):

> Give a [person] a fish and you feed [her/him] for a day. Teach a [person] to fish and you feed [her/him] for a lifetime.

Education skills are aligned with skills to collaborate with clients, and to design learning opportunities and resources for diverse experiential, rote, didactic, or other learning styles. Occupational therapists are particularly skilled in the educational use of simulated occupations in hospitals or other settings designed to offer therapy apart from the natural environment (Townsend, 1996). Where occupational therapy facilities have been created, client education may involve demonstrating or practising simulated occupations before clients transfer their learning to their own home, work, or other environments. Clients, from individuals to organizations, may learn through doing with instruction in performing or organizing routines of occupations, or in adapting the environment, for instance, in the home, community, or business.

One of the ways in which occupational therapists can educate populations is through mass and electronic media. For example, the occupational therapy site www.otworks.ca provides background information about occupational therapy and information, links, and resource information, all directed to a broad Canadian population. The Web site www.iamable.ca was designed as part of a research study to examine the effects of integrating rehabilitation in a primary health care setting to meet the needs of adults with chronic illnesses. The Web site offers community-specific information, but also has links and resources on topics of interest to the population of people with chronic illnesses being served through the study.

Electronic and Web-based education resources have become common in most parts of the world. While legitimate concerns have been expressed about the ability of people in marginalized groups to access these resources, great strides have been made through public libraries and community portals to make Internet resources more equitably accessible to the Canadian public. Certainly, there are limits to any population-based approach to education, yet the Internet offers one route to reach a large number of people with relative efficiency. Education in use of the Internet may prepare clients to engage in *communities of learning* (Lave & Wenger, 1990). Electronic technology is increasingly used in *communities of practice* for learning to use Internet information searching, on-line courses, on-line support groups, and e-mail.

Enablement to educate others lies at the core of fieldwork education with student occupational therapists. Occupational therapists educate by drawing students into practice as collaborators who are learning to refine their enablement skills. A range of educational methods are used; for instance, observation, demonstration, practice, simulation, planning, and evaluation. Education follows the action and reflection cycle made popular by Kolb (1984): students engage in practice by reflection on their performance and learning in informal meetings with an occupational therapy preceptor, as well as through formal mid-term and final evaluations. The educational context will be the variety of practice settings in which students have fieldwork education experiences. Enablement skills will include coaching students who are in new situations, guiding students to adapt their learning styles for efficient practice, and engaging students in real practice experiences.

Education skills are also used with occupational therapy support personnel. Depending on their formal or informal background in occupational therapy, the occupational therapist will enable support personnel to develop enablement reasoning. Education in the basics of occupational and enablement reasoning shapes the use of technical skills with a client-centred focus on occupation and awareness of effective and ineffective enablement. Support personnel may start with experiential, on-the-job training, which could be supplemented, if desired, with a certificate or diploma program. An increasing number of occupational therapy support personnel start their education with a certificate or diploma program, which includes fieldwork education (see chapter 14).

Related enablement skills are to prompt rote and repetitive learning, to enable instrumental learning, or to spark transformation through a learning cycle that integrates action and reflection (Kolb, 1984). Also related are facilitating, guiding, prompting, listening, reflecting, encouraging, and supporting, as identified in the 1997 definition of client-centred practice (CAOT, 1997a, 2002). Instrumental education may involve instruction, teaching, training, tutoring, informing others, and evaluating outcomes. For instance, Caretto, Topolski, Linkous, Lowman, & Murphy (2000) describe the role of occupational therapists in educating parents on infant feeding in a neonatal intensive care unit. Transformative education may be integrated with advocacy and coaching, including consciousness raising and critical reflection for client enlightenment and empowerment. Occupational therapy education is based on occupational analysis. The first steps in an occupational analysis are to understand how to "break down" or analyze learning, then to design/build a program with a series of steps for actions to realize goals. Client-centred education may be individualized or targeted at communities, organizations, populations, and the public to promote health, well-being, inclusion, and justice through occupation.

Engage

Engage is an historical cornerstone of occupational therapy and is the enablement skill to involve clients in doing, that is to say, in participating, in action beyond talk.

Engage means to draw into, involve others, involve oneself or become occupied (Answers.com). In the *Profile of Occupational Therapy Practice in Canada* (CAOT, 2007), occupational therapists engage others through the core competency role as *expert in enabling occupation.*

The enablement skill to engage is essential to build therapeutic alliances so that clients can voice their perspectives, choices, and decisions in therapeutic processes. Client-centred practice is founded upon the ability to engage clients, from individuals to organizations. Clients are not an object of concern, but active subjects with decision-making power.

Engagement is also an essential enablement skill for occupational therapists given that the domain of concern is with occupation. Occupation requires cognitive, emotional, spiritual, and/or physical engagement in the environment, as portrayed in the CMOP-E (see section I). Whether a client is an individual or an organization, occupational therapists look beyond a client's current capacity and analyze the underlying personal and environmental influences that impact on engagement in occupations. The TCOP (see figure 1.1) and the ICF (see figure 1.3) are also tools to chart the analysis of occupations, persons, and environment as a basis for enabling engagement. The ICF highlights engagement in the definition of participation as *engagement in valued social roles* (WHO, 2001).

Occupational therapy skills in the engagement of others can be understood from several perspectives. Occupational engagement promotes health and well-being by involving people in *performing* everyday occupations (Law, et al., 1998; Whiteford, Townsend, & Hocking, 2000). For instance, Schmidt Hanson, Nabavi, & Yuen (2001) demonstrated that sports participants scored significantly better than non-participants on four out of five subsections of the Craig Handicap Assessment and Reporting Technique (CHART), which measures physical independence, mobility, occupation, and social integration in everyday life. In a study by Orlinsky, Graw, & Parks (1994), client engagement, contrasted with doing things to or for clients, was found to relate to positive outcomes across different psychotherapeutic approaches.

Wilcock (2006) argues from another perspective, that occupational engagement may be for *being, becoming,* and *belonging*, as well as for *performing* or *doing* occupations. Engagement for being, becoming, and belonging may focus on mental or spiritual participation to counter a client's disinterested, uninvolved or disconnected stance. Occupational therapists who work within models of psychiatric rehabilitation are well acquainted with the need to assess client readiness to engage clients emotionally and intellectually before assessing resources and performance in physical function (Cohen & Mynks, 1993). Clients who are not at a high level of readiness may need to be engaged in building trust with their service providers (Cohen, Anthony, & Farkas, 1997). Enablement would aim to engage client awareness to develop a belief that life and systems could indeed be different, confirming clients of the positive benefits of change.

Occupational therapists engage individuals, families and groups, communities, organizations, and populations through occupation. The focus on occupation orients occupational therapists to engage clients in the determinants of health, including

Enablement: The core competency of occupational therapy

education, employment, housing, and transportation. Given that gender, social class, race, sexual orientation, and other characteristics are also health determinants, occupational therapists who work in population health would extend their engagement of clients and stakeholders well beyond the health sector. Occupational therapists may find themselves heading into new practice and funding territory to engage groups who want to address population-based determinants (see chapter 13): for example, Letts (2003a) found that engaging a community through organizing in the context of municipal restructuring sparked a joint initiative with senior citizens in Toronto. While occupational therapists do not typically study municipal structures, Letts and her students engaged a group of people who developed a community needs assessment and a new seniors' organization that wanted to address issues of importance to the seniors' population in the city core.

Enablement skills are used to advance occupational engagement. Engagement of those with occupational challenges will press the boundaries of normal expectations in society. Engagement of clients may also engage the occupational therapist in doing with, in order to demonstrate occupations. For instance, the occupational therapist may participate in shopping and cooking with individuals, or in facilitating community participation in a needs assessment. The occupational therapist acts, as in participatory research, as both an outsider with professional expertise and an insider who is engaging alongside the client. Challenging expectations of engagement in one's life or society may produce resistance. Clients and others may have become comfortable with limited possibilities, standardized norms, and expectations. Therefore, occupational therapists may need to combine engagement skills with collaboration skills in dispute resolution, mediation, and coordination skills to bring together diverse perspectives and competing interests. We must be aware in engaging others that some people and groups do not wish to fit an occupational therapist's or society's norms (Morris, 1991).

Specialize

Specialize is a key enablement skill which refers to the use of specific techniques in particular situations, examples being therapeutic touch and positioning, the use of neurodevelopmental techniques to enable children to participate in occupations, or psychosocial rehabilitation techniques to engage adults in their own empowerment. In the *Profile of Occupational Therapy Practice in Canada* (CAOT, 2007), specialize is a composite of enablement skills that contributes to the competency role of *expert in enabling occupation*.

Skills to specialize carry the imperative of enablement with clients, to ensure that clients understand, agree with, and participate, as they are able and wish to, in specialized approaches. With specialize as a key enablement skill, occupational therapists need to critically reflect on client and therapist expectations of top-down professional experts in light of a commitment to being client-centred.

One area of specialization includes skills to facilitate body function by applying hands-on techniques to support people physically. This includes the technique of scaffolding, which may require touching to support physical action and doing by presence or being with clients (Fearing & Clark, 2000). Skills to specialize draw on specialized theoretical or conceptual frameworks, such as assertive community treatment, community-based rehabilitation, counselling, driver rehabilitation, ergonomics, group therapy, hand therapy, psychosocial rehabilitation, sensory integration, or neurodevelopmental techniques.

At the population level, specialization may be in falls prevention and safety. Richardson et al. (2006) describe the Stovner Safe Community Project in Norway, in which an interdisciplinary team worked on a population-based initiative to prevent injuries in older adults. The intervention involved educating home care providers and physicians in identifying and addressing issues that might result in injuries. The occupational therapist made a safety equipment kit for home care workers to teach their clients how to prevent falls and injuries. Evaluation data demonstrated that the rates of upper-hip fractures were cut in half from 1990 to 1995.

Notes on generic enablement skills

Occupational analysis — to identify, classify, and interpret the personal and environmental factors that influence occupation — is one example of an enablement skill that underpins all occupational therapy. As well, all occupational therapy practice draws on skills associated with two competency roles in the *Profile of Occupational Therapy Practice in Canada* (CAOT, 2007): the roles of *professional* and *scholarly practitioner*.

Additional process skills are to analyze, assess, critique, develop relationships, empathize, evaluate, examine, implement, intervene, investigate, listen, plan, or critically reflect. Each action point in the Canadian Practice Process Framework (CPPF) (see chapter 10) requires analysis, assessment, critique, listening, and so on through processes to enter/initiate services, set the stage, assess/evaluate, enable agreement on objectives and plans, implement plans, monitor/modify, evaluate outcomes, and conclude/exit. Generic process enablement skills tap motivation for clients to engage and collaborate based on their own experience, knowledge, and skills. Related skills are to use evidence, develop critical perspectives, evaluate programs and services, generate and transfer knowledge.

The *professional* competency role and skills are to comply with ethical and moral codes, and with professional regulatory requirements, and to document practice and other information. The *scholarly practitioner* role and skills are the basis for integrating scholarship and evidence in everyday practice.

4.8 Enablement continuum

As stated throughout this chapter, occupational therapy enablement is complex. Occupational therapists are always balancing supports and limits to enable best practice and the best possible outcomes. Critical reflections on the CMCE point to a continuum of possibilities from ineffective to effective enablement (see figures 4.4 and 4.5). Discussions to develop the Canadian Model of Client-Centred Enablement (E. Townsend, G. Whiteford, H. Polatajko, J. Craik, & J. Davis, personal communication, July–September 2006) also prompted discussion about an enablement continuum.

Enablement: The core competency of occupational therapy

Figure 4.4   Enablement continuum

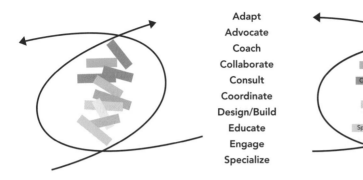

Adapt
Advocate
Coach
Collaborate
Consult
Coordinate
Design/Build
Educate
Engage
Specialize

Ineffective Enablement   Effective Enablement

Townsend, E. A., Whiteford, G., Polatajko, H. J., Craik, J., & Hocking C. (2007). Enablement Continuum. In
E. A. Townsend and H. J. Polatajko, *Enabling occupation II: Advancing an Occupational Therapy Vision for
Health, Well-being, & Justice through Occupation.* p. 129 Ottawa, ON: CAOT Publications ACE.

Figure 4.5   Four decision-making points on a disablement–enablement continuum

Ineffective Enablement
- negative & potentially destructive
- knowing best with limited input
- co-dependence
- alienation through expert dominance, overbearing zealousness, misunderstanding
- fractured relations, value clashes
- incongruence, non-resonance, unresponsiveness, irrelevance
- potentially offensive
- ineffective use of resources
- accountability skewed to interests for cost cutting, safety, etc., little mediation of client interests

Missed Enabling
- mutual agreement of no need for professional enablement
OR
- missed opportunity, vision, conditions for enabling
OR
- insufficient resources: human or financial
- unsuitable sociocultural, physical, and/or emotional conditions
- unsuitable accountability for what might have been done

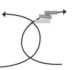

Minimal Enablement
- non-generative
- single-issue focus
- mechanistic, prescriptive, risk averse to just-right-challenge
- over-reliance and faith in expert's definition and prediction of risk
- socio-cultural restrictions
- minimal resource allocation
- accountability stresses technical interventions

Effective Enablement
- positive and generative
- mutual & valued process
- mediated, negotiated values, beliefs, etc.
- congruence & resonance
- seizing opportunities, new possibilities
- balance risk taking, just-right-challenges
- appreciative of limited knowledge regarding risk
- shared expertise & responsibility
- grounded in hope
- attentive to structured inequity, diversity, injustice in enabling individual & social change
- accountability for enablement conditions, processes, & outcomes

Townsend, E. A., Whiteford, G., & Polatajko, H. J. (2007). Four decision-making points on a disablement–
enablement continuum. In E. A. Townsend and H. J. Polatajko, *Enabling occupation II: Advancing an Occupational
Therapy Vision for Health, Well-being, & Justice through Occupation* p. 129 Ottawa, ON: CAOT Publications ACE.

The continuum has four main points of decision making and action, from ineffective to effective. The draft continuum put *disablement* at the other end of a continuum with enablement. This dichotomy has been described in the critical disability literature and the classic critique of *disabling professions* by Illich, Zola, McNight, Caplan, & Shaiken (1977).

Discussion eventually produced four points on an enablement continuum: effective enablement, minimal enablement, missed enablement, and ineffective enablement (see figures 4.4 and 4.5). There may be variations within a single occupational therapy practice. There may be different degrees of effectiveness with different clients, or there may be missed or minimal enablement opportunities because of service boundaries. With critical reflection, occupational therapists may change ineffective enablement, with recognition that complex practice conditions as well as therapist choices determine possibilities for enablement.

Effective enablement

The Enablement Continuum portrays one end as best practice — as positive, effective enablement. The CMCE portrays an ideal vision of effective enablement (described above). A key factor in effective enablement is to mold a practice context that supports enablement, focused on occupation. In the field, practitioners would establish workload and staffing levels required to enable clients to meet goals within the mandate of a particular program; practitioners would establish networking and referral systems for seamless services to meet client goals for occupational engagement; clients would be invited to make choices and decisions to ensure that enablement efforts are sensitive to sociocultural diversity and what is meaningful to them; and accountability for enablement would include occupational outcomes that matter to clients and managers. Client participation would be respected and included in setting visions of possibility for change with consciousness of power-sharing and justice. Effective enablement would result, for instance, in some of the following outcomes: organization clients would be delighted with new occupational routines established to be more inclusive and safety conscious without extra cost; community clients would be energized to overcome occupational deprivation or other challenges that citizens experience; families and groups would learn about occupations and enable positive occupational development and transitioning of their members; individuals would indicate satisfaction with occupational outcomes, based on recognition of what is useful and meaningful to them. In other words, enablement would be effective first and foremost from the client perspective. However, occupational therapists, managers, funders, and policy makers would agree that enablement is based on sound financial management and accountability to promote health, well-being, and justice through occupation.

Minimal enablement

Minimal enablement may occur despite good intentions for enabling occupation effectively. In the reality of difficult practice conditions, the occupational therapist may be unable to realize enablement possibilities. Perhaps assistive devices are provided, with neither a commitment nor mandate and resources for occupational therapy follow-up. Both client and occupational therapist may underestimate the potential for enablement. Assessments may be done without the occupational therapy resources for implementation and program evaluation. The use of standardized, prescriptive protocols may minimize the enablement potential of using more flexible tools. The ratio of occupational therapists to support personnel may mean that clients miss enablement because of insufficient access to professional expertise, despite good supervision of the support workers. With the emphasis in institutional health services on self-care, funds may not be available to enable clients to return to work, develop the routines and supports for living outside institutions, or advocate for accessible transportation. As health services focus more on acute, medical procedures, funding may be scarce for occupational therapy enablement of daily living with diverse clients. In today's cost-conscious world, funding bodies may not readily provide the resources needed to effectively enable occupation. Occupational therapists may choose not to ask for more resources, either out of deference to the demands of others, lack of confidence, or fear of losing the resources they have.

Missed enablement

Missed enablement occurs when lack of opportunity, resources, or vision result in unnecessary losses to others in health, well-being, or justice. With individuals, families, or groups, missed enablement may occur when persons, for example, are given medication without a referral to occupational therapy to address the occupational routines and habits required to integrate medication taking into daily life. Families or groups with members who live with severe and persistent mental illness may have funding to access psychological counseling and social work, but no funding for occupational therapy to enable daily living. Missed enablement may occur if institutional and community health services have not yet included occupational therapy in admission and discharge planning, when assessment of occupations to remain in the community may have cost benefits. Maybe school programs have integrated children with disabilities without including occupational therapy in their special needs teams except to measure wheelchairs for students who struggle with mobility. In probation programs for young offenders, there may be referral access to occupational therapy in mental health services, but no access to occupational therapy to develop the occupational potential of young offenders in the community. Primary health care programs now exist across Canada. Where occupational therapy is not included, there are missed enablement opportunities to develop and manage primary health programs with an occupational perspective — for seniors' safety in the home or for education on habits and routines to reduce obesity in children and adults. Missed enablement may be a matter of insufficient awareness to allocate resources for enabling occupation, or missed opportunities for occupational therapists to be more proactive.

Ineffective enablement

Ineffective enablement is at the opposite end of the continuum from effective enablement and may have negative effects — psychologically, physically, cognitively, or spiritually. If real harm occurs, of course, there will be redress from clients and the profession through regulatory or legal bodies. Without causing harm, however, enablement may be ineffective to the point of being disabling. The concept and critique of disabling professions was highlighted by Illich et al. (1977), a critique from which occupational therapy is not immune. Morris (1991, 1992), for instance, pointed to disabling and oppressive practices based on narrowly defined norms or expectations for persons with disabilities. Occupational therapy has not been visible in many social critiques of professions, but Maxwell and Maxwell (1983), and Abberley (1995) pointed to the potential for occupational therapy to be highly ineffective. Professional lack of awareness, education that lacks critical perspectives, emotional codependence between clients and professionals, or avoidance of tough dilemmas may be more disabling than enabling (Rotunda & Doman, 2001). As an example, Beattie (1992) pointed to ineffective enablement in the face of codependence that perpetuates substance abuse. Ineffective enablement is both a reflection of the context of practice and of individual occupational therapist choices. There is no blame attached to ineffective enablement, although the question is: What can occupational therapists do in difficult circumstances to be effective? Bonnie Sherr Klein described her frustration with occupational therapy in case 1. Her therapy following a brain stem stroke was to make potholders instead of working on the half-completed film, which was her driving passion. The practice setting may not have fostered effective, meaningful enablement, and the occupational therapist may have had the best of intentions. Yet ineffective enablement may also occur by omission, when occupational therapists fail to explain why occupations, such as making potholders, may be therapeutic, or forget to find out what occupations are meaningful to clients and use them as therapy. Standardized protocols and routine practices may be problematic if occupational therapists are neither encouraged nor personally motivated to ensure that enablement is effective. Unconscious bias, such as racism or sexism, may also result in ineffective enablement, as may professional naiveté. Our tireless optimism and visions of possibility may cloud our awareness and vigilance.

4.9 Reflections on enablement

Enablement is now front and centre in the lexicon of occupational therapy language. An important point to take from the chapter is that the early descriptions of occupational therapy as a client-centred practice have evolved. We now describe occupational therapy's core competency as client-centred enablement. We also describe occupational therapy values, beliefs, ideas, and concepts as enablement foundations. The Canadian Model of Client-Centred Enablement (CMCE) builds on those foundations and displays the enablement of individual and social change in a client-professional collaboration that draws upon a spectrum of enablement skills. The enablement continuum encourages us to raise critical perspectives about the pitfalls and opportunities of occupation-based enablement and to consider the "humanness" of occupational therapists who, like clients, bring diverse perspectives on ability, age, ethnicity, social class, and other characteristics as noted in text box 4.7.

Enablement: The core competency of occupational therapy

Chapter 5

Enabling individual change

Elizabeth A. Townsend
Barry Trentham
Jo Clark
Claire-Jehanne Dubouloz-Wilner
Wendy Pentland
Susan Doble
Debbie Laliberte Rudman

CASE 5.1 Catherine's story: Enabling individual change

Catherine's 20-year career as a professional concert pianist and recording artist was in serious jeopardy when the sudden onset of pain and immobility in her right hand put an immediate halt to her piano playing due to osteoarthritis of her thumb metacarpal (CMC) joint. Recognizing the importance of hand function to her career and the uncertain potential outcome from surgery, a hand surgeon immediately referred her to occupational therapy.

The occupational therapist made a custom-molded circumferential hand-based thumb CMC stabilizing orthosis constructed from 1/16-in. (1.6-mm) thick low-temperature thermoplastic. Although it alleviated Catherine's symptoms somewhat, it limited joint mobility too much to allow her to play the piano. Catherine also found it unattractive. The next attempt to help Catherine involved a prefabricated Rolyan® Neoprene Wrap-On Thumb Support that was trimmed down to free the thumb metacarpophalangeal joint and reinforced with thermoplastic, which was bonded to the outside of the orthosis and adjacent to the CMC joint. The neoprene was sufficiently flexible to enable the freedom of movement needed to play the piano and supportive enough to prevent pain. While the blue color was acceptable for piano practice, Catherine found it unsuitable for concert situations.

Further collaboration between client and therapist led to a custom-made black neoprene orthosis with thermoplastic reinforcement. This satisfied Catherine's functional, cosmetic, and comfort requirements for concert hall performances.

Catherine's career continued to flourish. Three years later she was still using the orthoses — the black neoprene orthosis for performances, the blue neoprene orthosis for piano practice, and a more stabilizing thermoplastic orthosis for other activities. A collaborative, client-centred approach ensured that the orthoses met both Catherine's biological needs (joint protection and pain relief) and occupational needs, enabling her to continue the pursuit of her livelihood and passion.

Catherine was overjoyed: "My hands are my life. I am so grateful to my therapist for listening to what I wanted and needed. Without these orthoses, my career would have been over. I call them 'my friends'. They enable me to continue performing at the highest technical level."

— By Pat McKee

5.1 Introduction

*Occupational therapy is the art and science of ... **enabling people to perform the occupations that foster health and well-being** ...*

Chapter 5 focuses on the person component of the occupational therapy definition introduced in chapter 1. To illustrate the Canadian Model of Client-Centered Enablement (CMCE), chapter 5 considers enablement foundations and skills, change models and examples of asset-based enablement with individuals, families, and groups. Enabling individual change lies on a continuum and is interconnected with enabling social change (chapter 6). As individuals, families, and groups experience change, they seek local or broad social change to support their individual and collective pursuits.

5.2 Enablement foundations and skills with individuals, families, and groups

Catherine's story of enablement is about her success to continue performing and participating as a citizen in earning a living. She risked losing income and social status and, potentially, her primary occupation. Her story briefly illustrates enablement foundations and skills for working with individuals, families, and groups (see table 5.1). The points drawn from her story about enablement foundations and skills, illustrate enablement at the micro level, reaching out to influence the local environment.

The primary enablement skills that Catherine's therapist used were to adapt and to design/build her immediate environment. In this case, the design and building of assistive technology involved a series of orthotic hand and finger splints and

Table 5.1	Enablement foundations and skills: Catherine's story
Enablement foundations	**Illustration from Catherine's story**
Client participation	Readiness to participate was established and her drive as a performing artist was identified
Visions of possibilities	Possibilities were known by the therapist because of knowledge and experience in splinting, orthotics, and occupational performance; possibilities were a driving, motivational vision of the client
Change	The therapist enabled environmental change, specifically by using assistive technology. Possibly, change was guided by the Health Belief Model which reminded both therapist and client that the real threat to her livelihood was outweighed by the perceived benefits of the new behaviour of wearing a splint while playing
Justice	Enablement was to prevent potential injustice, should she have lost her paid occupation and had to rely on reduced income with the potential for little support from a limited disability pension
Collaborative power-sharing	Collaboration was in shared decision-making about therapeutic goals, preferred orthoses, and in the schedule of therapy sessions
Skills	**Illustration**
Adapt	Adapt orthosis; adapt routines of playing, rest, use of ice
Advocate	Advocate for client's own belief in her potential to change
Coach	Coach client in new routines to accommodate orthosis
Collaborate	Collaborate with client through stages of orthotic design
Consult	Consult with client and other musicians about feasibility
Coordinate	Coordinate with client, physician, and rehabilitation team
Educate	Educate client and team on possibilities to support hand
Engage	Engage client in playing with an orthosis
Design/build	Design/build series of orthoses
Specialize	Specialize in materials science/biomedical engineering

ergonomic adjustments for the piano and Catherine's positioning. Enablement also included collaboration with the pianist to develop the greatest comfort and stabilization to avoid pain. She was consulted about colour, design, and her emotional response to wearing the orthosis in public. There was continual advocacy with Catherine, coaching to determine timing for wearing the orthosis or leaving it off, and education about repetitive motion injuries and their impact on occupational performance. Enablement focused particularly on her paid occupation, which was also her passion. Catherine participated, expressed her own voice, and shared power with the occupational therapist in making choices to realize a vision of possibility that she could continue as a performing artist.

At the micro level, enablement starts with individuals, families and groups, and it may reach out to change their local environment. Client participation starts by enabling clients to have a voice as a matter of respect and fairness. Competency to enable individuals, families, and groups to express their voices will integrate many enablement skills. One listens to and advocates with and for clients for their voices to be expressed, heard, considered, and included in decision making. With power sharing and justice as an explicit or implicit backdrop, enabling change with individuals, families, and groups requires the inclusion of their voices both in occupational therapy and in their own life.

The enablement skill of engaging clients as participants in practice is of central importance. Enablement of client voice extends throughout all practice processes, yet the enter/initiate starting is critical, as is setting the stage before identifying occupational objectives and plans (see the Canadian Practice Process Framework in chapters 9 and 10). Some clients are reluctant to voice their ideas, or they may have cultural expectations that they should remain silent and comply with a professional expert.

Enablement of people to voice their perspectives and priorities reflects a cultural emphasis on the individual. Canadians tend to value individualism (see text box 4.2), thus emphasize individual autonomy, self-knowledge, and agency. In the Canadian context, an individualistic practice would gauge client readiness to voice interests and priorities with a professional, even if the individual's perspectives differed from those of the professional. One should actively listen to clients' non-verbal and verbal communication. It is essential to establish trust, openness, understanding, empathy, and mutual respect. Individuals may also be encouraged to stretch beyond former ways of thinking and doing. Time and openness may be needed to give voice to experiences of changing identity and to integrate new assumptions and perspectives (Sinnott, 1994). As noted in chapter 4, the enablement skill to engage may need to start by sparking readiness to participate. If individual, family, or group clients express a lack of readiness, developing readiness may become the primary goal of therapy or services may not proceed unless the client is willing.

Enablement skills may be needed to adapt or design/build the environment so that individual, family, or group voices are more likely to be heard. Professional teams may need to name individuals as fully participating members throughout all processes of practice so that their voices carry weight in decision making beyond occasional input by invitation. Their voices, with those of their family or support groups, ideally influence the directions and priorities, goals, objectives, and targeted outcomes named for enabling change. One goal may be for individuals, families or groups to rediscover their own voices before they can assume an active role with professionals.

Occupational therapists specialize in enabling clients to express their emotions, ideas, thoughts, and opinions. Enablement may support client participation in either standardized or non-standardized assessments so that clients themselves discover and name their priority occupational issues. Enablement with individuals, families, or groups may draw on creative occupations such as art, music, gestures, writing, and handcrafts. Individual or group work might use specific technologies, such as specialized computers and symbols, to augment communication when verbal expression is limited. A range of enablement approaches might be used to engage individuals, families, and groups in expressing their voices. Approaches already used in occupational therapy are diary methods, video-journaling, photo-voice recording, participatory evaluation strategies, and narrative interviews (Clouston, 2003). When language, culture, or physical capacities limit expression, occupational therapists might start to engage clients by using creative media, non-verbal gestures, role plays, or visual cues. With clients who are able and ready for verbal expression, one may simply ask individuals, families, or groups to state and prioritize what they need, want, or are expected to do.

The processes experienced by clients can be both systematic and open to client voices and world views (Hendry & McVittie, 2004; Pollard, Smart, & the Voices Talk and Hands Write Group, 2005). Approaches need to be selected in ways that match the preferences and capabilities of various clients, demanding flexibility on the part of service providers based on the realization that one approach will not fit all (Hendry & McVittie, 2004). Enablement with individuals, families, or groups may involve coaching them to develop the self-confidence and self-knowledge to express and advocate for help in their priority, meaningful occupations. Individual clients may be encouraged to identify when and how family members, friends, and others might participate in helping them. One might also consult with and educate families or groups to understand what silences some voices and gives prominence to others within the family or group. Setting the stage may require skill to coordinate and manage the expression of an individual, family, or group voice. Where the interests of individuals are not known, ethical and legal arrangements will be needed for a legally-designated proxy.

Clients and occupational therapists may have different perspectives on the processes for working together on anticipated outcomes, both in terms of what they see as important and how they assess what has occurred (Backman, 2005; Laliberte Rudman, Hoffman, Scott, & Renwick, 2004). In considering outcomes related to individuals' subjective experiences in quality of life and well-being, Hendry and McVittie (2004) point out that the use of instruments that do not attend to individual understandings of the concept being addressed can "lead to the neglect of wider and more meaningful aspects of individual health" (p. 962). Therefore, it is important to elicit client voices on their experiences of exclusion and injustice beyond functional expectations in occupational performance (Kronenberg, & Pollard, 2005; Townsend & Wilcock, 2004a).

A real challenge in enabling the inclusion of individual, family, and group voices in the short-term services of today's health system is to find efficient and effective methods. If individuals are not ready, there may be too little time to wait to hear their voices unless occupational therapists form alliances to advocate that client voices are essential (see text box 5.1). There seems to be growing recognition that efficiency and cost benefits accrue when individual client voices are present in deciding priorities. Examples are when hospital and other services increase consumer representation on boards of directors and consumer advocacy groups emerge. Further research is needed to understand the economic and social costs of not enabling, or benefits of enabling, individual, family, and group voices to influence services.

Text box 5.1

Reflections on client voice

Enabling the expression of client voice is central to enablement reasoning. How can occupational therapists do this effectively when clients are unwilling or unable to express their voices?

When have you felt unwilling or unable to express yourself? What made you feel that way? What (if anything) helped you to express yourself?

How do you enable people to have a voice even when they cannot easily express themselves or convey their true interests because of illness or disability?

Sometimes cultural ways of being can make people reluctant to express themselves to a health professional. At other times, a client may be intimidated by the occupational therapist's perceived social status or class, education level, ability to articulate. How could you as an occupational therapist reduce potential intimidation?

— By Brenda Beagan

5.3 Change models for enablement with individuals, families, and groups

Numerous theoretical models of change may inform occupational therapy enablement with individual, family, and group clients. Five models are cited: Health Belief Model, Attribution Model, Transtheoretical Model, Social Learning or Cognitive Theory, and Transformative Learning. Each offers guidance for enablement to maintain, prevent losses, or enhance occupational engagement. The five models are congruent with asset-based enablement through occupation. Given a lack to date of a social theory of change through occupational enablement, we offer examples of change models from fields outside occupational therapy.

One step in setting the stage may be to elicit client motivations and beliefs about change. For instance, the Health Belief Model (Lewis & Daltroy, 1990; Rosenstock, 1990) proposes that change occurs if a threat is perceived and if the proposed change is perceived to result in benefits that would outweigh the costs of engaging in the new behaviour. The Attribution Model (Lewis & Daltroy, 1990) highlights the need to acknowledge how clients attribute causes to certain behaviours or outcomes prior to change.

The Transtheoretical Model of Health Behaviour Change (Prochaska & Velicer, 1997) can be of particular assistance in outlining optimum entry points. Collaborating to identify client readiness for change might draw on Prochaska and Velicer's 10 processes in five stages of change, including pre-contemplation, contemplation, preparation, action, and maintenance.

Social learning or Social Cognitive Theory (Bandura, 1986; Baranowski, Perry, & Parcel, 1997; Lave & Wenger, 1990) suggests that enabling individual, family, and group change is related to how people learn and change as a result of others in their environment. Individuals are thought to learn most from others if the models are seen to be like them in some way. Enabling necessarily involves education and learning to develop skills for change (Christiansen, Baum, & Bass-Haugen, 2005). It is important to note that enabling adult learning differs from enabling learning in children (Knowles, 1973; Knowles, Holton, & Swanson, 1998). Knowles championed this distinction by noting that, unlike children, adults can draw on the rich resources of life experiences and on role models, self esteem, and self-confidence.

Transformative Learning Theory is defined as a social process of adopting, construing, and appropriating "a new or revised interpretation of the meaning of one's experience … as a guide to action" (Mezirow, 1994, pp. 222-223). Mezirow (1991) suggested that complete and durable change occurs when an individual transforms her or his meaning perspectives through critical reflection. Transformative learning is the process, "by which we transform our taken-for-granted frame of reference (meaning perspectives, habits-of-mind, mind sets) … to become more inclusive, discriminating, open, emotionally capable of change and reflective" (Mezirow, 1994, p. 7). Enabling positive transformation individually or collectively requires a change in conversation and open dialogue focused on an exploration of possibilities. Mezirow's work resonates with occupational therapy in the belief that "learner empowerment is both a goal and a condition for transformative learning" (Cranton, 1994, p. 72).

5.4 Asset-based enablement with individuals, families, and groups

Pierre's story (case 5.2) about the interdependence of enablement spans his own personal transformation and the gradual inclusion in the economy and society of those living with a mental illness. The primary occupational therapy enablement skills were collaboration and advocacy, which enabled Pierre to experience himself as an active participant instead of a passive medical patient. Other foundations for his transformation were his vision of a possible life, and his interest to have choices and control in his daily life. (see table 5.2)

The stories of Catherine (case 5.1) and Pierre are both about enabling individual change, with attention to their local environment, and with awareness of the interde-

CASE 5.2 Pierre and the interdependence of enabling individual change

Pierre knows how mental illness can change everyday life. As a teenager, he recognized that his emotions and experiences of life were different than those of his adolescent friends. Since an early age, he could remember mood swings and times when he sensed that he was not fully in touch with reality. In his late teens, Pierre was confronted with hallucinations and delusions that prompted hospitalization and strong medication to deal with what was then diagnosed as schizophrenia. For over 10 years, he was in and out of hospital. He felt totally alone and withdrew from his friends and family until he was truly alone most of the time. He was assertive in trying to minimize his use of the strong medications that clouded his ability to interact with others. One day, after many hospital admissions, Pierre, in his early 30s, was referred to a psychosocial rehabilitation program in the community. Pierre's participation in the program changed his life.

The Psychosocial Rehabilitation Program is publicly funded as part of the provincial mental health services system. It emphasizes enablement of change through adult, social learning. Oriented to client-centred, asset-based enablement, staff and members collaborate to support members to build on the strengths of participants, with conscious awareness of all people involved and their environment. The aim is not independence, rather it is interdependence. Pierre began to accept that he needed others to help him, and that he felt better when he helped others. He participated fully in the program by joining the household management and cooking part of the program, as well as the research team, which gathered statistics and stories to evaluate the program. He began to see that he could work in an office to pay the bills and volunteer to help others with a mental illness.

Pierre now has a part-time job with accommodations of time outs and flexible breaks for stress relief. He attends the program the rest of the time for the support that he needs to give and receive. He speaks publicly about the necessity of a team of professionals and consumers who know how to enable the community to accept those with mental illness and to enable those in need to live as fully as possible with their illness.

— *Composite by Elizabeth Townsend*

pendence of all individuals. The Health Belief, Attribution, or Transtheoretical Models may guide enablement to deal with Catherine's perceived threat to her primary occupation, her need to attribute a cause to her repeated pain, and her acceptance of an orthosis as an optimum entry point for change. Enablement with Pierre would particularly draw on social learning and adult education as models that emphasize personal engagement and environmental change. Three asset-based strategies, outlined below, were evident: appreciative narrative inquiry and coaching were enablement strategies in both cases; with Pierre, enabling change drew particularly on transformative learning.

Table 5.2   Enablement foundations and skills: Pierre's story

Enablement foundations	Illustration from Pierre's story
Client participation	Pierre's readiness to participate in the Clubhouse grew as he became involved in doing something meaningful after many years of frustrating treatment focused on pharmacological intervention
Visions of possibilities	Pierre had sustained a vision of a possible life, although he hoped for a life without mental illness. He needed enabling experiences in which he could test out real-life possibilities for work, relationships, and symptom control
Change	Pierre gradually identified possibilities for personal transformation, and change in his performance in the occupations of the Clubhouse and daily life
Justice	Enablement, through occupation in the Clubhouse environment and through community work projects, restored Pierre's hope for greater justice and inclusion of people with severe and persistent mental illness
Collaborative power-sharing	Collaboration was in shared decision making that underscored Pierre's realization that often the best life includes interdependence, since independence implies that one can go it alone

Skills	Illustration
Adapt	Adapt Clubhouse environment and Pierre's expectations
Advocate	Advocate with Pierre for supportive employment options
Coach	Coach Pierre to manage symptoms during occupations
Collaborate	Collaborate with Pierre, his service team, and his supporters
Consult	Consult to plan with Pierre and other Clubhouse members
Coordinate	Coordinate Pierre's individual program with outreach
Educate	Educate the community and Pierre about interdependence
Engage	Engage Pierre in reshaping his life and local community
Design/build	Design/build programs, and the Clubhouse environment
Specialize	Specialize in psychosocial rehabilitation in a clubhouse

Asset-based enablement differs from problem-based practice, which focuses on deficiencies. A problem-based practice can deflate energy and rapport, and may not motivate and inspire people to change. In contrast, asset-based enablement aims to stimulate positive growth, insight, rapport, and energy. From the onset one mediates a common focus on goals and works to amplify positive opportunities. Important foundations for asset-based practice are client participation, visions of possibility (including the possibility of change), and an ethical commitment to justice, equity, diversity, and collaborative power sharing. Also important are values, beliefs, and assumptions about the power of optimism and hope to bring about change in individuals, families, or groups.

Appreciative narrative inquiry

Asset-based appreciative inquiry (Cooperrider & Whitney, 1999; Cooperrider, Whitney, & Stavros, 2003) incorporates both the philosophy of appreciative inquiry and the Mindset Model (Learner versus Judger) (Goldberg, 1998). Appreciative inquiry is a strengths-based approach to change, originally developed in the field of organizational behaviour: it involves story telling to inspire the soul by focusing on desired futures. The rationale for a focus on the future is that people are more likely to achieve what is in their conscious sphere of attention. The Learner and Judger mindsets named by Goldberg (1998) form an important basis for a psychotherapeutic approach. The Mindset Model describes two states of mind always present in all of us and asserts that we are able to choose one over the other at any time in viewing the world. Each mindset results in a vastly different orientation, focus, and perspective for the client, and ultimately her or his choices and outcomes. The Learner mindset is typically more useful because it is open-minded, flexible, solution-seeking and accepting of the self and others. The Judger Self, on the other hand, tends to be inflexible, reactive, controlling, problem-focused, defensive, and blame-seeking. Use of the Mindset Model facilitates self-awareness and allows individuals to make more skillful and informed cognitive, behavioural, and relationship choices.

Asset-based appreciative inquiry is fundamental to occupational therapy enablement. A longstanding premise of occupational therapy enablement is the opportunity to coach others to develop their individualization, uniqueness, and self-determination, through occupation. Typical occupational therapy storytelling seeks to draw out assets (strengths and resources) as well as liabilities (challenges and problems) for everyday living. On first meetings with people, occupational therapists collaborate to draw them into a mutual narrative inquiry about their occupations; for instance, about their occupational performance and satisfaction or their occupational dreams.

Using asset-based appreciative inquiry with awareness of the Mindset Model, an occupational therapist would learn about and appreciate — not judge — client narratives that tell the taken-for-granted stories of daily life: What did you do today? What does a typical day (week, month, year) look like? What do you need or want to do? What are you expected to do and what choices do you have or not have? What do you do that you find most meaningful and least meaningful? Clients are prompted to narrate chronicles of events that stand out for them. A powerful part of occupational therapists' appreciative inquiry is to listen to, document, and analyze the ordinary, taken-for-granted events, experiences, values, roles, routines, occupations, context, contributing factors, and perceptions of daily life.

Enabling may interweave facilitation, coaching, and demonstration of the telling of appreciative stories. One might demonstrate how to tell a brief story about daily life, then facilitate client storytelling by asking the following questions: What is going well? What used to go well? What would you like to experience more of in your life? One might also facilitate clients to respond to probing questions on what they need and want to do. The narrator-client would be prompted to offer her or his analysis of the personal and environmental forces that are influencing her or his life.

Retrospective, problem-based storytelling would focus attention on the present by using events and experiences from the past. Prompts would enable the storyteller to highlight current issues, concerns, and limitations that may specifically direct the course of subsequent assessment and intervention. In encouraging asset-based storytelling, one is always wary that focusing on the past, problems, and limitations could be shame-provoking, discouraging, and disabling — which would be minimal or even ineffective on the enablement continuum as noted in text box 5.2.

Reflections on assets, deficits, trust, and risk

Occupational therapists may be unfamiliar with the assets of diverse communities. Many Canadians do not have strong connections with groups who differ
from themselves in terms of race, ethnicity, sexual orientation, class, etc. In fact,
we often see diverse communities primarily in terms of perceived deficits. For
example, working-class communities are seen as lacking money, not as having
unusually strong family ties. What resources could you draw on (people, media,
research, other) to develop an understanding of the assets of diverse people?

Eliciting narratives and stories from people entails risk for them, in part,
because the occupational therapist becomes the holder of their information.
Moreover, many social and cultural groups have had collective and historical
negative experiences with health care providers and may have good reason to
fear disclosing stories. People with disabilities have not always been treated
well by health care (for example, the history of eugenics in Canada); people of
African heritage still recall the intentional harm done to them through health
care (for example, the Tuskeegee syphilis experiments); homosexual and bisexual people have long been harmed through health care (for example, the inclusion of homosexuality in the Diagnostic and Statistical Manual [DSM] used in
psychiatry until the 1970s and the history of electroshock "treatment").
Occupational therapists are asking for trust when eliciting stories; clients may
need evidence of trustworthiness.

— By Brenda Beagan

Narrative meaning is elicited to enable people to order daily events into meaningful
experiences through reflection and analysis (McKeough, Davis, Forgeron, Marini, &
Fung, 2005). Collaboration in narrative explorations allows clients and occupational
therapists to gain greater overall comprehension of personal and environmental factors within the plots, settings, conflicts, and interpretations of the story (Mattingly &
Flemming, 1994; Mattingly, 1998). The storytelling movement in occupational therapy seems to emphasize raising consciousness around individualized forms of
enablement and their effectiveness. The unconscious side of storytelling is that the
balance of power may continue to sit with professionals. We are the recipients and
holders of stories, by virtue of the story we ask a client to impart. We professionals
are also the persons who create the official record of client stories.

Transformative learning

Occupational therapists might apply enablement skills with an understanding that
transformative learning enables a complete and lasting change of actions when basic
underlying premises are critically examined (Mezirow, 1990, 1991, 1998, 2000).
Learning new ways of functioning in daily life is a central challenge for individual
clients and may necessitate processes of personal change. Enablement skills, particularly skills to adapt, coach, collaborate, consult, educate, engage, and specialize,
could draw on the theory of transformative learning, which is organized around four

constructs: meaning perspectives, distortion in meaning perspectives, meaning schemes, and critical reflection. Transformative learning will be most effective with those who can be drawn into self-reflection.

Meaning perspectives

Meaning perspectives are made up of higher order beliefs organized in a "belief system for interpreting and evaluating the meaning of experience" (Mezirow, 1991, p. 4). Personal core values, beliefs, goal orientations, and knowledge direct a person's view of her/his world, learned through personal, social, and cultural experiences (Mezirow, 1991). Meaning perspectives are the constituents of a personal paradigm and consist of the core personal values, beliefs, feelings, and knowledge that guide daily actions. Mezirow (2000) highlighted the conditions necessary for adults to make autonomous and informed choices and to develop self-empowerment for transformative learning. Occupational therapy enablement with individuals, families, and groups may focus on transforming meaning perspectives around performance of the body, autonomy, choice, and identity (Ashe, Taylor, & Dubouloz, 2005). For individuals, families, and groups, transformation may be a "process of reflection on systems of meaning, in light of changing abilities or conditions, and the reconstruction of new personal or collective story-lines that engage their resources and foster hope" (Ashe et al., p. 282).

Meaning perspective distortion

A meaning perspective distortion occurs when a person experiences a personal crisis; for example, a serious illness that challenges some personal meaning perspective, such as one's personal definition of independence. Distorted meaning perspectives are barriers to new learning. To resolve distorted meaning perspectives, individuals engage in critical self-reflection to redefine their core meaning perspectives. The new learning from self-reflection can enable personal change (Mezirow, 1998).

Meaning schemes

Meaning schemes are composed of specific knowledge, beliefs, value-judgments, and feelings that define rules for interpreting the meaning of habitual actions in daily life situations. Enablement involves listening to and coaching people to reframe and adapt their thinking and actions. The aim is for them to reconstruct their meaning schemes to incorporate chronic illness, disability, or other personal crisis.

Critical self-reflection

Critical self reflection underlies all transformative learning. Critical self-reflection guides occupational therapists and clients to reflect on personal presumptions that, at times, may contribute to a distorted or biased vision of reality. This may help occupational therapists and clients to challenge distorted meaning perspectives and to explore new ones. Perspectives can change because they are learned and because meaning is composed of cognitive-, emotional-, and volition-related dimensions — beyond a way of seeing things (Meizirow & Marsick, 1978). Critical reflection in transformative learning may lead to propositions to re-interpret and reframe existential feelings beyond what one experiences intellectually (Mezirow & Marsick, 1978).

Occupational therapists who are interested in enabling transformative learning may draw on a study of adults experiencing myocardial infarction. Dubouloz, Chevrier, and Savoie-Zajc (2001) report participants' identification of three key moments essential to change during three and six months of working with an occupational therapist. The moments were sparked by critical reflection and involved a deconstruction of old meanings. Participants created space for new meanings that gave a sense of coherence between feelings, thoughts, and actions after experiencing myocardial infarction. Although key moments were unique for each person, they occurred at the following times: first, when a principal meaning perspective was clearly distorted in light of the current situation; second, when a new replacement value emerged to fill the void of giving up a principal meaning perspective; and third, when the new meaning perspective provided a sense of coherence. During transformation, the participants experienced Lewin's three stages of change (Lewin, 1951). The *thaw* or deconstruction of a meaning perspective was like a shell cracking or an egg hatching. *Movement* was a phenomenon of emergence and the reconstruction of a new meaning perspective. *Crystallization* was needed to maintain the new meaning. In a study of the meaning perspectives of four adults with multiple sclerosis, Dubouloz et al. (2002) found that enablement of critical reflection produced a profound transformation in the definition of self — a prerequisite before each could discover a new meaning to life.

Additional lessons for enablement with individuals, families, and groups can be taken from another study of transformative learning with people with rheumatoid arthritis. Critical reflection based on knowledge of the illness acquired through occupational therapy contributed to three strategies which emerged in various ways for all participants (Dubouloz, Laporte, Hall, Ashe, & Smith, 2004). First, critical reflection on the diagnosis and period of rehabilitation enabled participants to recognize self-continuity and self-acceptability in illness, and allowed them to develop a new, principal meaning perspective of self-respect. Second, a new meaning perspective of self-caring evolved to replace a distorted meaning perspective that lack of activity was a matter of personal laziness and limitations. Feelings of incompetence became feelings of self-responsiveness. Third, participants experienced a transformation from a meaning scheme of dependence to a meaning scheme of interdependence. Thinking about interdependence made pacing, instrumental help, and social support seem acceptable. When participants integrated these three strategies into their daily occupations, they found that they could still feel productive.

A conceptual design for enabling a meaning perspective transformation (see figure 5.1) illustrates the complexity and dynamism of enablement skills to:
- Recognize the client's struggle with the meaning of her/his new occupational reality;
- Support the client toward self critical reflection related to her or his occupations;
- Support the client during the temporary disorientation that occurs during transformation;

- Assist, guide, support, and encourage client self-reflection to discover distorted meaning perspectives;
- Lead and suggest areas of exploration for meaning perspective transformation related to the client's occupations;
- Explore new meaning with the client during self-reflection on her or his occupations;
- Support the transformation of new meaning perspectives;
- Support the emergence of new meaning perspectives by facilitating shared experiences with others;
- Facilitate new meaning schemes through new rules of conduct in new occupations.

Figure 5.1   Enablement of a meaning perspective transformation process

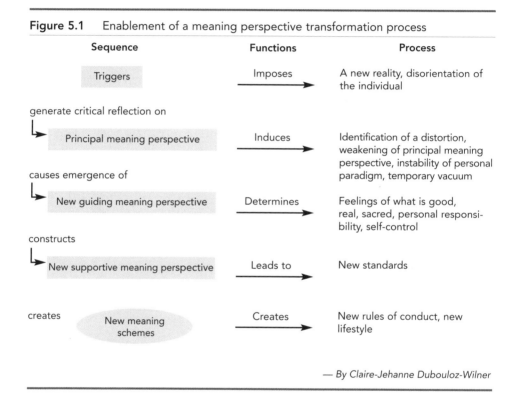

— By Claire-Jehanne Dubouloz-Wilner

Coaching

Certified, professional coaching[1] is a relatively new addition to the occupational therapy spectrum of enablement skills, although coaching has been part of the occupational therapy repertoire since the profession began. Coaching is not only one of the 10 key enablement skills, but is also a formal approach to asset-based enablement. The inclusion of coaching in chapter 5, beyond the brief description of coaching as an enablement skill in chapter 4, profiles an asset-based approach that is particularly useful with individuals, on their own or in couples, and groups, including families. The International Coach Federation describes professional coaching as:

---

[1] Coaching is described here as an enablement skill distinct from its specific use in sports. Coaching of clients to engage in occupations has always been part of occupational therapists' enabling tool kit. Certified, professional coaches use specialized approaches to facilitate change.

"... an ongoing partnership designed to help clients produce fulfilling results in their personal and professional lives, improve their performance and enhance their quality of life. Coaches are trained to elicit solutions and strategies from the client; they believe the client is naturally creative and resourceful. The coach's job is to provide support to enhance the skills, resources, and creativity that the client already has" (2006).

Coaching is a powerful asset-based, appreciative set of skills for enabling lasting occupational change with clients. The origins of coaching for enablement are in organizational behaviour to maximize human performance in the workplace. Like most of the human service professions, coaching borrows theoretical foundations from a range of fields, including human development, psychology, philosophy, and education. The coaching process is highly client-centred, fosters self-directed learning, and is grounded in self-assessment, personal values, and recognition of strengths. Research has shown that coaching is highly effective with clients who have an illness or disability, and with the general population in promoting health and wellness.

As with appreciative narrative inquiry and transformative learning, coaching includes specific strategies for facilitating change from a current state to a more desired future state. Coaching goes beyond the use of checklist tools. It involves specific skills and strategies to assist clients in identifying what they really want and to expand the client choices around what is possible. The focus is on enabling clients to choose, implement, integrate, and sustain the desired changes in their occupational lives.

The hallmark of coaching is a conversation-based partnership. Occupational therapists' coaching would focus on daily life; that is, on occupation. Coaching helps clients to discover and prioritize what is important to them, access their strengths and creativity, and then choose and design a plan of action to achieve agreed upon objectives. The approach is fundamentally about facilitating change that will lead to desired results, and easing movement from a current state to a more desirable future state. Coaching is not therapy or counseling; the participant is not cast in the role of a patient or sick person. Clients are viewed as creative, resourceful, and whole.

Certified professional coaching is an emerging field with literature and other evidence dating back to the 1960s (Grant, 2003; Stober & Grant, 2006). Coaching appears to be highly effective in enabling various populations to make occupational lifestyle changes. Research is increasingly finding positive effects of coaching; for instance, with adults with heart disease (Vale, Jelinek, Best, & Santamaria, 2002; Vale et al., 2003), HIV/AIDS (Garfinkel & Blumenthal, 2001), and addictions (Shafer, Kiebzak, & Dwoskin, 2003). Studies have found positive effects of coaching with families in crisis (McGoldrick & Carter, 2001) and with persons diagnosed with diabetes (Joseph, Griffin, Hall, & Sullivan, 2001; Whittmore, Chase, Mandie, & Roy, 2001). Coaching research also extends to obstetrics where coaching with new mothers and families has produced positive outcomes for mothers and infants (Hadikin, 2001). Coaching has been used to improve the performance of executives (Kampa-Kokesch & Anderson, 2001) and to promote the health of new immigrants (Irwin & Morrow, 2005). Other studies have found that coaching may result in stress reduction and boost the productivity of underproductive workers (Yen, Edington, McDonald, Hirschland, & Edington, 2001), and can improve the quality of life of older adults (Holland, Greenberg, Tidwell, & Newcomer, 2003; Lynch, Morse, Mendelson, & Robins, 2003).

In recent years there has been an explosion of interest in coaching in a variety of fields. Applications of coaching are wide reaching, from coaching for behavioural change and optimal performance, to coaching for health and fulfillment. Once clients clarify their strengths, values, and vision of what they really want to achieve, they begin to take action. Progress (and lack of progress) associated with coaching has been examined from a learning perspective using the action-reflection-learning approaches described by Kolb (1984) and Schön (1987). Research on human flourishing has helped to shed light on the features of a positive context for coaching (Aspinall & Staudinger, 2003; Emmons, 2003; Frederickson, 2003; Isaacowitz, Vaillant, & Seligman, 2003; Keys & Haidt, 2003; Ryan & Deci, 2001; Seligman, 2002; Snyder & Lopez, 2002).

Coaching draws on detailed accounts of human strengths, resilience, the importance of values, and the role of meaning in well-being. Coaching also incorporates positive psychology and authentic happiness as proposed by Seligman (2002). He proposes the minimizing of negative emotions and the maximizing of positive emotions. Seligman emphasizes engagement, which he says is generated when individuals find opportunities to use their strengths in daily living. He also emphasizes the importance of meaning in life, to involve individuals using their strengths in service to a cause that they find meaningful, often one that is greater than themselves.

Coaching is asset-based, not problem-focused. Coaching holds that the negative energy and emotion of identifying, analyzing, and correcting weaknesses is not sufficient to transform people or enable them to move in new directions. The use of a problem-solving approach typically leads one to expect correction of the problems. Coaching doesn't ignore problems; rather, it shifts the focus from problems to strengths and possibilities, from deficiency to potential, growth, and learning. The aim is to elicit energy and positive emotion. Ideally there is a growing sense of empowerment, motivation, commitment, and aspiration. By clarifying strengths, values, and resources, clients choose what changes they want to make, and are encouraged to make choices about their own lives and to take responsibility for their own choices, learning, and change. The leverage for the change is client-centred; that is to say, client-based and intrinsic rather than expert-based and extrinsic.

These are some typical coaching questions: Who am I at my best? What is most energizing and meaningful to me? What do I want to do with my life? How can I go about creating the life I want? Coaching is essentially about helping people to discover how to bring their choices and actions more in line with their unique best self. A coach enables people — individually and in families or groups — to connect more creatively with their deep human desire to make a contribution to the betterment of humanity. A coach recognizes that the quest for meaning and satisfaction has a paradoxical tension between self-differentiation and unique self-expression on the one hand, and community integration and connection on the other hand (Cooperrider & Whitney, 1999; Csikszentmihalyi, 1990, 1993, 1997; Frankl, 1985; Kegan, 1982, 1994; Page, 2005; Vaillant, 2002). Skill in coaching can help occupational therapists to focus on enabling meaningful and satisfying occupation.

Health professionals like occupational therapists may choose not to become certified, professional coaches. However, coaching schools accredited with the
International Coach Federation sometimes offer short courses specifically for professionals who wish to learn and enhance their coaching skills. Increasingly, coaching
is included in occupational therapy education and practice. Occupational therapy
coaching would be distinguished by its focus on occupation. Coaching may be integrated with engagement in occupations, or may reflect on occupations, as is done in
Kolb's (1984) experiential learning cycle.

The illustrations of enablement with individuals, families, and groups in chapter 5
will speak in some way to the majority of occupational therapists in Canada and
worldwide. Examples of change models, asset-based approaches, and enablement
skills offer occupational therapists background knowledge to articulate what the profession offers in many settings. The Canadian Model of Client-Centred Enablement
offers guidance to enable individual change, with awareness that the outcomes of
enablement are not only personal but also cultural, economic, and social.

Text box 5.3

Reflections on enablement across the scope of practice

In reflection on Catherine's story, how might practice based on client-centred
enablement using a splint as assistive technology differ from practice that is
funded only to provide a splint? Reflections on the scope of practice and the
occupation-based mandate of the profession raise questions about the funding
for diverse practice settings, clientele, and approaches. In mental health services, what different change models and asset-based strategies would be used
in acute-care, out-patient, day program, and community mental health services?

In reflection on Pierre's story, how might asset-based strategies be used
to enable Pierre to advocate for himself and others living with a mental illness?
How might he and others learn to advocate collectively so that the onus for
advocacy is not only on individuals? What choices, risks, and responsibilities is
Pierre taking when he speaks publicly? What enablement skills would be used
most in working with Pierre and others to enable individual change in an
interdependent context?

— By Elizabeth Townsend

Enablement: The core competency of occupational therapy

Chapter 6

Enabling social change

Elizabeth A. Townsend
Lynn Cockburn
Lori Letts
Rachel Thibeault
Barry Trentham

CASE 6.1 Bintu's story: Enabling social change

Bintu can barely contain her excitement. Still, like the other child mothers, she remains remarkably attentive. Breast-feeding or rocking their babies in the shaded courtyard, these 20 girls are survivors of Sierra Leone's brutal civil war. On average, they have spent eight years of captivity in rebel camps, where they were reduced to sexual slavery and subjected to systematic abuse. Yet they still have enough life in them to dream of a future.

Aged from 12 to 17 years, they have just come out of the bush: illiterate, unskilled, HIV positive, addicted to drugs, traumatized, and with children from rape. Many have had breasts, arms, ears, and legs amputated when they tried to escape. Those kidnapped in infancy do not remember their communities of origin and have no social anchoring, and the older girls are too ashamed to attempt contact with their families. All crave to belong. Despite the pain and the past, today there is laughter and hope in their voices: they will make themselves heard and get the help they need.

For the Canadian occupational therapist involved in the project, the challenges are clear, although the sequence of intervention is less so. What will the girls choose to tackle first? Poor parenting skills? Addictions? Physical disabilities? Trauma? And how? The culture gap is substantial and the relationship with this vibrant, but profoundly wounded group is still fragile. Drawing on principles of client-centredness, the occupational therapist starts with community consultation. With the girls, she explores not only what matters most to them, but also how they would go about pursuing their goals. And because her own background is so different, she calls in local female mentors to act as sounding boards and cultural brokers. She guides the process in a low-key way that allows natural leaders to rise and take charge.

For 10 days, discussions are held with the girls, mentors, community leaders, social agencies, and government officials. Pivotal issues are identified and plans are drawn. The girls themselves decide their priorities. They request assistance to develop good parenting skills, give up drugs, become literate, address their disabilities, undergo vocational training, secure micro-credit, and launch micro-businesses. They know the hurdles ahead, but they also know the road to their own enablement.

For the first time, they feel the pride of making their own decisions and believe they can find their place in tomorrow's society. Healing is on its way, fueled by their competence and will.

— By Rachel Thibeault

6.1   Introduction

Occupational therapy is the art and science of ... **enabling a just and inclusive society so that all people may participate to their potential in the daily occupations of life.**

Enablement: The core competency of occupational therapy

Chapter 6 focuses on the environment, as captured in the second part of the occupational therapy definition introduced in chapter 1. To illustrate the Canadian Model of Client-Centered Enablement, chapter 6 considers enablement foundations and skills, change models and examples of asset-based enablement with communities, organizations, and populations. Enabling social change lies on a continuum and is interconnected with enabling individual change (chapter 5). Change in communities, organizations, or populations influences the individuals involved.

Practice that focuses on enabling social change at the macro level looks beyond psychological or other individualized explanations for human behaviour and targets **social structures, systems, culture, and the built and natural environment.** There is recognition that the practice and societal contexts determine what people think and do and that they even shape what people imagine is possible. Local, micro, social change may be targeted at the immediate environment of individuals, families, and groups. Alternately, practice may seek macro change in communities, or the provincial, national or international context.

Around the globe, including in Canada, huge inequities that persist in everyday occupations are justified on the basis of differences in (dis)ability, age, culture, gender, race, and religion (Waring, 1988). Bintu's story opens chapter 6 in part because Canadian occupational therapists are involved in countries like Sierra Leone, contributing where they can to enable social change in the face of difficult everyday circumstances. The story also brings home important enablement issues about conditions of abuse, poverty, and exclusion that marginalize some Canadians (see table 6.1).

Occupational therapy has a long, yet relatively unknown history in community development (Cockburn & Trentham, 2002; Friedland & Rais, 2005; Reitz, 1992; Townsend, 1993, 1998; Trentham, Cockburn, & Shin, 2007). Early Canadian occupational therapists enabled social change with government and the medical field by advocating for policies to include all people in community life (Friedland, 2003). Occupational therapy leaders, such as Helen Levesconte, recognized from the beginning that occupational therapists needed to understand social and economic policy and legislation (Friedland & Rais, 2005). An implicit social vision of justice seems to have driven the formation of occupational therapy with concerns for macro level social change as well as micro level individualized therapy (Kronenberg & Pollard, 2005; Thibeault, 2002; Townsend, 1993; Wilcock, 2006).

Occupational therapy is not well known for enabling social change, environmental level initiatives, or justice. This chapter encourages occupational therapists to make alienation, deprivation, inequity, imbalance, exclusion, oppression, and marginalization in everyday life more explicit, and to engage in social change.

Occupational therapists' interests in justice are in the social inclusion of difference, with equitable opportunity and required resources for all to participate in a just and inclusive society. Occupational justice is strongly aligned with Young's (1990) call for a politics of difference.[1] Outcomes of interest to occupational therapists in enabling social change may be to advance occupational rights — rights for all to

---

[1] Iris Morton Young's (1990) argument for a politics of difference prompted the concept that occupational justice is concerned with inclusion regardless of difference in everyday occupations — a justice of difference.

experience opportunity, meaning, participation, choice, empowerment, and balance in everyday life (Stadnyk et al., in press). We know that policy and other social change strategies may be positively oriented to enhance opportunity and inclusion for all as a matter of justice (Cockburn & Trentham, 2002). The following discussion of enablement foundations, skills, and change models provides some "exact details of our methodology" (Driver, 1968, p. 59) as noted in the opening quote of section I, Introduction.

6.2 Defining communities, organizations, and populations

Community can mean many things. To some, community has warm and friendly associations. An ideal Western view of community may be of a place where all people realize their unique value to contribute to the collective good; a place that fosters a sense of connectedness, belonging, and relationship. Although utopian views of community prevail in many discussions, community can also be a place of denial and repression. Some communities are most concerned with the collective, not with individuals. And communities may not welcome all individuals.

Some definitions of community refer to a group of people living within a geographical area who share common services or facilities. Other definitions of community refer to a group of people who share common interests, such as the worldwide occupational therapy community, or a common identity; such as children living with disabilities and their parents (Lotz, 1982; Lyon, 1989).

How, then, are populations and communities different? The *Oxford English Dictionary* defines the word *population* as "all inhabitants of a place" and "a particular group within this" (1989). We often talk about the full population of a country, but we also talk about populations within a country; for instance, we refer to seniors as a population and the population of new Canadians. Population health has been defined as "the health outcomes of a group of individuals, including the distribution of such outcomes within the group" (Kindig & Stoddart, 2003, p. 381). The focus tends to be on health indicators or outcomes at the population level.

Populations may be known by their citizenship or outcomes at the population level. Populations may be known by their physical abilities, age, or socioeconomic status, but individuals within a population may not perceive themselves as being members of it. Rather, they may view themselves as being members of the general population without aligning themselves with any population in particular.

While distinctions between communities and populations are unclear, one difference between them may be the sense of shared experience that is implied in the word *community*. Shared experience may be based on geography or some other commonality, such as disability or gender. The sense of shared belonging within a community or population is on a continuum, and is dynamic and changing. Members of a community may have one or more characteristics in common beyond a sense of shared belonging.

Enablement: The core competency of occupational therapy

In grouping community, population and organization clients in this chapter, it can be seen that organizations are clearly unlike the other two categories.

Organizations are social structures created to manage simple or complex functions. Organizations may be clubs, agencies, small businesses, corporations, professional bodies, government functions, or non-governmental organizations. Each will differ in their interests and structures.

Occupational therapists generally practice in the highly complex organizations that manage health. To a lesser degree, occupational therapists are found in the insurance, education, transportation, housing, employment, natural resources, and industrial sectors. Occupational therapists may work with clients who are involved in virtually any organization — from a self-help group to an international business — and within diverse organizational structures, from the public services to all manner of private entrepreneurship. Private practitioners create their own organizations with funding from insurance, contracts, or individuals.

6.3 Enablement foundations and skills with communities, organizations, and populations

In Bintu's story about child mothers in Sierra Leone, initial enablement efforts may have been targeted to address the mothers' disabilities — both physical and psychological. However, the girls wished otherwise and rooted their choices in their cultural reality: they knew what was essential for survival, and the tacit rules and expectations of their society. By respecting local knowledge, the occupational therapist instigated a healthy relationship with the group and fostered a sense of agency and participation in the girls. She cultivated power-sharing conditions conducive to long-term community acceptance of the program that was implemented to enable change. In Sierra Leone, most influential stakeholders had been consulted and included in the program, but one oversight nearly brought the process to an end: the traditional healer, who had been unintentionally excluded, threatened to turn the local population against the girls, something well within his power. After he was given a role in the project, not only did it move forward again, but it also gained broader community support and greater momentum. An unintentional, missed enablement opportunity was transformed, through awareness and action, into effective enablement. The most positive enablement intentions may sometimes result in unavoidable confrontation: as their micro-businesses grew, the girls could not secure credit from the banks, to which they were legally entitled. Going to the media, lobbying, and putting pressure on local elites became necessary steps. With reference to Bintu's story, table 6.1 briefly illustrates enablement foundations and skills for working at the macro level with communities, organizations, and populations.

Enabling social change will require collective participation and visions of possibility. The power of collective social groups will require explicit attention. Where the concern is to enable increased participation in society from particular groups, enablement aims to equalize their power for social inclusion and justice particularly in working with non-dominant, marginalized, or oppressed communities or populations. Networks,

Table 6.1   Enablement foundations and skills with communities, organizations, and populations

Enablement foundations	Illustration from Bintu's story
Client participation	Bintu became ready to participate soon after the Canadian occupational therapist arrived; she learned how to listen, reflect, and support the emergence of readiness in others
Visions of possibilities	Visions of possibility transformed energies with new meaning perspectives replacing visions of abuse. Collective talking and reflecting strengthened common vision, hope, belief in community power, and conscientization
Change	The therapist enabled community and population change based on recognition of the dynamic, driving power of culture. Possibly, change was guided by grassroots and locality models of community development with an emphasis on asset-based approaches of engaging people collectively in shaping their destiny through their chosen priority occupations
Justice	The occupational therapist was explicit about the injustice of abuse, terror, and exploitation of child soldiers, and affirmed the population's own awareness that life had been unjust
Collaborative power-sharing	Collaborative power-sharing was a new experience of leadership and community driven energies, with Peter and Lucy identified as natural leaders; the near oversight of a traditional healer illustrated the imperative to understand and take account of cultural power structures

Skills	Illustration
Adapt	Adapt nominal group techniques
Advocate	Advocate with Bintu and the other girls for micro credit
Coach	Coach the girls in leadership skills
Collaborate	Collaborate with the girls, traditional healer, and others
Consult	Consult with the girls, leaders, and funding agencies
Coordinate	Coordinate development agency and community efforts
Educate	Educate Canadians, local African government, and the girls
Engage	Engage the girls in "learning through doing"
Design/build	Design/build with others the plan for a non-governmental organization and micro credit
Specialize	Specialize in international community-based rehabilitation

partnerships, and solidarity are needed to enable change in social structures, systems, culture, and the built and natural environment.

Sustainable, positive change occurs when a population, community, or organization shares power to own both problem and solution, and to build capacity and leaders in the process (Khan, 1991). Enabling social change is recognized as a shared political process (Freire, 1970). It includes political strategizing, although this element is rarely expressed explicitly and often overlooked in occupational therapy (Kronenberg, 2005). Almost all occupational therapists are involved in supporting, changing, or actually writing policy that changes micro or macro social structures. To date, occupational therapists have written very little about this aspect of practice (Barbara & Whiteford, 2005).

Power-sharing in enabling social change starts with a client-centred commitment to listen, understand, and include the voices of each social group, particularly those of non-dominant groups. Typically community development takes a grassroots, ground-up approach, although-top down community development can be done effectively (Rothman & Tropman, 1987). Organizational development and population health are often viewed as top-down approaches, although some consultative, participatory models may operate from the ground up. Being client-centred and occupation-based, the trademark of occupational therapy enablement in social change will be to include client perspectives, engage people in occupations or use data on occupations, and be collaborative in advocating with and for clients. In all approaches, power and sociocultural differences between the enabler and the population, community, or organization need to be acknowledged and accommodated, likely with mediation of competing, or at least different, perspectives and interests.

In enabling social change, the backgrounds of the occupational therapists may be far removed from those of whom they hope to help, as in Bintu's story (see text box 6.1). In these cases, bridges need to be built; for instance, with cultural brokers. Enabling social change often requires individuals who can highlight the most culturally relevant and sensitive occupational issues, prevent clashes, and contribute to the creation of local networks. Cultural brokers enhance the possibility of success by working with and on behalf of the professional to enable deeper cultural awareness of the values, beliefs, routines, and systems already in place (Wright-St. Clair & Seedhouse, 2005).

Text box 6.1

Reflections on power-sharing with diverse communities

Is Bintu's story about a group, community, organization, or population? What differences about power-sharing and models of change would occupational therapists want to understand in working with small Canadian communities — for example, in a rural area where teen suicides are extremely common? How might power structures and resources differ in rural areas than in a complex, urban hospital?

— By Brenda Beagan

When clear communication lines have been established, enablement can then truly serve the community in need, mobilizing its informal leaders, supporting the goals identified by its members, and following the course of action chosen by the community members. Enabling power-sharing with communities will make or break programs and must be considered with utmost care. In some instances, power relations can be used to collective advantage. At other times, they must be challenged. Sustainability is largely defined by a judicious identification and nurturing of the right networks and partnerships (Thibeault, 2002).

Key occupational therapy enablement skills are to educate others through group facilitation (Letts, 2003b) and to draw on the political skill of advocacy, which encompasses policy analysis and community organizing (Kronenberg & Pollard, 2005; Trentham & Cockburn, 2005). Advocacy to plead in support of a cause or proposal requires a thorough knowledge of the occupational issues and the ability to present a persuasive case that may be in conflict with opposing group interests. To communicate and collaborate at the community, organization, or population level, one may gather strong occupational stories (Raeburn & Rootman, 1998) or specialize in using art-based, creative occupations like drama, music, art, writing, handcrafts or photo-voice recordings. Enabling may engage public support, through rhetorical and media communication skills, or knowledge of governmental and other social structures. It would also involve collaboration, to draw upon as many voices as possible. Enablement may be to design/build programs and services, to adapt existing services or buildings, or to coordinate and manage change in the built or natural environment. Typically, social change involves networking and the enablement skills to actually engage all stakeholders as active participants. Collaboration might also entail coalition building, depending on the change issue being advocated. Power-sharing could involve mediation and negotiation to encourage communities, organizations, or populations to come to a consensus around occupational issues and strategies to address them. In case 6.1, the story of working with Bintu, the occupational therapist's reflections on power were key to finding a community leader and advocating for the project.

Social change may be through occupational therapy knowledge transfer (KT) to educate communities, organizations, or populations on the everyday life consequences of impairments in body function, and on techniques to facilitate occupational development, for instance through playground designs to include children with disabilities within a community. Public education for prevention and primary health care may mean taking occupational therapy knowledge of medical conditions — from arthritis to schizophrenia, anatomy to neurophysiology, and occupations to occupational justice — to public events, such as community evening courses on falls prevention.

6.4 Change models for enablement with communities, organizations, and populations

When working with communities, organizations, or populations, occupational therapists borrow theories and practice for sharing power in social change from a variety of fields: community development (Krupa, Radloff-Gabriel, Whippey, & Kirsh, 2002; O'Neill & Trickett, 1982); community-based rehabilitation (Helander, 1992; Krefting, 1992); health promotion (Labonte, 1994; Seedhouse, 1997); and organizational development (Sinetar, 1991). Each of these fields contributes to occupational therapy awareness and practices in power-sharing with reference to concepts such as citizen participation, empowerment, population health, health determinants, community resilience, organizational change, equity, inclusion, and justice.

Many questions may guide occupational therapists in selecting a model for social change: What are the goals of social change? What forms of social change are possible to improve everyday health, well-being, and justice? What environment factors will influence change — either to resist or support change? What occupational therapy competencies are required for enabling social change in a particular situation? What diversity issues need attention?

6.5 Asset-based enablement with communities, organizations, and populations

As with individuals, families, and groups, asset-based enablement with communities, organizations, and populations is designed to inspire and stimulate change. With a positive view of the potential to enable change in communities, organizations, or populations, enablement rests on the values, beliefs, ideas, and concepts described in chapter 4 as enablement foundations.

Approaches to community development

John's practice (case 6.2) illustrates asset-based community development in which an occupational therapist is engaging groups of "people to develop the skills they

---

CASE 6.2 John and enablement with a community service

John has worked for over 10 years with a community-based occupational therapy service. With an interest in community development, John has encouraged the service to take contracts working with consumers and community members. One community agency for youth has maintained a contract for the last four years. The project aims to draw youth who are living on the street into a pre-employment skills development program. John has been representing the community-based occupational therapy service on this project.

In responding to a contract for consultation with the community agency for youth, John has organized workshops on writing advocacy letters for affordable housing. He has also worked with the youth to organize a kitchen party; that is, a gathering in the kitchen of the community agency for youth. The kitchen parties always start with role plays with the youth who are learning to speak in public about their lives. The parties end with the youth and coaches, such as John, playing music and cooking something to eat together.

Throughout the four years of the contract, John has been involved in enabling the youth to develop mutual support systems, to identify common issues, and to develop strategies for youth who are interested in participating in social action. John has been on hundreds of committees, written letters and proposals, and worked with many politicians and other decision makers. Youth have almost always been included as participants in these activities and the overall occupation of advocacy for themselves. Each activity is designed to demonstrate their assets — in contrast to their portrayal in the media as needy and uninvolved. John has developed proposals with boardinghouse owners, organized Web-based access to information at the community agency's drop-in centre, mentored occupational therapy and other students to learn about community development, and developed cases to encourage occupational therapists to seek out contracts with community agencies.

— By Lynn Cockburn

---

need, and removing the structural barriers that prevent them from achieving their full potential as members of the community" (Hoffman & Duponte, 1992, p. 21). He is funded to educate youth in advocacy skills because of his value-based foundations and skills for enablement. John is continually consulting and coordinating with many agencies to learn about funding opportunities and to develop community support networks. His coordination is likely linked with his enablement to design proposals and reports, using documentation as a strategy to organize community services with others.

Asset-based community development draws out resilience: the ability to bounce back given that "a resilient community is one that takes intentional action to enhance the personal and collective capacity of its citizens and institutions to respond to and influence the course of social and economic change" (Colussi, 1999, p. 11).

There are tensions between asset-based and needs-based approaches in community development. Occupational therapists will want to recognize not only needs, but also capacities and assets. Enablement ideally highlights the assets, capacities, and skills of individuals and groups within communities, and the assets of communities themselves. A community assessment might analyze the community's capacity to provide services, organize community occupations for different groups, and advance goals through sound leadership. Enablement would aim to build community enablement skills in community members.

A common challenge for enabling social change through community development is to discover entry points into the community that may not be clearly marked. Enablement without a known referral or predictable process may require creativity and comfort in departing from the formal, structured health services environment.

One community model stands out as particularly interesting for occupational therapists. Freire's model of community development is grounded in a social critique that takes the standpoint of those who are oppressed in society, as most famously expressed in his book, *Pedagogy of the Oppressed* (Freire, 1970). Freire's critical perspectives focus on conscientization: consciousness raising through adult literacy and community development. He started from his belief that people know about oppression through their subjective experiences of living. He then educated community members in consciousness raising about past and present actions so that they would understand how systems and structures, not their own failure to act, produced their oppression. Discussion to reflect on the effects of systems and structures was an important step before engaging citizens in planning and implementing change. Freire's educational method of conscientization has been adopted by adult educators, public health officials, community developers, occupational therapists, and others throughout the world.

In occupational therapy, use of Friere's (1970) model would be interpreted as a form of client-centred practice. The client perspectives and interests would be identified as the centre point of practice. Typical populations of concern would be people with disabilities, people living with a mental disorder, or seniors — all of which have experienced oppression from a population perspective, even if some individuals do

Enablement: The core competency of occupational therapy

not. Depending on the location of practice within a health context or the community, client engagement may be to develop competence through simulated or real occupations (Townsend, 1998). Freudenberg et al., (1995) offer a caution against putting too much emphasis on building competence among community members, however. They are mindful of the need for a sociopolitical process to change governing bodies to support more equitable opportunities, for instance to include students with disabilities in schools, and to distribute resources more fairly to achieve greater equity.

In addition to Freire's (1970) model of community development, Rothman and Tropman (1987) provide a useful framework of three models: locality development, social planning, and social action. Each model is characterized by particular assumptions about where to start and where to focus in enabling change in micro- and macro-level structures.

Locality development

Locality development is, by definition, local. A variety of people, often within the boundaries of a geographically defined community, are involved to determine goals and an action plan. A high emphasis is placed on shared planning, and the development of common values and community connections.

Social planning

Social planning is a top-down approach. Issues and problems are defined most often by the state through its agencies. Courses of action are, to a large extent, predetermined. Community members are encouraged to buy into the process of participation. With this approach, a high emphasis is placed on outcomes and goal completion.

Social action

Social action is characterized by grassroots, or bottom-up, initiatives driven by the efforts of charismatic leaders who energize members of groups and communities. The social action tradition requires a social analysis of diversity related to such factors as ability, class, gender, race, and sexual orientation. A high emphasis is placed on activism, which may generate conflict between opposing views, and between those who have power and those who do not.

Locality development is the most prevalent social change model used in occupational therapy to date. Enablement at the local level can address both capacities and barriers to community participation (McColl, 1998). An occupational therapy framework for locality development is the Client-Centred Strategies Framework (Restall et al., 2003), which emphasizes diverse perspectives, collaborative planning, and client, family and community education. Enablement involves multiple advocacy actions by clients, their family, groups, social networks, and professionals within a geographically defined locality, such as a town or city neighbourhood.

Another locality development model used by occupational therapists is the Community Development Continuum Model (Jackson, Mitchell, & Wright, 1989) (see table 6.2). The model identifies five levels that link enablement for individual and social change.

Table 6.2   Community Development Continuum Model

1. **Developmental casework**
   - develop individual capacities to make informed decisions
2. **Mutual support**
   - connect to others
   - self-help, mutual aid
3. **Issue identification**
   - assist people to connect to others on issues of common concern that go beyond the personal to the social, political, or community level
4. **Participation and control of services**
   - membership on boards, committees, etc.
   - the building of new organizations
5. **Social movements**
   - increased control over resources and decisions through creating or joining social movements
   - may be cooperative or confrontational

Reprinted with permission from Jackson, Mitchell and Wright. (1989). The Community Development Continuum. *Community Health Studies* 13 (1), 66-73.

An occupational therapist using the Community Development Continuum Model might use developmental casework in enabling individuals to develop their capacities to make informed decisions at the micro level. Enablement might continue toward social change by engaging and educating individuals to connect and assist each other in mutual support and issues identification. At these levels, localized community development may be possible by enabling change in individualized services and funding structures. Enabling participation and control of services, and participation in social movements would likely occur in conditions where occupational therapists are funded to work with community or non-governmental organizations. Enablement skills at this end of the continuum may range through advocacy and mediation to find common ground. Collaboration in coalition building and consultation with multiple groups and potential allies would be important processes throughout. Enablement would also include coordinating and managing teams that include diverse community partners.

Public education as well as education with participating communities and organizations would be ongoing to ensure that all are included. It is extremely important to engage everyone, particularly to draw out the voices of marginalized populations. Actions may be to develop mutual aid groups and partner in coalition building on large-scale social change projects. Enablement skills would be used to engage new voices in processes of reflection to develop new personal or collective storylines that identify resources, spark visions of possibility for building new types of communities, and foster hope.

Also emphasizing locality development, community capacity building (CCB) has been very popular with North American community health workers over the past decade. Enablement based on CCB contrasts with methods that foster dependence on professional experts to solve community problems (Kretzman & McKnight, 1997) and instead draws on the capacities or assets of a community. This asset-based approach highlights the importance of developing informal community associations (Kretzman & McKnight, 1997). The CanChild Centre for Childhood Disability Research (2005) lists the five key aims of CCB:

Enablement: The core competency of occupational therapy

- Create community awareness of neighbourhood strengths and needs;
- Strengthen neighbourhood helping networks;
- Strengthen professional helping networks where professionals act as advisors of a community-directed process that is led by community citizens;
- Form links between lay and professional helping networks;
- Link lay/professional helping networks in the macro system through an integrated database of services, plans, funding bodies, and policies.

Social planning may draw on design and mapping skills to gather all relevant information, although mapping what people do may not capture power inequities. Consultation may be needed to examine existing epidemiological databases that provide information on the prevalence of health conditions and other demographic information. For example, enablement may involve collaboration with those who can provide information from public health departments. In Canada, contact would be with the Public Health Agency of Canada, Health Canada, and community development associations, such as the International Association for Community Development. Enablement may also mean collaborating and coordinating efforts to organize community forums as a way to elicit information using a nominal group technique (Tague, 2004). Information to guide enablement may also be gathered using techniques such as surveys, key informant interviews, and focus groups.

To apply a social action approach in community health, one might consult PATCH (Planned Approach To Community Health) (http://www.beatricene. com/patch/what _is_patch.htm) for more details. PATCH is a community health planning tool developed by the Centre for Disease Control in the United States. It is congruent with the WHO definition of health and health promotion as outlined in the *Ottawa Charter for Health Promotion* (WHO, 1986). The approach supports the use of a wide variety of data gathering methods and also emphasizes the active involvement of community members in all aspects of assessment and planning.

Organizational development

Organizational development is a major concern in enabling organizations to be effective and efficient. Occupational therapy enablement in this context draws on many of the same enablement skills used with individuals, families, and groups. The locality, social planning, and social action approaches may be applied in the same way as in community development. Enablement is concerned with macro systems change, yet the individuals in the organization, and various groupings need to have a voice.

Enablement in case 6.3 started with top-down decisions which require bottom-up education, consultation, and collaboration. The first step in engagement was to determine readiness and to create space for staff to have a voice. Nettie, the occupational therapist, needed to identify key stakeholders with diverse perspectives who would work with her to design a plan with a timeline and targets that reflected her commitment to the organization. Collaboration was the key, and engagement of the staff in occupations was her trademark occupational therapy approach to change management.

CASE 6.3 Nettie: Enabling organizational development

Nettie, an experienced occupational therapist, was contracted to enable a large-scale Canadian health organization of more than 4000 employees to shift its operations from a medically-based model to a community-based, chronic disease management model. She is to evaluate, redesign, and implement a new state-of-the-art ambulatory care program based on evidence-based practice.

Research on community-based, chronic disease management has shown positive results towards enhanced integration of health and health-related services, better and more efficient service delivery, and improved staff and client satisfaction. After a tour of the organization and a brief meeting with the executive management team, Nettie is aware that staff members are concerned that the community-based model will undermine the scientific rigor of modern medicine.

The management team has shared the vision for change with staff throughout the organization. Nevertheless, most departments seem to be very resistant to change. With awareness of impending changes, many middle managers have changed jobs or chosen early retirement. Although Nettie is primarily a consultant, she is the key-point person to help the organization develop effective communication and strategies for change management. She is responsible for enabling staff to coordinate resources and collaborate in adapting a broadly defined model that they can adapt to their specific departments.

Nettie plans to listen to all levels of staff when she studies the strengths and challenges of the organization, then coach those in the organization through the change. She plans to engage staff to work through this change as an opportunity for new occupational dreams.

— By Judy Quach

Occupational therapists, like Nettie, who take on organizational development as a manager, consultant, or researcher, can continue to practice occupational therapy. Nettie's enablement included listening to diverse perspectives. She coordinated change by posting plans, progress, and outstanding issues for all to see. She enabled groups within the organization to set up collaborating teams to propose initiatives to positively manage change in their own area of the organization. She met with both top-level and ground-level leaders to consult on different strategies that would be thought appropriate by the various staff groups. In managing change, Nettie used her enablement skills by engaging staff actively in the work to adapt and redesign policies, rather than Nettie drafting them in the isolation of her office. She developed workshops, retreats, planning days, and celebration events as occupations that would enable staff to develop a sense of community as a basis for talking through changes in funding structures and everyday work conditions. She coached some staff individually and in groups. Her locality development approach educated staff and other managers about change and the importance of meaningful occupation for all members of the organization. Her occupational perspective was employed in setting up a daily routine for stress management exercises with a lunch break.

Enablement: The core competency of occupational therapy

Enablement in case 6.4 had several components of organizational development. Traditionally, children affected by Developmental Coordination Disorder (DCD) are referred to school-based occupational therapy for help with difficulties in printing or writing. While this is helpful, the children's other occupational issues are not often addressed. Moreover, appropriate resources for parents and teachers are not accessed when DCD is not recognized.

In occupational therapy, education was provided in large and small group sessions to family physicians and primary care pediatricians. Specialized multimedia information packages were developed and used. The study occupational therapist provided personalized, just-in-time outreach education with individual children and their families, and with groups of physicians. Physicians were encouraged to refer children suspected of having DCD for an occupational therapy assessment, which could be carried out in their offices. Family meetings were held where the physician and occupational therapist could discuss the motor assessment findings, and recommend resources and next steps. The study occupational therapist also provided parents with resources, including information sheets from the CanChild Web site (CanChild Centre for Childhood Disability Research, 2005) to give to teachers, coaches, and community workers. The therapist also acted as a link between the health and education systems.

The physicians and parents reported that occupational therapy had been a tremendous resource. On hearing the results of the demonstration project, one group of physicians decided to include an occupational therapist in their proposal for services

---

CASE 6.4 Practice and research as an agent of social change

A project to enable children to live more fully with Developmental Coordination Disorder (DCD) illustrates systems level enablement. Approximately 5% of school aged children are affected by DCD, a developmental disorder characterized by difficulty learning new motor skills. The impact of this condition on a child's occupational performance is profound: occupational issues are typically with self-care, sports and other physical performance, and likely result in these children being ostracized by peers. Secondary issues, such as obesity and depression, are common. Yet, the occupational issues of these children are rarely recognized as part of an identifiable syndrome, and parents are often sent from professional to professional to find an explanation for their child's difficulties.

An occupational therapy researcher, in collaboration with a speech-language pathologist researcher, developmental pediatrician and others, implemented a systems-level intervention to improve the recognition, diagnosis, and management of children with DCD. The study occupational therapist coordinated a demonstration project and worked directly with the children involved (Gaines, Missiuna, Egan, & McLean, 2006).

— By Mary Egan

within a new family health team. The local children's hospital developed specialized services for preschool children with DCD. Plans are being made to include services for children with DCD in a new, university-based, interprofessional, health clinic designed to address the needs of individuals in the region.

Cases 6.3 and 6.4 briefly illustrate enabling change through organizational development and systems-level change. In both cases, enablement would focus on the environment; that is, on enabling social change in structures, systems, policies, and funding. With an occupational perspective, the occupational therapist would attend to what people need and want to do. The therapist would consider what people perceive as meaningful, and develop systems-level supports. A top-down social action strategy would be combined with a locality development strategy, by engaging those involved in occupations. An important part of systems-level enablement is advocacy, collaboration, and coordination to design and implement programs, funding, policy, evaluation, and research. Partnerships and alliances may be had with any stakeholder within and beyond the health system.

Population health

Enablement skills used for working in population health are applicable whether working outside Canada, as in the case of Lucy and Peter (case 6.5), or inside Canada but outside a comfortable and familiar cultural zone. Engaging Lucy and Peter in nominal group techniques means engaging them to brainstorm issues with agreement that no idea is rejected. Discussion of each idea is without judgment before members rank them.

Using nominal group techniques and other methods, occupational therapists may raise awareness of population issues. Throughout, important questions to continually ask are: Who has a voice and whose voice is not clearly heard? Whose perspectives are present or absent in decision making? What advocacy is needed and how might professional expertise interfere or help?

Often, population clients are not well enough organized to be an occupational therapy *client* per se. It is not easy to put boundaries around a population. For occupational therapists interested in working with populations, one of the first challenges is to identify the key stakeholders. While there are examples in which population representatives come to the occupational therapist (McComas & Carswell, 1994; Neufeld & Kniepmann, 2001), there are more instances when this is not the case. As well, occupational therapists need to be cautious to ensure that a diversity of interests and stakeholders are consulted in identifying who will be involved in a population-based partnership.

With rising interest in Canada on the determinants of health and primary health care, discussion often leads to population-based initiatives. Population health places emphasis on *upstream* or root causes that result in challenges to health (Scriven & Atwal, 2004). Health is understood from a socioenvironmental perspective. The focus is on environmental risk conditions and psychosocial risk factors that influence health (Labonte, 1993). Examples of risk conditions include poverty, limited education, unemployment, and hazardous community, transportation, living, or working condi-

Enablement: The core competency of occupational therapy

CASE 6.5 Lucy and Peter, and population health

Leaning on their crutches, Lucy and Peter are ready to lead their African community needs assessment meeting. They have been trained by an occupational therapist in nominal group techniques and now face over 200 people with disabilities associated with HIV/AIDS who have come to the needs assessment meeting. People cough loudly, flaunting their disregard of public displays of coughing and other symptoms of HIV/AIDS, a disease and population that are taboo for public discussion.

The meeting was officially called for people with disabilities. Many who attend the meeting have tuberculosis, a disease that is almost always associated with HIV/AIDS, but is far more socially acceptable in their country.

Nearby, the occupational therapist has been dishing out food at a frantic pace for hours. There is no complaint: this good turnout will help to identify more accurately the needs and wants of this community. Today's question is short and to the point: What is most important to us and how can we secure it?

The process was enlightening. The occupational therapist had expected the group to demand antiretroviral drugs. After that, it was expected that they would press for access to health care, followed by proper housing and transportation. Study after study had emphasized these priorities.

With facilitation by Lucy and Peter, the opening plenary meeting closes on stunning conclusions: This community has priorities that do not match the established profile for HIV/AIDS priorities.

First, they want food security. Noticing the occupational therapist's surprise, Lucy explains that antiretroviral drugs do not work if sufficient food isn't given: "No point throwing drugs at us if we're not fed." Second, they want education for their children: despite their semi-denial, they know their chances of survival are slim, and they want to see their children educated before they die. They rank employment third, to promote self-sufficiency. And, lastly, they point to their own needs for health care and drugs.

Listening, truly listening to this community has yielded a radically different picture than the occupational therapist and public had imagined. This different picture is hard to reconcile with governmental and non-governmental organization mandates: the community realizes how difficult it will be to find a supportive agency when its needs are so much at odds with official policy.

The community members create their own lobbying force, a non-governmental organization devoted to meeting their priorities. As a team, they plan the project, identifying each member's role. The people with disabilities have the expertise and competence to be their own advocates, but they openly recognize the power differential between them and the occupational therapist when it comes to negotiating with institutions to obtain seed money. The occupational therapist can open doors which they can't open. They choose to use this power differential to their advantage and define what they want the occupational therapist to do.

— By Rachel Thibeault

tions. Psychosocial risk factors include such things as isolation, stress, and limited social networks. Determinants of health are those factors that influence health, including income, education, social support, environmental conditions, gender, race and ethnicity, disability, and health services (Hamilton & Bhatti, 1996).

Occupational therapists readily understand the underlying values and interests of population health, including socioenvironmental approaches to health and determinants of health. In working with individual clients, occupational therapists observe and are sometimes frustrated by systems-level barriers. For example, occupational therapists know that attitudes, policies, and economic targets limit people with disabilities from finding meaningful, paid employment. Not surprisingly, occupational therapists are looking to address such barriers by working in prevention, health promotion, community development, and primary health care programs (Cockburn & Trentham, 2002; Letts, Fraser, Finlayson, & Walls, 1993; Scriven & Atwal, 2004; Trentham et al., 2007). Practice in these areas involves working with communities and groups to identify the issues that need to be addressed. Enablement includes collaboration in developing, implementing, and evaluating strategies to address the issues at hand. A key component of any population-based strategy is working in partnership with communities.

Enabling change with populations requires information- or data-gathering to identify the occupational issues affecting a population. Population health data can help policy makers identify the major factors that undermine health in a population.

Occupational therapists can use population health data to identify and demonstrate key health needs with occupational implications. One useful dataset, largely untapped by occupational therapists, is the Statistics Canada Participation and Activity Limitations Survey (PALS) (Statistics Canada, 2001). Access to PALS and other datasets is limited to researchers who register with Statistics Canada. Use of such data often requires literacy and numeracy that may not be common in the populations with whom the occupational therapist is working. Therefore, power imbalances to access this information and interpret it may occur. Occupational therapists with skills to analyze large datasets can access and synthesize available data and then work with members of the population who can interpret the data and enrich it with narratives about everyday experiences.

In population health, there is continual interplay between a population and the individuals associated with it. Populations are abstract notions. For example, we may talk about the population of older adults in a particular city or country, or we may discuss specific marginalized groups such as the population of people who are homeless or living with HIV/AIDS. With these populations, there is seldom a single list of all members of the population.

While individuals or groups within a population may not be referred clients, there is little doubt that relationships and therapeutic alliances are likely to form with individuals. As with the slogan from the environmental movement to *think globally, act locally,* global or community initiatives combined with local, individual initiatives, may result in population-based change. Relationships formed with individuals and communities can naturally lead to links and networks within a population.

Enablement: The core competency of occupational therapy

Chapter 6 cases and illustrations for enablement at the macro level with communities, organizations, and populations are, like those in chapter 5, asset-based approaches for enablement focused on occupation. The illustrations are of enablement foundations and skills at the systems level. That is, practice is directed toward changes in social structure rather than to the issues of individuals, families, or groups. The Canadian Model of Client-Centred Enablement offers guidance for enabling social change in the influence of cultural, institutional, physical, and social factors in the environment as depicted in the CMOP-E. We are reminded to listen to the culturally-based stories and priorities of communities, organizations, and populations, whether in Canada or else-where. It can be challenging to ensure that the diversity of the population and social conditions is represented in population networks (see text box 6.2).

Text box 6.2

Reflections on the diversity of populations and social conditions

What does diversity mean in enabling social change? How might an occupa-tional therapist attend to diversity in asset-based community development in an inner-city housing development? How might diversity be taken into account by an occupational therapist engaged in organizational development with a busi-ness that wishes to become more inclusive in hiring persons with disabilities? What issues of diversity might occupational therapists raise in population health with seniors in various neighbourhoods within an urban area?

— *By Brenda Beagan*

Enablement: The core competency of occupational therapy

SECTION III

Occupation-based enablement

Introduction

Occupational therapy is the art and science of enabling engagement in everyday living, through occupation; of enabling people to perform the occupations that foster health and well-being; and of enabling a just and inclusive society so that all people may participate to their maximal potential in the daily occupations of life.

Figure Section III   Occupational Enablement

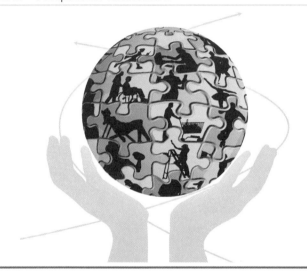

With the adoption of this definition of occupational therapy, Canada is advancing a vision of an occupation-based, enablement practice. The call for an occupational perspective has been long standing: many early and contemporary writers have advocated for it (Clark, 1993; Kielhofner, 1997; Nelson, 1988; Polatajko, 1994; Reilly, 1962; Yerxa, 1967). Indeed, as early as 1967, Yerxa (1967) argued that occupational therapy is only "authentic" (p. 1) when it is occupation-based. Nonetheless, occupation-based practice has been slow to emerge (Schell, 2003). As Wilcock (1991) noted, somewhat disheartened, "Occupational therapists do not view the world, or work with their clients, from an occupational perspective" (p. 86). It is the purpose of section III to enable occupational therapists to enact an occupation-based practice.

Starting with a description of the practice mosaic that is occupational enablement, section III integrates the old with the new and traces the evolution of our practice from one focused on the therapeutic use of activity to one that embraces an occupational perspective. In chapter 7, the breadth of occupational enablement will be given attention and an occupational perspective will be specified. The mosaic of practice will be given meaning through the use of exemplars drawn from experienced practitioners. In chapter 8, five essential elements that characterize occupation-based occupational therapy will be explicated. An aid for understanding occupational challenges, the Fit Chart, will be introduced along with a process to identify the best, the most likely, and the most acceptable solutions for enabling change. In chapter 9, the new Canadian Practice Process Framework, which is comprised of context and process components, is introduced. In chapter 10, each of the eight action points that comprise the practice process will be amplified. Chapters 9 and 10 are punctuated by a series of cases, figures, tables, and text boxes to guide occupation-based enablement.

Vision

To enable our clients to benefit from the full potential of a practice focused on occupational enablement.

Purpose

- To bring structure and form to occupation-based practice;
- To describe the *how* of occupational enablement.

Objectives

- To establish the breadth of occupation-based practice;
- To identify the essential elements of occupation-based enablement;
- To introduce a new practice framework that highlights the context and process of practice.

Practice implications

Section III reaffirms the power of occupation as means and end — occupation is the means or medium of therapy, and also the desired outcome at the end of therapy. The section offers cases, exemplars, figures, tables, and text boxes as tools for understanding occupational issues and identifying solutions. With this section, you are encouraged to adopt the Canadian Practice Process Framework — be you a clinician, educator, researcher, administrator, manager, consultant or other type of practitioner, or a reader who is not an occupational therapist. You are encouraged to immerse yourself in frameworks and examples for evidence-based, client-centred, occupation-based practice.

Chapter 7

Occupation-based enablement: A practice mosaic

Helene J. Polatajko
Noémi Cantin
Bice Amoroso
Pat McKee
Annette Rivard
Bonnie Kirsh
Debbie Laliberte Rudman
Patty Rigby
Nancy Lin

CASE 7   Daniel and the hoop shot

My first job as an occupational therapist was as a self-employed school-based therapist, receiving referrals from a local agency contracting services from community care access centres (home care). A lot of the children with whom I worked were referred for occupational therapy because of fine motor challenges. The children were typically referred in grade 1, when difficulties learning to print became evident, or in grade 3, when they seemed to struggle with learning handwriting. This is why I was intrigued when I received a referral for Daniel, an 11-year-old boy who had fine motor issues.

Daniel lived with his parents and three siblings in a small community. He was enrolled in grade 6 at the local school. According to Daniel's teacher, the legibility of Daniel's written output was poor. However, Daniel's father said his son was doing fine in school and that his teacher was exaggerating his difficulties. I subsequently met with Daniel to complete the *Canadian Occupational Performance Measure* (COPM) (Law et al., 2005) and get his opinion on his occupational issues. According to Daniel, his main issue was his inability to shoot a basketball. Basketball was the focus of his current gym class, and a sport played by his older brother. After some discussion, Daniel agreed that if his teacher had difficulty reading his handwriting, then maybe it was also an issue worth considering. Daniel and I therefore agreed to work on two occupational goals: shooting a basketball and handwriting.

In deciding how to work with Daniel on his goals, I considered my options: I could focus on his underlying fine motor issues or concentrate on his occupations. Using current evidence to guide my assessment and intervention decision, I chose the latter. Specifically, I chose to use the *Cognitive Orientation to daily Occupational Performance* (CO-OP) (Polatajko, & Mandich, 2004) approach, a performance-based approach that has good evidence supporting its use with children with motor issues. While his teacher and case manager thought that basketball was an unusual therapy goal, especially given Daniel's reason for referral, I explained to them that basketball would be a way for me to teach Daniel a global problem-solving strategy that he could apply to other occupations. I further explained how enabling Daniel's performance in an occupation meaningful to him would likely have many positive effects in his life at home and school. It did not take long for this to happen. Within a few sessions his teacher said to me: "Whatever you are doing, it is working! Daniel is less disruptive in class, his confidence is up, his outlook more positive … and his handwriting is more legible! Whatever you are doing, keep doing it."

— By Noemi Cantin

Occupation-based enablement

"Those who are enamored of practice without science are like a pilot who goes into a ship without a rudder or compass and never has any certainty where he is going. Practice should always be based upon a sound knowledge of theory."

(Leonardo da Vinci, 1452–1519)

7.1 Introduction

With the publication of *Enabling Occupation* (1997a, 2000), the profession undertook to define a practice that captured the full potential of occupation. As discussed in chapter 1, the evolution from diversional activity, to the therapeutic use of activity, to occupational enablement was the natural outcome of our historical focus on occupation and our basic assumptions about the importance of occupation to human health, well-being, and justice (see figure 1.2).

For many years, in keeping with the medical model, much of our practice focused on reducing impairment, typically through the therapeutic use of activity, based on the assumption that impairment reduction assured occupational engagement. However, as newer models of health, such as the *International Classification of Functioning, Disability and Health* (WHO, 2001) indicate, impairment reduction in and of itself does not necessarily enable participation or occupational engagement. Indeed, as the Canadian Model of Occupational Performance and Engagement (CMOP-E) portrays, human occupation is the result of the complex interaction of a number of factors related to person, occupation, and environment. Further, there are circumstances other than health conditions that limit occupational performance and engagement. Thus, a practice focused on occupational enablement must extend beyond impairment reduction in order to enable occupation.

A focus on occupation requires a significant expansion of the nature and scope of occupational therapy (Burke & Kern, 1996). As Wilcock (2002) noted, we need to shift our thinking from a medical perspective to an occupational perspective. We also need to shift our thinking from a treatment perspective, doing things to and for people, to an enablement perspective of collaborating with clients, as illustrated in the Canadian Model of Client-Centered Enablement (CMCE) (see chapter 4).

The case of Daniel (case 7) demonstrates both occupational and enablement perspectives. As indicated in the case, the therapist who is faced with a child with occupational issues has a decision to make: how to enable change. The options discussed by Daniel's occupational therapist represent two distinct perspectives; the traditional medical/therapeutic use of activity perspective and the newer occupational enablement perspective (see figure 1.4). Opting for an occupational enablement perspective, the therapist chose to focus on Daniel's occupational issues as a means for him to improve his handwriting skills. Interestingly, within an occupational perspective, the therapist had numerous options: to advocate for the teacher to be more accepting of Daniel's handwriting; to adapt the occupation by replacing handwriting with a voice recognition program; to convince Daniel that he didn't really want to play basketball; to adapt the rules of basketball so that they were more compatible with his skill level; and so on. Some options may seem far-fetched, but they are all within the scope of a practice framed in occupational enablement.

The purpose of this chapter is to describe occupational therapy based on the full range of enablement, from the specialized therapeutic use of activity for impairment reduction, to the use of advocacy to promote greater occupational inclusion and justice. This will be done by specifying an occupational perspective and describing the mosaic that is occupation-based enablement. First, however, the breadth of a practice framed in occupational enablement will be made explicit.

7.2 The breadth of occupational enablement

In the broadest sense, it can be said that almost any person and any environment can enable occupation. Our day-to-day experiences provide us with endless examples of ordinary enabling events (see table 7.1). As described in chapters 2 and 3, culture, institutions, societies, built and natural physical environments, occupational opportunities and possibilities, and person factors such as growth, development, life transitions, and losses all influence human occupation. All have the potential to enable and, by extension, to disable human occupation. When human occupation is limited and enabling requires special skills, occupational therapy becomes essential.

Put simply, occupational therapy is necessary when solutions to engagement in the occupations of everyday living become a challenge, or are at risk of becoming a challenge; when solutions to performing or engaging in desired occupations become difficult.

For much of our history, as discussed in chapter 1, our approach to occupational enablement was focused primarily on working with individuals who had experienced

Table 7.1	Occupation enablers
Occupation is enabled when...	
A parent	gives an infant a rattle
A nursery schoolteacher	sets up a play station
A friend	teaches his friend to rollerblade
A school counselor	discusses career options
An optometrist	provides reading glasses to an aging person
A surgeon	does a tendon transplant
A dentist	provides dentures
A community	creates a safe park
A bus company	puts in a public transportation service for persons with disabilities
A city council	approves the budget for curb cuts
A policy maker	institutes equal opportunity employment
A legislature	creates antidiscrimination laws for the workplace
An occupational therapist	enables a client to overcome occupational issues, when finding solutions to engagement in the occupations of everyday living become a challenge

Occupation-based enablement

a health condition, injury, disease or disorder that resulted in an impairment of body function or structure and activity limitations (Polatajko, 2001). Occupational therapy skills in the therapeutic use of activity were applied to reduce an impairment by engaging an individual in activity. Essential to this process were our skills at activity selection, adaptation and grading, and our ability to create supportive environments. The therapeutic use of activity continues to be an important component of the occupational therapist's tool kit.

As occupational therapy evolved, our occupational enablement perspective has broadened. We now work with people to reduce the impact of their health condition on activity and participation. Occupational therapists become involved when a health or social condition results in an "actual or potential issue (or problem)" (adapted from Fearing and Clark, 2000, p. 184) in the ability to choose, organize, and satisfactorily perform or engage in meaningful occupations (adapted from CAOT, 1997a, 2002, p. 30). Our skills in the therapeutic use of activity have been augmented by our skills in enabling occupational performance and engagement. Accordingly, we expanded our focus beyond the activities of individual clients to effect individual, occupational, and environmental changes when individuals, families, groups, communities, organizations, or populations identify occupational issues. Occupational issues are challenges to occupational engagement or to inclusive and just participation in occupations, including, yet not limited to, issues of occupational performance, alienation, balance, development, deprivation, or marginalization.

Embracing the full scope of an occupational enablement perspective may include the following: any circumstance that may lead to an occupational issue; any health condition that may result in occupational losses or transitions; any environmental factor that may restrict occupational engagement. The full spectrum of enablement skills may be required for impairment reduction, adaptation, accommodation, skill acquisition, or social reconstruction. Bonnie Sherr Klein, the Burundian refugees, Emma, Joshua, Catherine, Bintu, Daniel, and many others portrayed in the book's cases may all benefit from practice that embraces occupational enablement.

In sum, our occupational and enablement perspectives have broadened our understanding and articulation of occupational therapy's domain of concern and core competency (see figure 7.1). First, occupational enablement makes explicit that our client group is not limited to individuals with impairments, and includes families, groups, communities, organizations, and even populations with occupational issues. Second, occupational enablement makes explicit our interests in health, well-being, and justice for the human population. Our occupational enablement perspective spans orthotics, seating, equipment adaptation, environmental redesign, and social reconstruction.

Figure 7.1   The breadth of occupational therapy focused on enablement

Clients

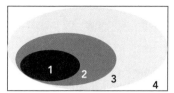

Targets

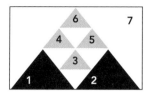

1. Individuals with impairments related to injury, disease, disorder, or disability

2. Individuals with occupational performance issues related to injury, disease, disorder, or disability

3. Individuals, families, groups, organizations, communities, or populations with or potential occupational issues

4. The human population

1. Impairment reduction

2. Adaptation (P, O, E)

3. Accommodation (E)

4. Skill acquisition (P)

5. Social reconstruction (O,E)

6. Health, well-being and justice

7. Occupational enablement

P = Person, O = Occupation, E = Environment

7.3 Characteristics of occupation-based enablement: Specification of an occupational perspective

An occupational enablement perspective demands dramatic shifts in the way we think about our clients and our practice (Yerxa, 1998). One shift is away from seeing clients only as injured, diseased, or disabled individuals to seeing them as occupational beings. Another shift is away from a focus on impairment reduction to a focus on the universe of human occupation and its enablement. An occupational enablement perspective is apparent in Daniel's case (case 7) when the occupational therapist chooses to address his occupational issues, rather than his impaired handwriting.

Occupational gains have an impact on health and well-being beyond a single occupational issue, as in Daniel's case. A critical review of studies looking at the relationship between occupation, health and well-being by Law et al. (1998) found significant evidence that occupation has a positive impact on both physiological and functional measures of health and well-being. The profession has understood the positive relationship between occupation, health, and well-being since its founding (Reilly, 1962; Rogers, 1983; Yerxa, 1991a), but various influences have limited the profession from exercising a broader practice until present day.

Over our history, the profession has considered occupation in two ways: occupation as the medium (means) of therapy (active doing), and as the goal (outcome) (Christiansen & Baum, 1997; Gray, 1998). Occupation as means refers to the use of occupation as the medium of change (Trombly, 1995; Thibeault, 2002). Occupation as end refers to occupation as the goal of therapy. While the former involves the use

Occupation-based enablement

of therapeutic activities, the latter is conceptually different and involves the therapist as an enabler (Rebeiro & Cook, 1999). The combined occupational and enablement perspectives can encompass both means and end.

7.4 Characteristics of occupation-based enablement: Specification of a practice

Seeing our clients as occupational beings

Occupation-based therapists conceptualize individual, family, and group clients as occupational beings with occupational needs, interests, expectations, and goals. With community, organization, and population clients, occupation-based therapists interpret issues from an occupational perspective. With all clients, occupation-based therapists seek to determine how best to enable performance of and engagement in desired occupations. An occupational perspective requires us to rethink the specifics of our practice, starting with the assessment process (Hocking, 2001). Occupation-based practice starts by establishing occupational goals and identifying occupational issues. This is best done in a client-centered fashion, as it is the meaning that clients ascribe to occupations and the experiences associated with them that makes these occupations such powerful tools in the occupational therapy process.

Hocking (2001) suggested a framework for using occupation-based assessments in practice. There is accumulating evidence that evaluations that centre on occupation help to identify positive, real life outcomes (Fisher, 1994; Trombly, 1995). The therapist first attempts to understand those involved as occupational beings. The therapist then gathers data to understand the function (purpose) of occupations, such as their significance and impact on life for those involved. Third, the therapist notes observable dysfunction in occupational performance or engagement, as well as limiting and facilitating resources. At this point, the analysis of occupational issues would include analysis of components of performance or environmental elements. Examples of occupation-based assessments include the *Canadian Occupational Performance Measure* (Law, Baptiste, et al., 2005) (used with Daniel), the *Assessment of Motor and Process Skills* (Fisher, 1994; Fisher, Liu, Velozo, & Pan, 1992), the *Activity Card Sort* (Baum & Edwards, 2001), and the *Paediatric Activity Card Sort* (Mandich, Polatajko, Miller, & Baum, 2004). Many more assessment tools are in development.

A focus on the universe of human occupation and its enablement

A focus on the universe of human occupation and its enablement is increasingly supported by research. The landmark Well Elderly study by Clark and colleagues (Clark et al., 1997) provided an excellent example of an occupation-based intervention. The study demonstrated that preventative occupational therapy, centred on lifestyle redesign, decreased the health risks of older adults. Using a randomized clinical trial of a large group of seniors, Clark and colleagues showed that preventative occupation has the potential to maintain and improve health status.

Passmore (2003) showed the impact of leisure engagement on mental health outcomes and the mediating factors of self-efficacy, competence, and self-worth in a large population of (healthy) adolescents. The adolescents completed a leisure questionnaire and a perceived self-efficacy scale. The findings indicated that participation in leisure has an important value and positive link with mental health, self-efficacy, and competency in teenagers.

Mee and Sumsion (2001) studied the value and personal meaning of occupation from the perspective of adults who live with a severe mental illness in the community. Some of the issues addressed in the study were clients' motivation for attending programs, the feelings they experienced while engaged in occupation, the significance of being engaged in occupation, and the personal value of participation in occupation. The findings showed that involvement in productive occupations generated a sense of purpose, promoted socialization, and helped alleviate feelings of boredom and isolation. Furthermore, engagement in occupation enabled study participants to organize their behaviours in adaptive ways and gain a sense of improved quality of life.

Mandich, Polatajko, & Rodger (2003) carried out a qualitative study to examine children's experience of living with a Developmental Coordination Disorder (DCD). The parents reported that the children's new-found skills had a significant impact on the children's lives; the children subsequently increased their self-confidence, were willing to try new things, were more likely to persist in their goals, develop new social contacts, and were privy to new opportunities. In the words of one parent the new skill (bike riding) was "a lifeline into the social community, and a lifeline so far as his self-esteem, it has definitely grown. It sort of was a rite of passage ..." (Mandich et al., 2003, p. 588). As with the project in case 6.4, children who had participated in an occupation-based program showed improvement in their self-identified occupational goals.

McGuire, Crowe, Law, & VanLeit (2004) examined the occupational roles of mothers with young children with disabilities. The mothers of children with disabilities reported spending extraordinary amounts of time doing self-care activities for their children, such as dressing and feeding. The mothers stated that the time spent taking care of children's needs did not allow them to meet their own needs for sleep and leisure. Engagement in occupations was an important determinant of health and well-being for these mothers. They reported positive benefits from doing occupations that met their own interests and roles outside of mothering. They enjoyed the time, such as family trips, and engaged in typical family-related activities with their children. They learned about themselves and their own expectations of motherhood through their experiences in mothering children with disabilities. By understanding their identities, capabilities, and challenges in the occupation of mothering, they were able to achieve positive self-esteem and well-being.

These few studies illustrate Reilly's (1962) argument that occupations, not activities, hold therapeutic power, and that the role of occupational therapists could be much broader than the therapeutic use of activities aimed at improving body functions.

7.5 Characteristics of occupation-based enablement: A practice mosaic

The characteristics of a practice that sees people as occupational beings who need occupation for health, well-being, and justice are indeed broad (see table 7.2). Using the CMOP-E to discern the full scope of occupation-based practice suggests that any interaction of person, environment, and occupation is of interest; that we can address the occupational issues, actual or potential, of any person and in any environment with respect to any occupation. Further, acknowledging that occupational engagement is not solely an individual matter, as outlined in section II, occupational enablement can happen at several levels: person, family, group, organization, community, and population. Finally using the CMCE, we can discern a broad spectrum of skills that can be used to effect enablement. As a result occupation-based enablement will form a true practice mosaic (see table 7.2).

A profession with as broad a scope as occupational therapy is best characterized as a mosaic, with some essential commonalities to be sure, but a mosaic nonetheless. As discussed above, the longest standing form of practice in the mosaic is focused on impairment reduction, primarily drawing on the therapeutic use of activities.

Impairment reduction and occupational enablement

Therapeutic use of activities

The primary vehicle for impairment reduction in occupational therapy has been the therapeutic use of activities (Reilly, 1962; Yerxa, 1967; Meyer, 1922, 1977; Mosey, 1986). For much of our history, the term occupation was used only to name the profession (Polatajko, 2001); the term activity was used to characterize the practice (Holm, Rogers,

---

Table 7.2   Characteristics of occupation-based enablement

Who	Clients of all ages, stages and walks of life, individually or as a family, group, organization, community, or population
What	Enable engagement in everyday living through occupation; that is, enable people to engage in self-care, productivity and leisure occupations, and enable participation in society; that is, to enable a just and inclusive society
When	Whenever the performance of, or engagement in, the occupations of everyday living become, or have the potential to become, an issue, or when community, organizational, or population conditions inequitably restrict engagement in necessary or desired occupations
Where	Wherever clients perform or engage in occupation: home, school, community, workplace, institution, etc.
How	Working in a client-centred enablement framework, drawing on occupational knowledge, and using a spectrum of enablement skills, the occupational therapist, in partnership with the client, puts in place a practice process to address the client's occupational issues
Why	Satisfy the human need for occupation, foster the health and well-being of individuals and promote occupational justice and inclusion

---

& Stone, 2003). The distinction between activity and occupation was unclear, but we wanted to escape the difficulties that arose from using the term occupation (Polatajko, 2001). Using the terms activity and occupation to distinguish between our therapeutic medium (means) and our targeted outcomes (ends), respectively, is in keeping with the distinctions made between the two terms in the Taxonomic Code of Occupational Performance (TCOP) (Polatajko et al., 2004) (see chapter 1). Accordingly, for the purposes of this book, the term activity will be associated with its therapeutic use.

Activities have a number of characteristics that make them an attractive therapeutic medium for occupational therapy. Activities are concrete and tangible as they frequently involve interaction with elements of the environment (Mosey, 1986). In performing an activity, there is a clear objective, and the individual is required to focus her or his attention on the task at hand until all steps are completed. The performance of activities thus elicits and organizes behaviour in a fairly predictable manner, especially when the activity is familiar to the client (see text box 7.1) (Mosey, 1986).

Text box 7.1

Reflections on familiar activities

Impairment reduction through therapeutic use of activity often engages clients in familiar activities to enhance abilities. What impact might it have if a therapist uses what are familiar activities to her/him that are not, in fact, familiar to the client due, for example, to the client's cultural background or poverty? How might this affect assessment and intervention? Is the client likely to tell the therapist the activity is unfamiliar? We often underestimate the impact of shame.

— By Brenda Beagan

Activities are comprised of elements that can be analyzed (Llorens, 1986; Mosey, 1986; Crepeau, 2003). Through activity analysis, those elements inherent to the activity are identified. The focus of the analysis is determined by the selected frame of reference or perspective taken. For example, using the TCOP (Polatajko et al., 2004), activity subsumes voluntary movement or mental process, actions, and, tasks. Accordingly, activity analysis would focus on identifying the specific voluntary movement or mental process, actions, and tasks, that comprise the activity.

Because activities can be analyzed and broken down into components and parts, they can also be synthesized (Mosey, 1986; Trombly, 1997). Following activity analysis, activity synthesis — consisting of combining elements in an activity — can be used to create an assessment of function and dysfunction, and to design intervention.

Numerous assessments have emerged using activities. Activities are used to elicit behaviours known to be indicative of function and dysfunction within a specific domain of concern (Mosey, 1986; Trombly, 1997). For example, activity analysis indicates that drawing and copying shapes requires, in part, visual motor integration skills. Accordingly, Beery and Buktenica (1989) assess visual motor integration skills by asking children to copy a sequence of developmentally appropriate shapes. Difficulties are considered to be indicative of visual motor integration dysfunction.

Similarly, numerous approaches have emerged based on the premise of the therapeutic use of activities. While approaches differ in their specifics and are based on different underlying theories, they generally identify the elements of an activity that should be combined to promote an individual clients' progress to higher levels of function (Mosey, 1986). The structure and complexity of activities are graded to challenge a particular function or dysfunction, and its composing elements are manipulated to create opportunities for the remediation of the body function and structural impairments of an individual.

For example, an activity such as stacking cones was used historically to open or strengthen a client's grip or to increase range of motion, depending on the size, weight, and placement of the cones. The activity can be graded by gradually increasing the size, weight, or placement of the cones, or by increasing the number of repetitions needed to complete the activity (Trombly, 1997). Any number of activities can be, and have been, used in a similar fashion to reduce impairment and improve function.

From a therapeutic use of activity perspective, the first stage of the occupational therapy process for a child referred for handwriting difficulties, like Daniel, would be to evaluate the integrity of body functions and structures that underlie handwriting — such as visual motor integration, fine motor function, bilateral co-ordination, and mid-line crossing. Using standardized assessments of these performance components, the therapist would attempt to determine Daniel's difficulties. Once the deficit is confirmed, if for example, it is found that Daniel has poor visual motor integration, the therapist would collaborate with Daniel and his parents to develop a plan comprised of a variety of activities that specifically target visual motor integration, such as doing mazes or copying shapes. The expectation is that once visual motor integration skills are ameliorated, Daniel would be able to learn handwriting.

The therapeutic use of activity in Daniel's case is based on an interpretation of the relationship between activity, and body function and structure. A number of theories have been developed that provide more specific explanations and hence more specialized approaches to impairment reduction through activity. The more common among these are neurodevelopmental approaches, and sensory integration (Ayres, 1972) (see text box 7.2). Each of these approaches guide different methods to improve Daniel's handwriting using activities.

Combining therapeutic use of activities and occupational enablement

While impairment reduction through the therapeutic use of activity has been a mainstay, occupational therapy — a profession of occupation — is concerned broadly with occupational enablement. Accordingly, the therapeutic use of activities approach with Daniel might be expanded with physical development and skill acquisition approaches. The more common among these for addressing body function

Impairment-focused approaches

Neurodevelopmental approaches are comprised of four separated approaches that were first introduced in the mid 1950s and early 1960s: the Rood approach (Rood, 1954, 1956); neurodevelopmental therapy (Bobath, 1990); movement therapy of Brunnstrom (1970); and proprioceptive neuromuscular facilitation (PNF) (Voss, Ionta, & Myers, 1985). These all differ in their specifics, but share a similar understanding of the importance of sensory stimulation for motor control, and of the necessity of repetition for learning. The basic assumption of these approaches is that the central nervous system (CNS) is hierarchically organized and that movements are controlled by higher centres, in response to sensory input to lower centres. This CNS organization is thought to be essential to movements, and disorganization results in abnormal muscle tone, movement patterns, and reflexes that ultimately impede occupational performance. Neurodevelopmental approaches are used with clients with damage to the nervous system and with motor control impairments. While the focus is not on the therapeutic use of activities exclusively, activities are used to encourage appropriate movement patterns or to promote a posture that would affect the targeted impairments. Examples of such activities would be lying prone on a scooter board to promote prone extension, or mixing a cake preparation in a direction opposite to a flexor synergy to promote shoulder extension and external rotation.

Sensory integration (SI) approaches (Ayres, 1972) are based on the assumption that the successful integration of sensory input (especially vestibular, tactile, and proprioceptive) within our nervous system is necessary for the development of higher cortical functions (such as motor planning, cognition, or language) (Parham & Mailloux, 2001). SI impairment is identified through standardized assessments that test tactile processing, vestibular processing, practice ability, and visual perception by using a series of activities (such as design copying or walking balance) that target each domain (Dunn, 1997; Fisher, 1994). SI intervention aims to remediate the identified impairment through the use of graded activities that provide ongoing sensory experience to elicit adaptive motor responses. A typical SI session may incorporate the use of swings, scooter boards, or balance activities challenging the child's impairments.

— by Noémi Cantin

impairments are the acquisitional, biomechanical, cognitive-perceptual, and sensorimotor approaches (see text box 7.3). For instance using letter templates for writing, tracing, writing letters with shaving cream, and developing a fun-based home program with his family would draw on these approaches. The therapeutic use of activities plus physical development and skill acquisition approaches might be further expanded with psychosocial and community-based approaches. Daniel's awareness of his writing difficulties may require attention to his emotional, psychosocial experience. Community-based approaches may be helpful to ensure

Therapeutic use of activity and occupational enablement approaches

Acquisitional approaches have been used mainly by occupational therapists working in mental health. The approaches are based on the assumptions that inadequate learning, interaction, or environmental responses may lead to an inadequate repertoire of skills and abilities, and that specific skills and abilities are required for competent occupational performance (MacRae, Falk-Kessler, Julin, Padilla, & Schultz, 1998). The domain of concern includes social interactions, cognitive functions, and performance skills. The various acquisitional approaches can be differentiated from each other by their theoretical foundations. Nevertheless, all focus assessment on identifying those skills and abilities required for competent occupational engagement. For example, an observation of a client at work may indicate that he has difficulties with task initiation, interpersonal skills, or time management skills. The focus of intervention is to enable the individual to acquire skills and abilities through the use of activities. For example, an intervention for a client who has difficulty initiating tasks may start with simple activities, which are initiated by the therapist and finished by the client (Mosey, 1986).

Biomechanical approaches are based on the assumption that musculoskeletal capacities underlie function, and that impairments in range of motion, strength, or endurance can interfere with competent performance. These approaches are used with a large variety of clients with biomechanical impairments, intervention methods being adjusted to the underlying pathology. Assessment consists of objectively measuring the integrity of underlying biomechanical body functions and structures. Unlike other approaches where activities are used for the assessment process (for example, copying design to evaluate visual motor integration skills), range of motion, strength, and endurance can be measured directly through the use of a goniometer, dynamometer, and ability to sustain activity (intensity or rate), respectively. Intervention focuses on prevention of deformity, maintenance of abilities, remediation of impairments, and compensation for impairments. A variety of media are used to achieve these objectives including splints, adaptive aids, physical agents, and therapeutic activities. Examples of activities used for intervention could be completing a puzzle positioned to promote elbow extension and challenge current range of motion, or weighting down woodworking tools to increase hand muscle strength.

Cognitive-perceptual approaches are based on the assumption that perceptual and cognitive functions are essential to performance and that impairment in those functions can interfere with competent performance. These approaches are used primarily by therapists working with clients who have experienced a central nervous system insult. The identification of impairments is done through standardized assessments that use a series of activities and movement patterns to challenge perceptual and cognitive functions. For example, praxis is assessed by asking a client to perform familiar gestures (for example, brushing teeth), and visual neglect is assessed by asking a client to draw a clock or dial a phone number. Intervention focuses on

Continued ...

remediation or compensation of impaired functions. Remediation makes use of a wide range of activities to retrain perceptual and cognitive functions, or train adaptive skills to compensate for impairments. Activities are analyzed to determine their perceptual and cognitive demands and graded to challenge the client's current abilities. For example, a client with visual neglect may receive scanning training using paper-and-pencil activities or real-world activities that require scanning (for example, finding a can of soup in a cupboard).

Community-based approaches are based on educational beliefs that people learn through doing in real life contexts (Dewey, 1990; Dewey & Bentley, 1949). Community development principles and processes support practice that is context relevant, learner-centred, participatory, and consciously attentive to sociocultural diversity (Cockburn & Trentham, 2002). Examples of community-based approaches are extra-mural hospital services, health promotion, home care, primary health care, school-based rehabilitation, and community-based rehabilitation (CBR). Hammell (2007) highlights the importance of bringing a critical perspective on client-centred practice in practice and research. Community-based approaches draw on "a specific philosophical, political and ethical approach to developing [and using] knowledge that is fundamentally concerned with realigning power" (Abstract, early on-line edition).

Psychosocial or biopsychosocial approaches refer to a cluster of holistic approaches to address the psychological, cultural, and spiritual aspects of life (Cara & MacRae, 1998; Cooper, Stevenson, & Hale, 1996; Stein & Cutler, 2002). Attention to psychosocial issues, including feelings, thoughts, values, beliefs, habits, values, rituals, and assumptions, is a central feature of all occupational therapy. These approaches are the cornerstone of mental health occupational therapy practice (CAOT, 1993). Psychosocial rehabilitation (PSR) (Cohen, Anthony, Farkas, 1997) is particularly of interest to occupational therapists who work in community mental health initiatives. PSR is highly client-centred, based on principles of client participation and engagement to develop skills and leadership with persons with a severe and persistent mental disorder. Asset-based appreciative inquiry (Cooperrider & Whitney, 1999; Cooperrider, Whitney, & Stavros, 2003) is another psychosocial approach that incorporates both the philosophy of appreciative inquiry and the Mindset Model (Learner versus Judger) (Goldberg, 1998).

Sensorimotor (SM) approaches loosely refer to a broad range of interventions that use some combination of sensory input with motor output to promote motor skill development. SM approaches, among the most common approaches used in paediatric occupational therapy, incorporate a variety of techniques to promote the coordination of sensory and motor information (Dunn, 1997). Impaired sensorimotor skills are typically identified through standardized activity-based assessments that tap fine motor, gross motor, balance, or coordination skills. SM interventions use multisensory activities that specifically target the impaired sensorimotor skills; for example, activities that provide vestibular, proprioceptive, tactile, or auditory stimulation while practicing a specific skill to support skill acquisition, such as writing letters in the sand, tracing sandpaper numbers, outlining one's shape in a mirror using shaving cream.

— by Noémi Cantin

Occupation-based enablement

good community integration given that Daniel's handwriting difficulties and involvement in occupational therapy make him different and vulnerable to social exclusion from his classmates.

Engagement of Daniel in basketball is a good example of a community-based approach, integrated with a skill acquisition approach, and the therapeutic use of an activity. Daniel is acquiring a skill in basketball and the emotional support that will enable him to connect and be a community member with his friends in a team sport. The choice of basketball is also excellent for developing the eye-hand coordination skills that he needs to improve his writing.

7.6 Occupational enablement: Six exemplars

Impairment reduction is a legitimate target for an occupation-based practice, but there may be no need to focus on impairment reduction at all. For example, in Daniel's case, the therapist's actual approach did not focus on impairment reduction, nor did it employ a therapeutic use of activities; rather the therapist focused directly on enabling occupation.

Our history as an occupation-based practice is relatively new. Although there is a small literature base describing the mosaic, there is an expansive potential for the mosaic in practice. Our mosaic is as broad as the occupational needs and contexts of the clients we serve, and as varied as the therapists who practice it. In the absence of extensive published literature, experienced practitioners have been asked to provide exemplars from their area of expertise. The six exemplars are in no way fully representative of all of the areas of occupation-based practice; rather, they illustrate a span from working with individuals to changing environments; they are in health, school, and industrial settings; and they are across the lifespan, from children to retirees. The exemplars presented here demonstrate that occupation-based practice is truly multifaceted in terms of client groups, practice targets, and enablement approaches (see table 7.3). The exemplars are first presented in order of client age, starting with children, and then in client groups, starting with individuals. We will start with more on Daniel, whom we met at the beginning of this chapter.

Practice exemplar 7.1: Enabling school-based competence by Noémi Cantin

Occupational therapy is provided in schools in some Canadian provinces, funded either by health services or education. The goal, generally, is to offer children of all abilities equal access to the publicly-funded education system. The role of school-based occupational therapists is not to provide full rehabilitation services, but to enable children's participation in the school environment. A continuum of service delivery models exist within the schools which range from the individual direct treatment model, where the child is taken out of the classroom, to the consultation model, where the child remains in the classroom and the therapist provides advice to the teacher (Case-Smith & Cable, 1996; McWilliam, 1995). Within the direct treatment model, the occupational therapist first conducts an evaluation to gain a better

Table 7.3   Practice exemplars: Our multifaceted practice mosaic

Occupation-based enablement	Clients						Practice targets						Enablement skills									
	I	F	G	O	C	P	IR	Adp	Acm	SA	SR	H/WB	Adp	Av	Co	Cl	Cn	Cr	D/B	Ed	En	Sp
7-1: School competence – Cantin	•							•	•	•		•	•		•	•	•	•			•	•
7-2: Orthotics – McKee & Rivard	•						•	•	•			•	•			•			•		•	•
7-3: Return to work – Kirsh	•							•	•	•		•	•	•	•	•						
7-4: Retirement planning – Laliberte Rudman			•	•							•	•			•					•		
7-5: Environmental design – Rigby	•			•	•		•	•			•	•	•			•			•			•
7-6: Institutional redevelopment – Lin				•		•	•			•	•	•	•						•	•		•

Clients: I – individual; F – family; G – group; O – organization; C – community; P – population.
Practice targets: IR – impairment reduction; Adp – adaptation; Acm – accommodation; SA – skill acquisition; SR – social reconstruction; H/WB – health and well-being.
Enablement skills: Adp – adapt; Av – advocate; Co – coach; Cl – collaborate; Cn – consult; Cr – coordinate; D/B – design/build; Ed – educate; En – engage; Sp – specialize.

understanding of the child's abilities, occupations, and environment. A program is then constructed — the main component of which is one-on-one intervention away from the classroom — and is supplemented by classroom recommendations for the teacher. Within the consultation model, the therapist conducts an evaluation but does not provide any direct intervention; rather, the therapist provides recommendations for intervention to the teacher, who is responsible for implementing them.

While there is much discussion in the literature about the evidence supporting the use of one model over another, integration seems to be the key concept that is emerging to describe effective school-based therapy (McWilliam & Scott, 2001a; McWilliam & Scott, 2001b). Evidence suggests that therapy focused on meaningful occupations (as opposed to foundational prerequisite skills), integrated into the routine and context of the classroom and developed in collaboration with the educational team, fosters better outcomes (Case-Smith & Cable, 1996; Kemmis & Dunn, 1996; Barnes & Turner, 2001; Nochajski, 2001).

An occupation-based perspective guides both my consultation and my direct service. Whether I work from a consultative or direct intervention model of service delivery, my assessments always focus on evaluating the child's current level of performance on the skills chosen as goals for the intervention, and my intervention focuses on improving the performance of those skills.

Within the consultation model, although I am asked to see particular children, I consider teachers to be my primary clients. During an initial discussion with the teacher, we collaborate to identify three specific occupational goals for the children with occupational performance issues. I then perform an initial assessment of the child's occupational performance and provide recommendations to be implemented by the

Occupation-based enablement

school. Depending on the nature of the occupational issues, there can be activity recommendations to practice certain skills, adaptations to specific occupations to enable performance, assistive technology or environmental adaptations to accommodate skill limitations. Once or twice a month, I provide follow-up visits during which I meet with the teacher to discuss the recommendations provided, re-assess their appropriateness, and modify them when necessary.

In my direct intervention, I consider the children to be my primary clients, and their goals become the focus of my intervention. The first and maybe most important step to enabling occupational competence in children is the selection of occupational goals that are relevant and important to them. My work with Daniel is an example of the direct intervention I provide using an occupation-based, *integrated* model within the school system. As indicated in case 7, my work with Daniel was guided by the CO-OP protocol, a performance-based approach that focuses on improving performance of ecologically valid skills identified by the client (Polatajko & Mandich, 2004). My aim is to ensure generalization and transfer of the newly developed skills.

In accordance with my occupation-based perspective and the CO-OP approach that I used with Daniel, I initiate direct intervention by explaining to the children that we will be working on things together that are hard for them to do, and that they want to do better. We spend our first meeting establishing the goals and determining their existing skill levels that relate to their chosen goals. As in Daniel's case, the printing difficulties in the school system were not solely a performance issue but rather were a manifestation of a desire to achieve a sense of mastery and competence over a desired occupation. Fitting in and having the same or better everyday skills as their peers is also important to a child's sense of self and sense of belonging (Mandich et al., 2003). In my experience, most teachers are interested and enthusiastic about occupational goals, such as playing basketball to connect him with peers, develop emotional self-confidence, and develop handwriting skills. An occupation-based approach works well when concepts such as enablement and occupational competence are explained to them; these resonate with teachers' own educational beliefs and values.

Practice exemplar 7.2: Occupation-based orthotic intervention by Pat McKee and Annette Rivard

Nick, a university student and avid amateur lacrosse player, was determined to continue playing despite pain and risk of further injury after spraining his thumb during a game. His specific needs were addressed with a custom-made thumb-stabilizing orthosis made from thermoplastic, thin enough to be worn under his lacrosse glove, which was acceptable to the game referees. Nick returned to the game, playing without pain and with confidence of avoiding re-injury.

Nick's story, like that of Catherine in chapter 5, illustrates an occupation-based perspective to orthotic intervention: one which both reduces the impairment and enables occupation (McKee & Morgan, 1998; McKee & Rivard, 2004). Orthoses are "externally applied devices used to modify the structural and functional characteristics of the neuromuscular and skeletal systems by applying forces to the body" (International Organization for Standardization, 1998, section 2.1.2). From an occupational perspective, orthoses are prefabricated or custom-made devices that apply forces to body structures that are impaired by acute injury, cumulative trauma, disease, surgical intervention, congenital anomaly, or degenerative changes. An orthosis is designed and built (a key enablement skill) to favourably influence circulatory nutrition, strength, mobility and/or stability to the body part, and ultimately to promote current or future occupational performance and engagement.

From an occupation-based enablement perspective, orthoses enable occupation by using a biomechanical approach (see text box 7.3) to reduce impairments in biological structures. We describe this as a bio-occupational approach which is also client-centred. The practice process of orthosis fitting involves identifying and addressing the body function and structure factors that underlie the activity limitations and participation restrictions experienced by the client. The intervention also requires the development of an orthosis that considers the complete client picture, including personal attributes, and occupational and environmental demands.

The guiding principles of a bio-occupational approach to orthotic intervention (McKee & Rivard, 2004) are as follows:

Occupational considerations
- Identify and address occupational goals
- Use an occupational perspective and promote client-centredness
- Optimize comfort, cosmesis, convenience
- Minimize occupational hindrance
- Use a *"less is more"* approach — design, fabricate, and finish an orthosis (or select a prefabricated orthosis) that imposes the least amount of hindrance and visibility possible
- Ensure client understands the purpose, as well as how to adjust and care for orthosis
- Consider client's environments

Biological considerations
- Identify and address biological goals and minimize biological harm

Mechanical considerations
- Incorporate sound mechanical principles

Follow-up
- Optimal benefits of orthotic intervention may not be realized if there is no funding or mandate for follow-up consultation

A client-centred, bio-occupational orthotic approach ensures that the central goal of intervention remains one of enabling current or future occupation rather than merely providing a splint. Routine use of functional outcome measures, such as the *Canadian Occupational Performance Measure* (Law et al., 2005), can facilitate client-centered, occupation-based orthotic intervention and provide evidence of its efficacy (McKee & Rivard, 2004). Orthoses that are thoughtfully designed with client input and carefully constructed with occupational needs in mind make an important difference in a person's occupational life by relieving pain, providing joint stabilization, protecting vulnerable tissues, and enabling valued occupations (Ford, McKee, & Szilagyi, 2004; McKee & Nguyen, 2007). Occupation is directly or indirectly enabled by addressing biological structures and their impairment.

Lynn, is a 26-year-old university student with spina bifida. She had no active range of motion of her ankles and no sensation in her feet, yet was able to walk with ankle braces and canes. Painful spasms disturbed her sleep and were causing progressive contracture that threatened her ability to continue to walk. Using the bio-occupational approach, Lynn's occupational therapist, Mary, worked collaboratively with her to design and create a unique custom-fabricated, ankle-foot orthosis for night use that met Lynn's requirements for comfort, appearance, and ease of use. Lyn's occupational requirements include — comfort, restorative sleep, and continued ability to walk — these were met by identifying and addressing the underlying biological conditions: muscle paralysis, muscle spasm, progressive contracture, and lack of sensation. Mary's knowledge of biological processes, such as promoting tissue growth, preventing tissue injury and controlling muscle spasm, ensured that the orthotic design applied appropriate forces. Follow-up visits enabled minor adjustments and verified usability of the orthosis, even two years later. In Lynn's words:

> "The orthosis allows me to rest more fully, reducing spasms and pain that would often go through my entire left leg. It makes my foot feel like a comfortable part of my body and I know it's not going to become stiff in a painful position."

Practice exemplar 7.3: Enabling return to work by Bonnie Kirsh

Return to work after injury or illness has become a major issue in society. There is growing awareness that loss of work has enormous humanitarian and economic costs. Unfortunately, research into return to work has, for the most part, been conducted in the absence of an occupational framework (Shaw & Polatajko, 2002). Vocational outcomes addressed in the literature also lack consistency, which makes comparisons and determination of best practice difficult (Kirsh et al., 2005). Fortunately this is changing, and systematic, occupation-based studies are beginning to emerge in a number of areas. Research includes methods of evaluating performance in response to physical, cognitive, and behavioural demands of the workplace (Johansson & Bernspang, 2001; Chappell, Higham, & McLean, 2003; Gibson, Strong, & Wallace, 2003); identification of prevailing trends and factors that determine the nature of services provided to clients (Lysaght, 2004); examination of approaches to clinical reasoning and decision making regarding return to work (Bootes & Chapparo, 2002); and, delineation of program characteristics that promote successful vocational outcomes (Kirsh et al., 2005).

An occupational perspective is uniquely suited for understanding, evaluating, and addressing interactions between the person, occupation, and environment in order to maximize return to work, retention at work, or entering the workplace for the first time. A range of assessments and programs exist to address these dynamic factors. Work hardening and work adjustment opportunities promote the development of work-related abilities and behaviours within the person. As well, workplace accommodation, support, and the promotion of healthy workplaces enable successful occupational engagement. Further, occupational choice, flexibility, and job matching ensure that occupations are tailored to suit needs and abilities. An occupational perspective on return to work encourages a comprehensive approach that considers these multilevel variables and their interactions. It also advocates that challenges and barriers to return to work are not a function of impairment alone; rather they are a complex dynamic of personal, occupational, and environmental factors.

Some service delivery models within the vocational realm are gaining recognition as best practice. Research into supported employment, for example, points to its effectiveness in helping people with severe mental illnesses to obtain competitive employment (Crowther, Marshall, Bond, & Huxley, 2001). Occupational therapists have embraced the supportive employment model (Moll, Huff, & Detwiler, 2003) and are well positioned to address its core features: occupational engagement, ongoing support, and occupational and environmental adaptation, such as workplace accommodation and education. Other best practices include on-the-job training, job matching, pay for work, problem-solving, and integration of services and systems (Kirsh et al., 2005).

Andrew is a 27-year-old man who lost his job four years ago when his mental illness gained momentum, and his behaviour and concentration became increasingly problematic. Although unemployed since then, he dreams of returning to a job he enjoys. However, Andrew is unsure of his ability to work and how to explain the gaps in his resume to a potential employer. Marcella, the occupational therapist working with Andrew, helps him identify and engage in occupations that reinforce his strengths and abilities. This increases his confidence and sense of self-efficacy, providing him with opportunities to reflect on work preferences, interests and aptitudes. Through this reflective process, Marcella encourages Andrew to self-evaluate, set goals, and identify potential job choices. A few weeks post training, with Marcella's support, Andrew accesses a supported employment opportunity based on his job preferences and enters the labour market without having to explain his history. The occupational therapist, Andrew, and his employer work together to adapt the workplace: they incorporate a quiet spot to work, flexible hours, as well as both written and verbal instructions, and regular feedback sessions with Andrew's employer. Andrew determines the pace and combination of his tasks so that he can match them to his ability and mood, knowing they must all get done by the end of the week. Marcella monitors the effectiveness of the return-to-work intervention through regular meetings with Andrew and the employer. Marcella also continues to support both parties for as long as needed in their work and in their ability to communicate with one another. The employer has learned a great deal about Andrew's competencies and no longer worries about a recurrence of Andrew's symptoms. Andrew is continuing to develop his work skills and confidence, and makes a significant contribution to the workplace. These interventions, targeted at providing a fit among person, occupation, and environment, have helped Andrew embark on a trajectory of hope, achievement, and productivity. At the same time, they have educated the work community about the potential contributions of persons with mental illness (see text box 7.4).

Occupation-based enablement

Reflections on stigma

Marcella's enablement of Andrew's occupational goals has been successful. Some further reflections on possible complications: What might she do if Andrew faced stigma from his co-workers because of his mental illness? What if he was living in poverty due to his disability, and thus did not have work-appropriate clothing? Or what if he lived in inadequate housing that made maintaining a schedule suited to a job difficult? What if he faced homophobia in the work setting, as a gay man? Where does Marcella's responsibility for enabling begin and end?

— By Brenda Beagan

Practice exemplar 7.4: Occupation-based retirement planning by Debbie Laliberte Rudman

With increasing life expectancy, greater female participation in the labour force, and general improvements in the health status of aging individuals, more Canadians are expected to live longer. Many Canadians will soon transition from employment to some form of retirement and are likely to live a substantial number of years as retirees (Schellenberg, 2004). Responsibility for retirement planning — particularly within the financial realm — has shifted in recent years. Although responsibility for financial planning was once accepted by governments and employers who managed pensions, today the responsibility has shifted towards individuals and their families. Not only are individuals faced with the responsibility of financial planning, but they also face complex choices given that the types of occupations people can and do participate in after retirement are also becoming more diverse. The traditional notion of retirement as a complete cessation from work is being dismantled, and new forms of retirement, including options that involve continued working in some capacity, are evolving (Denton et al., 2004; Laliberte Rudman, 2005). Within this social context, it is increasingly important for individuals to proactively plan for the transition. However, research suggests that substantial sections of the population are not preparing for retirement (Schellenberg, 2004).

Focusing specifically on financial preparation for retirement, research has demonstrated a range of factors that impact on the extent to which people engage in thinking about and preparing for retirement, including educational status, gender, health status, sense of control over one's life, time perspective, and occupational type (Andersen, Yaojun, Bechhofer, McCrone, & Stewart, 2000). One of the factors found to encourage financial planning is participation in retirement planning sessions (Kemp, Rosenthal, & Denton, 2005). In addition to encouraging financial planning, engaging in retirement planning has been found to increase positive attitudes toward retirement during the transition, and to significantly enhance retirement satisfaction (Elder & Rudolph, 1999; Reitzes & Mutran, 2004). Evidence suggests that although some retirement programs focused solely on financial planning and produced positive outcomes, they have still been criticized as being insufficient (Denton et al., 2004).

From an occupational perspective, moving into retirement is a time of occupational transition, involving a dynamic process of changing interactions among person, environment, and occupation. This process involves the restructuring of daily, weekly, monthly and yearly occupational patterns, and may involve changes in the meaning attributed to occupations all together (Jonsson, Kielhofner, & Borell, 1997; Jonsson, Borell, & Sadlo, 2000; Laliberte Rudman, 2005). In a longitudinal study of the retirement process, Jonsson et al. (2000) found that participants developed a new occupational structure in retirement and developed a slower rhythm of life. While retirees experienced positive outcomes, such as an enhanced sense of freedom, Jonsson and colleagues also found that many retirees would have preferred to have more regular occupations and their desire to do more occupations in retirement often did not become a reality.

Retirement is not a static state. As part of the dynamic process of aging, retirees frequently face continuing change. Aging is often associated with deteriorating functional abilities or the emergence of chronic disabilities (Health Canada & Interdepartmental Committee on Aging and Seniors Issues, 2002). Building a satisfactory occupational pattern in retirement can be challenging. When considering the link between occupational participation in later life, and health and well-being (Clark et al., 1997; Iwarrson, Isacsson, Persson, & Schersten, 1998; Lovden, Ghisletta, & Linderberger, 2005), there is great potential for occupational therapists to expand their role in this area and contribute to the development of more holistic retirement preparation programs that enable people to achieve a satisfactory and health-enhancing repertoire of occupations for retirement.

An automotive company has recently instituted an employee health and wellness program to enhance productivity and retention. The company wants to reduce employee sick leave and retiree medical benefit payments. Mitch, a private-practice occupational therapist, responds to the company's call for proposals. He determines that most of the factory workers are aged 40 and over and that the average retirement age is 60. A sizable proportion of workers make a transition from sick leave directly into early retirement. Based on these findings and research evidence, Mitch successfully proposes and constructs a retirement planning program to assist workers in optimizing their health through active participation in life during their transition to retirement and in their retirement years. The program extends beyond financial planning. An appealing feature to the company of Mitch's proposal is his plan to facilitate retirees to develop personally meaningful and satisfying occupational patterns that fit their personal preferences, resources, and context. Mitch frames the program using an occupational perspective, highlighting the connections between occupation and health.

The program is modeled after the Well Elderly Study Occupational Therapy Program (Clark et al., 1997, 2001; Jackson, Carlson, Mandel, Zemke, & Clark, 1998). This is a lifestyle redesign program that demonstrated the effectiveness of preventative occupational therapy in reducing the health risks of older adults. Mitch's retirement planning program extends over eight weeks and involves group participation. Attendees focus on the development of customized plans for transition into retirement and continued occupational engagement once retired. The program includes opportunities for peer exchange of local information and exposure to educational materials on the connections between aging, health and occupation, and on financial and occupational resources. The employees are encouraged to reflect on the significance of their current occupations, and to consider their personal and environmental resources and constraints. They develop personal occupational portfolios for retirement planning to increase their awareness of financial, social, occupational, and other resources. They also strategize ways of optimizing engagement and re-engagement in personally meaningful occupations. Mitch evaluates the program's effectiveness by tracking the workers' sense of preparedness for retirement and their planning behaviours. He examines the development of their occupational portfolios before and after the eight-week program. He also recommends that the company collect data to see if retired employees who were involved in the program use medical benefits differently than those who did not participate.

Practice exemplar 7.5: An occupation-based perspective on design by Patty Rigby

As the CMOP-E indicates, environments can support or restrict occupational performance and engagement. Occupation-based therapists have a unique set of skills for designing environments that can enable occupational participation. There is great potential for occupational therapists to provide consultation services to agencies concerned with creating people-friendly, inclusive environments (Ringaert, 2003).

The YMCA in a large urban community hired Jessica, a private practice occupational therapist. The contract is to provide recommendations for the design and construction of a new family development centre planned for an inner-city community with a large immigrant population. Using an occupational perspective, Jessica assessed the needs of the centre; she considered whom the centre would service (people), the services it would provide (context), and the occupations that would be performed there. Based on her needs assessment and her experience, Jessica proposed that the new centre be designed following the principles of universal design (The Center for Universal Design, 1997) with some enhancements. Universal design principles, used throughout the entire design process, ensured that the centre would be accessible to all potential users. The users of the new family development centre would likely include young children, parents with strollers, people with a mobility- or sensory-based disability, and those without English literacy skills (Story, Mueller, & Mace, 1998).

Jessica provides recommendations for the design of the building's interior, signage, centre resources, and the building's exterior, including landscaping. For the building's interior, she suggested that all routes connecting spaces within the centre be accessible with a path of at least 36 inches clear of furniture and other obstacles. Bathrooms for adults are to have doors with electric door openers, pedestal sinks, and toilet stall doors that swing outwards. All door openings will be a minimum 32 inches wide, and all doors and sinks will have easy-to-use levered handles. Jessica recommended the installation of bathrooms with toilets and sinks designed for children. She strongly encouraged the posting of signage for amenities, such as toilets and telephones, with a universally understood symbol. She urged the preparation of resources that are culturally sensitive and intuitive to use. She recommended simple colours and patterns, as well as colour coding to mark similar areas. Jessica recommended lowered public phones and drinking fountains to make them accessible to wheelchair users and children.

For the building's exterior, Jessica recommended landscaping with a ramped sidewalk from the street to create a level front entrance to the centre. Also recommended were power doors activated by motion sensors. Jessica actually participated in the planning of the accessible playground. She recommended materials and equipment that facilitated participation and the social inclusion of children with various disabilities. Her recommendations highlighted ways to promote children's safety, comfort, enjoyment, learning, and development on the playground. She emphasized that the playground must have accessible routes in and around the play area to make it easy to get around for everyone, including caregivers. Each play component included enough space to allow children to transfer easily in and out of a wheelchair and move around freely. She recommended that the play components be usable by children with a variety of abilities and skills and thus be flexible for multiple use. In selecting swings, for example, she recommended that they consider a glider swing where two or more people could swing, so a child with a disability could sit with another person who would provide assistance. Jessica recommended firm and stable play surfaces for easy access. She also recommended that areas where children may fall should have a cushion type of resilience; for example, surfacing with recycled rubber, to help prevent injury. The YMCA included funding for Jessica to stay on as a member of the final design team to oversee the integration of her recommendations in the overall design, and to guide their implementation during construction. Opening day offered an ideal opportunity for her to evaluate the success of her contract.

Practice exemplar 7.6: An occupation-based perspective on institutional site redevelopment by Nancy Lin

My practice as an occupational therapist is geared at the institutional level. My client is, in essence, my employer — a major mental health facility that has hired me to be part of the management team responsible for a major new initiative.

Located in a major Canadian city, the facility is currently undergoing site redevelopment aimed at fundamentally changing the delivery of addiction and mental health care. There is recognition from clinical experts, the community, and politicians that the current buildings, built in the 1970s, are no longer adequate environments for providing or receiving the best care. The new state-of-the-art buildings to be designed are intended to create an environment that fosters recovery, independence, and community integration for consumers of mental health and addiction services. Part of the redevelopment project involves the construction of "alternative milieu" buildings, which are four-storey apartment-like residences. In contrast to the traditional hospital ward where space is shared with many other individuals and access is controlled by hospital staff, the alternative milieu units will give residents their own bedrooms and bathrooms, and access to shared common areas — such as a lounge and dining room — with approximately four other residents. In addition, residents will have their own keys and the ability to control access to their living spaces.

The facility's redevelopment is a huge undertaking that involves many phases, and the coordination of many different departments and organizations. Funding must be obtained from the government, and private donors, and contracts must be awarded. The community, staff, and clients must be informed of construction disturbances, and the hospital must continue to provide leading clinical care. Clinical redevelopment transition managers have been hired to ensure that the clinical needs are met as the centre undergoes site redevelopment.

Transition management positions require a clinical background, which in my case is occupational therapy. The clinical redevelopment transition manager's clients are the front-line staff, program directors, and program managers. The manager must understand the needs of the mental health clients who use services at the facility. The manager assesses and determines the impact of environmental and clinical program changes on staff and clients, then devises and implements a plan to assist the staff in transitioning to a new way of delivering services. In addition, transition managers encourage staff to challenge the way they think about and deliver clinical care. The aim is to exceed best practice guidelines. The managers are required to understand concepts of change management and be skilled at helping individuals move through the stages of change. They are also required to be knowledgeable of the various stakeholders and their needs, and possess good negotiation, leadership, and management skills.

Occupational therapists, in my experience, are ideally suited for these positions. In choosing me to become a member of the management team, my background in occupational therapy was considered an asset. It was noted that occupational therapists provide a unique perspective to the clinical redevelopment transition manager role because they are able to readily determine the strengths, weaknesses, and opportunities of a situation. In addition, occupational therapists understand that the physical, social, institutional, cultural, and political environment affects an individual's ability to engage in meaningful occupation and to derive meaning from occupational engagement. Occupational therapists are equipped to navigate and create environments that enable and facilitate change, learning, growth, and skill development in staff. As a member of the management team, my contributions are influenced continuously, explicitly and implicitly, by my occupational perspective and enablement approaches.

Chapter 8

Occupation-based practice: The essential elements

Helene J. Polatajko
Jane Davis
Noémi Cantin
Claire-Jehanne Dubouloz-Wilner
Barry Trentham

CASE 8.1 Reflections on Martha: Learning from a second look

Occupational Therapy Interventions (OTI), a private company, provides community services in the workplace and medico-legal evaluations. A former client of the company, a small legal firm specializing in real estate transactions, requested a consultation to determine the factors affecting the occupational capacity and future employment potential of one of its employees, a paralegal by the name of Martha.

This was the second request regarding Martha. A year earlier, an OTI occupational therapist had carried out a comprehensive evaluation of Martha's occupational performance. That evaluation had resulted in a collaboratively developed occupational performance profile and a set of workplace recommendations. Occupational capacity enhancements were implemented using universal design principles and pain management techniques. However, despite these interventions, Martha's strong desire to work, and a supportive workplace, Martha's absenteeism had increased over the year.

To respond to this second request, the Hierarchy of Return to Work (HRTW)[1] (Dyck & Jongbloed, 2000) framework was used in conjunction with the Person-Environment-Occupation (PEO) model (Strong, 2002). The documentation from the original occupational performance profile was re-examined in light of a more detailed description of job demands and work flow provided by the employer.

This broader, second analysis produced a more comprehensive profile of Martha's interests and roles. It also indicated a capacity for administration. Martha's response contained descriptions of the occupational adaptations and compromises that had been put in place to sustain her productivity the year before. The first evaluation had focused almost exclusively on Martha's physical capacity. The second, more in-depth analysis identified a number of emerging psychosocial stressors, which including the following: not meeting her own high performance standards, an inability to sustain performance outputs during peak periods, an inability of coworkers to provide task support, and recurrence of depression.

The evaluation process substantiated the employer's concerns that Martha was at risk for increased deterioration of occupational capacity and worker role loss. The situation was also creating undue hardship for the employing lawyer. The employer was unable to make any further accommodations and in light of the findings from the evaluation, decided to work with Martha so that she could receive disability benefits.

The results of the second analysis caused the occupational therapist to reflect: Would the earlier use of a broader and longer-range prevention perspective, in conjunction with occupational choice exploration, have enabled Martha to achieve a better workplace fit? How often are documented psychosocial factors given limited attention in favor of the physical considerations of the person and the environment?

— By Sharon Brintnell

[1]The HRTW is a systematic evaluation of the client's occupational capacity that starts with current job, same employer, no accommodation or training, and continues through to new job, new employer with or without accommodations and training.

*It is the fundamental principle of cognition that the universal can be per-
ceived only in the particular, while the particular can be thought of only in
reference to the universal.*

(Cassirer, 1923, p. 86)

8.1 Introduction

As described in chapter 7, occupation-based practices form a true mosaic of enablement. At the core of this mosaic are some common characteristics of occupation-
based enablement, essential elements, that make occupational therapy unique, setting
it apart from the ordinary occupational enablement done by many others, as highlighted in table 7.1. The characteristics of occupational therapy enablement were
noted in table 7.2, particularly in describing the *who, what, when, where, how,* and
why of occupation-based enablement.

In chapter 7, and in the various cases and text within each chapter of this book, we
have seen occupational therapists become involved at various points in people's
occupational lives. The opening cases for chapters 1 to 8 have shown occupational
therapists using key and related occupation-based, enablement skills in various
ways:

- Engaging Bonnie Sherr Klein in playing shuffleboard to improve her balance
  (chapter 1);
- Educating Burundian refugees to negotiate between their own cultural values
  and the Canadian way of doing things (chapter 2);
- Consulting with a care facility on targeted options to engage Emma in occupations of her choice in recognition of Emma's occupational loss (chapter 3);
- Designing/building a home program to enhance Joshua's development and,
  with his mother, advocating with local officials for accessible transportation
  (chapter 4);
- Designing/building, then adapting an orthosis with Catherine for her to follow her passion and livelihood as a pianist (chapter 5);
- Collaborating with Bintu and her friends, the community, business, and
  government to reconstruct home and community so that Bintu and others
  could reclaim their lives (chapter 6);
- Coordinating the YMCA team in the design of a family development centre
  to meet the needs of an inner city community with a large immigrant population (chapter 7);
- Coaching Martha with specialized enablement in Hierarchy of Return to
  Work (HRTW) to identify the full complexities of her occupational issues to
  optimize her job performance (chapter 8).

Each case is unique; and all share a commonality, differing only in their specifics.
All cases contain the essential features of what Yerxa (1967) called "authentic" (p. 1)
occupation-based, occupational therapy.

This chapter will identify and examine the particulars of a practice mosaic of
occupational enablement, which spans from impairment reduction to social
reconstruction. It will pinpoint the essential elements of a practice that promotes

occupational health, well-being, and justice. By definition, these essential elements should be present in all practices in the enablement mosaic. Table 8.1 lists five essential elements of an occupation-based practice and relates them to the six practice exemplars from chapter 7. This table shows how essential elements are present across diverse practices. The elements identified in table 8.1 are generic to the examples in table 7.3, which show how the practice mosaic of occupational therapy spans diverse client groups, practice targets, and enablement skills.

Table 8.1   Essential elements of an occupation-based practice

	School competence – Cantin	Orthotics – McKee & Rivard	Return to work – Kirsh	Retirement plan – Laliberte Rudman	Environmental design – Rigby	Institutional redevelopment – Lin
1. Presence of an occupational challenge	•	•	•	•	•	•
2. Solutions that enable	•	•	•	•	•	•
3. Client-centred enablement	•	•	•	•	•	•
4. Multidisciplinary knowledge base	•	•	•	•	•	•
5. Abductive reasoning	•	•	•	•	•	•

8.2 Five essential elements of practice: Trademarks of occupational therapy

The "primary role of enabling occupation constitutes a necessary and sufficient condition for the practice of occupational therapy."

(CAOT, 1997a, 2002, p. 30)

When the above statement appeared in the original *Enabling Occupation* document in 1997, it was rather revolutionary. By describing occupational enablement as a *necessary* condition, the statement boldly declared that unless occupational therapists enabled occupation — regardless of what else may have been accomplished — that it was not occupational therapy. This statement expressed the breadth of occupational therapy enablement (see figure 7.1) and implied that impairment reduction alone is a missed enablement opportunity according to the enablement continuum (see figures 4.4 and 4.5).

Some may believe that the statement went too far by declaring that occupational enablement was not only necessary, but also *sufficient*. While articulating the breadth of our scope, we have not yet stated how to delimit it. The argument can be made that any practice that increases occupational performance and engagement would qualify as occupational therapy. That is clearly not the case.

Occupational enablement constitutes a necessary condition for occupational therapy, but it does not constitute a sufficient condition. As discussed in chapter 7, not all forms of enablement constitute occupational therapy; for example, winning the lottery enables a single mother to increase her occupational opportunities and those of her children, but it does not constitute occupational therapy practice. There are five specific elements that are **essential** for occupational enablement to qualify as occupational therapy.

The five essential elements

The specific elements that define our profession emanate directly from the *who, what, when, where, how,* and *why* of practice (see table 7.2). As already indicated in chapter 7, occupational therapy is necessary when engagement in the occupations of everyday living becomes a challenge or engagement is at risk of becoming a challenge. Thus, the presence or potential of an *occupational challenge* is the first essential element for occupational therapy practice.

1. Presence of an occupational challenge

The requirement of an occupational challenge emanates directly from the assumptions we hold about human occupation. As discussed in chapter 1, our focus on the human as an occupational being is based on the assumption that humans have a basic need for occupation. Occupation affects health and well-being, organizes time, brings structure and meaning to living, and is the everyday medium in which we do or do not experience inclusion and justice.

Occupational engagement is an anticipated state; absence of occupation or diminished engagement in it signals the presence of an occupational challenge because occupation is a basic human need.

2. Need for occupational enablement: Possibility of solutions that enable occupation

The need for occupational enablement as an essential element of occupational enablement emanates directly from the presence of an occupational challenge. The presence of activity limitations or occupational participation restrictions, or the risk of such limitations or restrictions, signals the need for occupational enablement. The need for occupational enablement calls for possible solutions that enable occupation. Accordingly, winning the lottery does not qualify as occupational therapy — whereas enhancing Joshua's development, improving Bonnie's balance, enabling Catherine to continue as a pianist, designing a centre that meets the engagement needs of an inner-city population, helping Burundian refugees adapt to life in Canada, and coaching Bintu and the girls to reclaim their lives, do qualify as occupation-based practice. Recognizing Emma's occupational loss also suggests the need for occupational enablement.

Our assumptions about occupational enablement indicate a third essential element.

3. Client-specific goals/challenges/solutions and client-centred enablement

Occupations are idiosyncratic, and people accumulate their own occupational repertoires and develop their own occupational patterns over the course of their lives according to their interests, values, and contexts. Therefore, practice must identify client-specific goals or challenges and enable client-specific solutions.

Client-centredness is an essential element of occupational enablement; practice must be client-centred, not prescriptive across individuals. As discussed in chapter 4, client-centredness has been a defining element of Canadian occupational therapy since the publication of its first national guidelines in 1983 (CAOT, 1991; DNHW & CAOT, 1983). Client-centred occupational enablement necessitates that practice is focused on client goals. Practice is conducted in collaboration with clients, responds to their needs, and respects their values, interests, and wishes, whether clients be individuals, families, groups, communities, organizations, or populations.

Our understanding of human occupation, reflected in our models, suggests two additional essential elements.

4. A multidisciplinary knowledge base

A multidisciplinary knowledge base is needed to understand the inherent complexity of occupational therapy. The need for multidisciplinary knowledge is due to the fact that human occupation is influenced by persons, environments, and occupations interacting with one another; each is complex in its own right.

5. A reasoning process that can deal with complexity

Human occupation is extremely complex and idiosyncratic with multiple possibilities that determine solutions for enablement, thereby requiring a reasoning process that can address complexity and can be informed by the client and by practice models, theories, and evidence.

The need for a multidisciplinary knowledge base and reasoning that can deal with complexity are essential elements of occupational therapy for understanding human occupation and enablement. To build complex reasoning, occupational enablement requires a multidisciplinary knowledge base and the use of abductive reasoning, drawing on occupational and enablement reasoning. A process is needed to consider the relative contributions of person, environment, and occupation variables to the occupational challenges experienced by the client, and to identify potential solutions.

8.3 Occupational challenges

To address the occupational challenges of our clients, it is important to understand the source of those challenges and how the strengths, resources, conditions and opportunities for enablement affect them. Models of human occupation (see chapters 1 and 2) suggest a number of potential sources of challenge and targets for change. Our Canadian model, the CMOP-E, identifies three major constructs related to human occupation: occupation, person, and environment. Our occupation-based practice is not only concerned with human occupation, but also with the context of that human and her or his occupation — the environment. As portrayed in the transverse view in figure 1.3b, occupation is our domain of interest, and our interest in person and environmental factors is delimited by their relevance to occupation.

The CMOP-E provides a visual expression of that relationship: it portrays human occupation as the result of the dynamic interaction of person, environment, and occupation. Behind this simple statement are idiosyncrasies and complexities for critical reflection, because occupational engagement is individual to each person, time, and place. Not every person will interact with every occupation in every environment. Indeed, a particular person may not interact with the same occupation in the same environment at all times. The CMOP-E is useful for identifying the variables to consider in understanding human occupation; however, this model does not suggest how these variables are put together. Just as one could have a list of ingredients for a specialty cake, but no recipe, the CMOP-E provides a listing of necessary variables to enable occupation, but does not give insight into how to combine these ingredients to enable occupation. The model is inadequate in demonstrating how the interaction of the three variables — person, environment, and occupation — results in occupational engagement in some instances, but not in others; that is, it does not explain client-centred enablement or occupational challenges.

The Person-Environment-Occupation (PEO) Model (Law et al., 1996) provides more explicit information on the nature of the interactions that result in optimal occupational performance. As the model portrays, the degree of fit between person, environment, and occupation determines the occupational performance. The PEO Model's Venn diagram[1] format indicates that there are four possible interactions: person-environment, person-occupation, occupation-environment, and person-environment-occupation. The model implies that the degrees of interaction could vary depending on the degree of fit between the variables. Rooted in the work of Lewin (1933) on environmental press and Murray's (1947) work on need-press, the PEO Model suggests that occupational challenges occur when there is poor congruence between the person's capacity, the occupational demands, and the environmental supports and barriers. This latter aspect creates the opportunity for enabling occupational change: understanding the fit or lack of fit between person, occupation, and environment, which provides the potential for identifying the source(s) of the occupational challenges and creating a plan and solution(s) that enable occupation.

Occupational challenges and the person-occupation-environment fit

As the CMOP-E and PEO indicate, understanding the fit — or lack of fit — involves comparing and contrasting the cognitive, affective, and physical abilities (CAP) of the person. As reflections on Martha's situation reveal, it is important to always con-

---

[1] Venn diagrams are illustrations used in the branch of mathematics known as set theory. They show the mathematical or logical relationship between different groups of things (sets). A Venn diagram shows all the logical relations between the sets.

sider all aspects of CAP, even if the occupational challenge identified would suggest considering only one dimension. Martha's case demonstrates that occupational performance and engagement is affected not only by the abilities of the person, but also by the occupation itself, and that the context and examination of fit can be very complex. The work of flow theorist Csikszentmihalyi (2003) provides some insight into how fit may be considered.

Csikszentmihalyi (2003) has carried out extensive investigation of the experience of individuals engaged in occupations. According to Csikszentmihalyi, the state experienced by an individual during engagement is determined by the match between opportunities to act and personal capacity or, in other words, the complexity of the challenges offered by the occupation and the capacity of the individual to meet that challenge. Csikszentmihalyi's work has demonstrated that when fit is high and when an individual's skill level is optimally matched with the challenge presented by an occupation, the individual reaches the highest level of happiness, satisfaction, and fulfillment; the individual experiences flow.

Indeed, Csikszentmihalyi (2003) has identified eight states of engagement (see figure 8.1), each related to the level of fit. The nature of the state attained can inform the likelihood that an individual will continue to engage in or re-engage in an occupation. If engagement results in positive states, such as control or flow, the individual will seek to achieve that state again and therefore is likely to engage in the occupation. This was seen with Bonnie Sherr Klein (chapter 1), when, despite her fragile health state and the wishes of her rehabilitation team, she felt "as if I was cheating on my rehabilitation work …" (CAOT, 1997a, pp. viii–ix); she spent her weekends working to finish her film. If the engagement results in negative states, such as apathy or worry, the individual will seek to avoid that state and therefore is likely not to re-engage in the occupation. This was seen in chapter 3 with Emma who was bored beyond measure and waited for each day to end.

Csikszentmihalyi's (2003) work demonstrates that some of the experiences of engagement promote the development and growth of an individual's capacity, whereas others hinder it. If the challenge is too great, or too small, the person may engage less and less in the occupation and subsequently deteriorate, as happened with Emma. As time passed, Emma ventured less and less outside her bedroom, sitting idly and crying as her anxiety and blood pressure rose while her weight and alertness dropped. If a challenge is within reach, an individual may engage more and more and subsequently increase capacity. This was seen in chapter 7 with Daniel, who, once he was supported in skill acquisition and began experiencing success, became less disruptive in class, gained confidence, and became more positive and productive.

Implicit in Csikszentmihalyi's (2003) work is support for the assumption of idiosyncrasy. The literature on Flow Theory shows quite clearly that capacity (ability, skill, and knowledge) alone is not sufficient for an individual to engage in an occupation, nor is the lack of capacity sufficient to stop engagement. As we learned from the Burundian refugees in chapter 2, the individual mediates decisions regarding engagement based on the motivation/interest and meaning that the individual holds for the occupation of interest in a specific context. Indeed, as Bonnie showed us, interest, motivation, and meaning can cause an individual to find solutions to over-

Figure 8.1 Map of everyday experiences

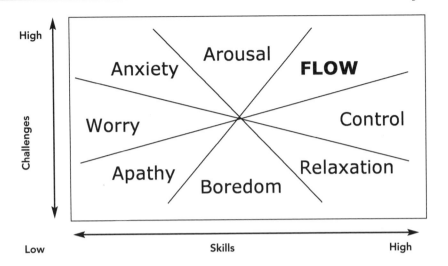

The Map of Everyday Experience, from *Good Business* by Milhaly Csikszentmihalyi, copyright 2003 by Milhaly Csikszentmihalyi. Used by permission of Viking Penguin, a division of Penguin Group (USA) Inc.

come capacity limitations. Conversely, Emma showed us that the lack of interest, motivation, and meaning can prevent engagement even where there is capacity.

The work of Bandura adds another dimension to occupational engagement and fit. Bandura's (1986) concept of self-efficacy indicates that belief about one's ability to perform a given occupation in a given situation will affect engagement in a particular occupation. Like flow, self-efficacy is related to the experience of occupational engagement and is context specific: it can be high in one domain and low in another. The degree of self-efficacy associated with a set of skills can predict the amount of effort devoted to learning a new skill. Self-efficacy affects the choices or willingness to learn a new skill, the amount of effort expended in trying to learn a new skill, the level of persistence when a difficulty is experienced, and the interpretation of that difficulty. Self-efficacy is diminished by repeated failure (see text box 8.1) and enhanced by success, especially where the success is attributed to one's own efforts. Thus, self-efficacy is a mediator in occupational engagement. We saw this with Daniel, whose confidence went up and whose outlook became more positive as his skills in basketball, and subsequently handwriting, improved.

A lack of fit for some clients — who may not even want to fit in — may raise questions about alienation, deprivation, exclusion, oppression, disempowerment, or marginalization. Research on enabling social change adds another important dimension to the considerations of occupational engagement: that of power relationships, justice, and inclusion. Rather than considering a fit between the person and the occupation and environment, knowledge about enabling social change must consider power relations along with social and other environmental conditions that influence justice and inclusion for particular social groups. Typically, occupational therapists who engage in enabling social change would work with groups, communities, or populations at risk for, or who are experiencing, occupational injustice. The occupational challenges

Reflections on flow and poverty

Notions of flow and self-efficacy appear on the surface to be highly individual. Yet social contexts have a direct impact on these aspects of the person. People who live in poverty often lack a strong sense of self-efficacy. They have often said that, in their experience, what they do in the world does not have an impact or make a difference — and that no matter what they do, things do not improve for them. They say that life is often precarious, seeming out of control: they struggle to make ends meet, then a child loses a shoe, so they have to buy new ones and cannot pay the rent — causing them to get evicted or lose their jobs because of an unstable housing situation. People who face racism may also experience low self-efficacy: they invest energy into higher education to improve their lot, yet are still not able to get a decent job due to racism.

The occupational under-engagement of individuals from specific social groups is commonplace. In the 1960s, gender roles and expectations in North America meant that women were routinely under-engaged and restricted to roles of homemaker and mother. This was such a poor fit for many women that the Rolling Stones wrote a song about "Mother's Little Helper" referring to tranquilizers frequently prescribed to help women cope with their dissatisfaction!

— By Brenda Beagan

of concern would be injustices related to such conditions as occupational alienation, occupational deprivation, occupational imbalance, or occupational marginalization. In Joshua's case (chapter 4), questions arise regarding the possibility of occupational marginalization when he attends school. With Bintu (chapter 6), we see occupational marginalization and deprivation that she and her friends have experienced because of war. Thus, when considering fit from a social perspective, the power relationships and related environmental conditions need careful attention.

Occupation-based models, such as the CMOP-E and PEO, or an enablement model, such as the CMCE, may be combined with teachings from Csikszentmihalyi's (2003) Flow Theory to understand occupational challenges. Also useful are Bandura's (1986) Theory of Self-efficacy, and theories of individual and social change (see chapters 5 and 6). To understand occupational challenges, one wants to understand occupation, and the person and environment influences. Occupations may be understood, for instance, through occupational classifications or occupational analysis. Also of interest are person capacity (including cognitive, affective and physical ability, and skill and knowledge) and the mediating variables (motivation, interest, meaning, and self-efficacy) that affect occupations; the capacity demands of the relevant occupations and environments and their mediating factors are of interest as well. Occupation-based enablement models provide us with the means to compare and contrast, and to determine the factors that support or restrict occupational engagement by particular people, families, groups, communities, organizations, or populations. Further, they indicate that the aims of occupational enablement would target changes that will improve the person-occupation-environment fit and reduce the occupational challenge.

The Fit Chart (see figure 8.2) identifies 18 distinct variables that characterize the person, occupation, and environment constructs and that interact within and across person(s), occupation(s), and environment(s). In keeping with the CMOP-E, person, occupation, and environment appear in the singular; however, it is understood that person represents the full range of occupational client groups — individuals, families, groups, communities, organizations, and populations. As was seen with Martha, it may not be sufficient to focus on a single variable to determine the source of the occupational challenge, so each variable must be considered. Perhaps most signifi-cant among these interactions are those between the capacity and mediator variables. Bonnie Sherr Klein, Hussein, Daniel, and the Burundian refugees all provide excel-lent examples of the mediating effect that meaning, motivation, interest, and self-efficacy can have on occupational performance and engagement.

The Fit Chart indicates that *lack of fit* and *fit* can be characterized along a continuum from low to high, and that the level of fit relates to the level of occupational engage-ment, occupational performance, and the experience states of Csikszentmihalyi (2003). In the case of Martha, using the Fit Chart would have indicated that occupa-tional performance and engagement were problematic, suggesting a lack of fit. And, as became apparent in the second interaction with Martha, the Fit Chart would have

Figure 8.2   Fit Chart

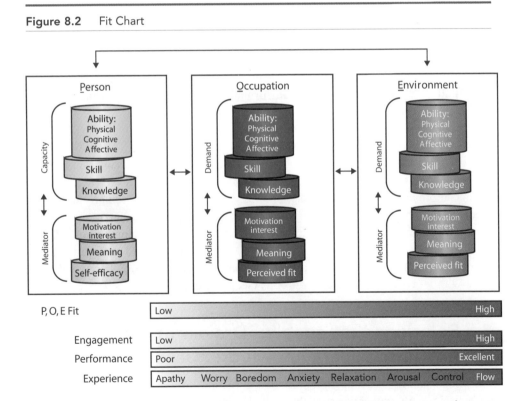

Polatajko, H. J. (2007). Fit Chart. In E. A. Townsend, & H. J. Polatajko, *Enabling occupation II: Advancing an occupa-tional therapy vision for health, well-being, & justice through occupation.* p. 213 Ottawa, ON: CAOT Publications ACE.

Occupation-based practice: The essential elements

indicated that variables other than physical fit needed to be considered in order to understand the occupational challenges she was facing.

It is a complex task to consider the interaction of 18 different variables that can vary independently and interdependently, especially due to both the subjective and objective variables that are involved. The variables also have great breadth and complexity, ranging from such specifics as grip strength to such amorphous concepts as institutional culture. A multidisciplinary body of knowledge is required to understand the full scope and complexity of the occupational challenges. Occupational therapists engage clients in setting client-specific goals, addressing their identified challenges, and determining solutions that enable their occupational performance and engagement.

8.4 Client-centred enablement: Client-specific goals/challenges/solutions

The CMCE guides client-centred enablement focused on occupation, with explicit attention to power sharing, diversity, and justice (see chapter 4). The CMCE is a guide for occupation-based enablement that meets the five essential elements of occupational therapy: (1) addressing occupational challenges; (2) using asset-based solutions to draw on strengths and resources; (3) ensuring that enablement is client-centred (not prescriptive); (4) using a multidisciplinary knowledge base; and (5) using professional reasoning that can deal with the complexity of occupational therapy. To realize client-specific goals, challenges, and solutions, the occupational therapist may draw on approaches for individual and social change.

One example for client-centred enablement to seek client-specific goals, challenges, and solutions may be in the use of transformative learning approaches based on the work of Mezirow (2000). Another might be to use community development approaches based on the work of Freire (1970), or Rothman and Tropman (1987). Solutions may also be in the empowerment of clients and their support networks. The occupational challenges of concern may range from body dysfunction to social exclusion and injustice in everyday occupations in particular contexts. Individual change approaches, with individuals, families and groups, are particularly important when occupational challenges restrict participation in everyday occupations. Social change approaches are particularly important when clients are communities, organizations, or populations. Local social change, for instance to install ramps in schools or locate funds to support caregivers, will be part of any occupation-based enablement with individuals, families, or groups (see chapters 4, 5, and 6).

8.5 Solutions that enable: Drawing on a multidisciplinary knowledge base

The understanding of occupation presented in section I of this book was based on a multidisciplinary knowledge base that included but was not limited to occupational science. Similarly, the understanding of enablement presented in section II drew

Occupation-based enablement

together numerous bodies of knowledge that included but were not limited to historical and present understandings of client-centred enablement in occupational therapy.
As was seen with the practice exemplars in chapter 7, occupational therapists draw
on a multidisciplinary knowledge base to address the types of occupational challenges their clients face. Without limiting the list, examples in which occupational
therapists use multidisciplinary knowledge include neurodevelopmental, sensory
integrative, sensorimotor, acquisitional, occupation-based, bio-occupational
orthotics, workplace accommodation, life-style redesign, universal design, site redevelopment, psychosocial, and community-based social reconstruction (recall summaries of sample frames of reference in table 7.3). An occupational perspective and
enablement skills are the unique contributions of occupational therapists in the integration of multidisciplinary knowledge.

Specialized knowledge bases, such as those listed above, are often called frames of
reference. As Rogers (1983) noted, a frame of reference "operates largely as a non-
conscious ideology in forming the pre-assessment image of the [medical] patient"
(p. 605). The therapist's frame of reference and perspective of the client are the
major determinants that influence the naming of occupational challenges. The interpretation flows from the naming of challenges, as do the objectives, plans, implementation, and evaluation in the occupational therapy program (Rogers & Holm,
1994). Frames of reference guide occupational therapists when deciding what will
be evaluated during assessment, and what will be done to implement objectives and
plans to reach a specific targeted outcome. As with Martha, when the occupational
therapist broadened her frame of reference to look beyond physical capacity to psychosocial factors and job demands, a more in-depth understanding of Martha's occupational challenges emerged.

A frame of reference can be described as the viewpoint, context, or set of assumptions within which a person's perception and thinking seem always to occur, and
which selectively constrains the course and outcome of action (Atherton, 2002).
Occupational therapy frames of reference are sets of interrelated theories, constructs,
and concepts that determine how specific occupational challenges will be perceived,
understood, and approached (Mosey, 1986).

The frames of reference used by occupational therapists are extremely diverse, targeting specific aspects of person, occupation or environment alone, or in combination.
Occupational therapists integrate approaches from a multidisciplinary array of knowledge. It is virtually impossible to identify all the frames of reference that can be used
by occupational therapists to explain and affect the fit between person, occupation,
and environment. Indeed, leading occupational therapy scholars such as Kielhofner
(1997), Mosey (1986), Trombly (1997), and Wilcock (2001b, 2002) have written eloquently about the breadth and complexity of occupational therapy. As discussed in
chapter 7, the majority of the approaches used to date in occupational therapy are
concerned with occupational challenges related to personal capacity. A physical
capacity focus is emphasized where the team and organizational emphasis is on
impairment reduction. An increasing range of occupational therapy frames of reference focus on the environment or social change. New approaches continue to emerge
as our occupational enablement perspective sharpens.

8.6 Solutions that enable: Using abductive reasoning

Each therapist is professionally responsible to determine the frame or frames of reference that offer the best possible solution for the occupational challenges that clients face. The professional reasoning of an occupational therapist must critically evaluate and reflect on the potential for multiple solutions to occupational challenges. This requires the use of abductive reasoning — a form of reasoning suited to complex situations and multiple solutions.

Evidence indicates that the reasoning process a therapist uses is a significant factor affecting the quality of client care (Rogers, 1983) and is important in obtaining the best outcomes for clients experiencing occupational challenges (Schell, 2003). Rogers (1983) stated that "the assessment of occupational competence requires a wide-angled lens" (p. 604), reinforcing the need for a broad occupational perspective in the occupational therapy process. Abductive reasoning supports that broad perspective.

Abductive reasoning is "a matter of utilizing the principle of maximum likelihood in order to formalize a pattern of reasoning known as the 'inference to the best explanation'" (Fetzer, 1990, p. 103). The purpose is to advance already existing conceptual ideas or theoretical understandings, or create new concepts that broaden current descriptions of phenomena (Aliseda, 2006). Abductive reasoning identifies the best explanation given a complex situation. It permeates scientific inquiry, medical diagnostic practices, common sense, and general problem solving (Aliseda, 2006; Magnani, 2001). Abductive reasoning also generates a possible explanation of an observed phenomenon based on the best understanding and experience. Further, abductive reasoning is used when a situation cannot be fully explained by theory, even when some aspects of the phenomenon are consistent with theory. Therefore, it is applied in situations which lack complete evidence. Explanations from abductive reasoning are what is very likely, or what is most likely true, meaning that explanations are open to change. Abductive reasoning occurs in opposite order to deductive reasoning, going from evidence to hypothesis. To distinguish it from inductive reasoning, abductive reasoning requires at least a rudimentary theory to support explanations with a high likelihood of confirmation.

Abductive reasoning is viewed as both a process and product (Aliseda, 2006). The outcome of the process of abduction is the product, which is the selected abductive explanation or the explanatory argument. The reasoning process involves both constructing possible explanations and selecting the best one from amongst these (Peirce, as cited in Aliseda, 2006). Reasoning describes the way in which possible explanations were constructed and how the best abductive explanation was selected. The inferences made in this process, or the inferential structure, influence the likelihood of confirmation or plausibility of the abductive explanation. The strongest inferences are those that are consistent with theory, can be tested, and are economical to pursue (Peirce, as cited in Aliseda, 2006).

Abductive reasoning in occupational therapy is a process of considering the relative contributions of person, occupation, and environment variables to the occupational challenges experienced by the client; then identifying potential solutions, as was done with Martha. Using abductive reasoning, an occupational therapist can revisit conclusions drawn and determine new alternatives, as was seen in Martha's case. Using abductive reasoning, the occupational therapist can, for example, determine which frame of reference is best to address occupational challenges and to identify the most likely solution, as was done in Daniel's case in chapter 7.

8.7 Solutions that enable: Determining the most acceptable solutions

The range of solutions can be as broad as the range of challenges. Indeed, it is rare that there is only one solution to improve occupational performance and engagement. Using the Fit Chart, it can be seen that any specific fit issue has at least three solutions: change the person, change the occupation, or change the environment. Abductive reasoning, coupled with factual evidence, identifies which solution is most likely to succeed. However, the best possible solution based on theory and evidence may not be practical in the circumstances, too demanding of resources, or, most importantly, not acceptable to the client. For Rick Hoyt's parents, institutionalization was not acceptable, nor was being banned from the Boston Marathon (chapter 1). Similarly, not working on her movie was not acceptable to Bonnie Sherr Klein (chapter 1). On a much smaller scale, working on handwriting was not acceptable to Daniel until it was put in relation to shooting hoops in basketball (chapter 7).

Unless the client is willing to enact the solution, there is no possibility that it will be effective. Therefore, the use of an abductive approach in occupational therapy must be based in client-centred enablement. Solutions may fall within or outside the scope of occupational therapy. For example, preparing Rick's father to run a marathon is well outside the scope of practice of occupational therapy, because his preparation does not raise any occupational challenges that require the multidisciplinary knowledge, abductive reasoning, and enablement skills of an occupational therapist. He is a self-enabler requiring the ordinary enabling that families and communities do all the time (see table 7.1). However, designing or adapting equipment so that Rick can be involved in the marathon with his father, consulting with Rick on his plan, and advocating for and with Rick to be allowed to participate is well within the scope. Thus, our occupational perspective (chapter 1) and client-centred enablement skills (chapter 2) are essential elements of occupational enablement. As well, the presence of occupational challenges, the need for occupational solutions, and the use of a multidisciplinary knowledge base and abductive reasoning define and delimit the scope of occupational therapy.

8.8 Solutions that enable: Effecting occupational change

Occupations vary tremendously from person to person, day to day, hour to hour, and — at times — even minute to minute. As individuals progress through life, we enable them to engage in life to their full potential in the face of occupational challenges. As communities, organizations, and populations evolve, we enable them to address occupational challenges and advance occupational solutions. The potential to effect variations in occupations, and the understanding of how the person and environment influence occupations, are grist for occupational therapy. To enable occupation, or more aptly, to enable occupational change — or prevent undesired change — it is important to understand the occupational change process.

Occupational change can occur in various ways. Occupations can be added, abandoned, or altered. Change can be enabled through the use of adaptive, restructuring, reframing, and reconstructing strategies that draw on the 10 key enablement skills. Regardless of the nature of the change, the imperatives drawn from section I indicate that change must address at least two aspects of occupation. The more superficial *instrumental* aspect is associated with the capacity variables on the Fit Chart, which are relatively easy to change. Examples of an instrumental change are to pad a spoon, prescribe a walker, provide information, hire a personal care attendant. The more deeply seated *meaning* aspect is associated with the person and environment mediator variables on the Fit Chart, which are relatively difficult to change. Examples of a meaning change are to shift meanings, values, beliefs, motivation, interest, and self-efficacy. Instrumental issues can be dealt with through adaptation or education; whereas, the meaning issues require personal and social transformation. Change in occupational performance and engagement may also require the social reconstruction of occupational conditions — social change. Where inequitable opportunities and resources restrict participation, funding, policy and legislative change may be required in local, regional, national or international structures, or in the physical environment.

Effecting occupational change requires the therapist to draw on the full range of enablement skills discussed in section II. For example, to effect change a therapist may need to design/build a social network, advocate for changes in physical spaces, use specialized skills to increase physical, mental or cognitive abilities, or adapt tools to enable performance in a desired occupation (Bontje et al., 2004). These enablement skills can be used to effect change to various degrees and at various levels. The change can be relatively circumscribed, affecting the performance of or engagement in only one specific occupation. Alternately, change can be pervasive, affecting occupational patterns, repertoires, or occupational life-course narratives and trajectories. Change strategies may be focused at the level of the individual or the level of society, that is to say, at the level of the environment, or at both levels simultaneously through occupation.

Further, effecting change may be to develop occupational potential, to restore occupational performance and engagement, to prevent occupational loss, or to promote occupational health, well-being, and justice.

Examples of developing occupational potential are in engaging children with attention deficit disorders or with other occupational issues to participate in school-based occupations, or designing inclusive living units with flexible space and staff support for people like Emma to have meaningful occupational opportunities.

Restoring occupational performance and engagement have been illustrated widely in the literature, including this book's reference to Bonnie Sherr Klein's return to filmmaking (chapter 1), and Catherine, the pianist's orthosis (chapter 5). Occupational therapists may use a community development approach to restore the occupational lives, for instance, of Bintu and her friends in Sierra Leone or Burundian refugees who have immigrated to Canada.

Occupational therapists prevent occupational deprivation, when advocating for fair occupational participation, as in the case of Rick participating with his father in the Boston Marathon. Prevention may be the focus in working with organizational clients, such as Nettie enabling organizational development to prevent stress during a major occupational change in the workplace.

Promoting health, well-being, and justice through occupation may be with the individual, the family, a group, a community, an organization, or population of clients. In one example, occupational therapists may bring occupational and enablement perspectives to the coordination of the YMCA team in the design of a family development centre for an inner-city community with a large immigrant population (practice exemplar 7.5). Occupational therapists may also educate workers and employers about return to work options for those with persistent mental illness (practice exemplar 7.3).

Transforming meaning

The process of transforming meaning is essential in effecting occupational change. As the Fit Chart demonstrates, meaning is an important mediator in the interaction of a person's occupations and their environment. For occupational change to be effective, it is critical to understand the personal and environmental processes of meaning transformation that need to accompany changes in instrumental and meaning aspects of occupational performance and engagement. Understanding client experiences in modifying their daily occupations assists occupational therapists to be more client-centered. This was seen with Catherine (chapter 5) for whom it took adaptation and redesign of several orthoses to meet her various needs.

A number of models and theories are available to understand occupational change (see chapters 5 and 6). These include and are not limited to the Health Belief Model, (Rosenstock, 1990), Attribution Model (Lewis & Daltroy, 1990), the Transtheoretical Model (Prochaska & Velicer, 1997), aspects of social learning theories (Bandura, 1986; Lave & Wenger, 1990; Baranowski et al., 1997), Transformative Learning Model (Mezirow, 1991), community development models (Freire, 1970; Rothman & Tropman, 1987), the Community Capacity Building Model (Kretzman & McKnight, 1997), community-based rehabilitation (Helander, 1992; Krefting, 1992); health promotion (Labonte, 1994; Seedhouse, 1997), and organizational development (Sinetar, 1991).

The Meaning Perspective Transformation Process (Mezirow, 1991) is particularly useful in linking the instrumental and meaning levels of occupational change. Mezirow's (1991) theory of transformation, described in chapter 5, notes that complete and durable change occurs when an individual's meaning perspectives are transformed through critical reflection. Meaning perspectives are the constituents of a personal paradigm and consist of the core personal values, beliefs, feelings, and knowledge that guide daily actions. Dubouloz and colleagues (Dubouloz et al., 2002; Dubouloz et al., 2004) explored Mezirow's (1991) premise and suggested that for true occupational change to occur it is important to assist, support, and encourage clients' self-reflection to guide the awareness of need for the transformation of their meaning perspectives.

Effecting change in specific occupations

Change strategies targeting individual occupations can address aspects of the person, the occupation or the environment, singly or in combination.

Enabling the person to change

One approach to occupational enablement is to enable a change in the person's capacity and mediators by addressing cognitive, affective, or physical abilities, and meaning, motivation/interests, and self-efficacy. Enabling a person to change will involve collaboration and client-centredness. Strategies to address capacity may involve enabling problem solving through coaching to deal with a cognitive loss. Strategies may also focus on affective change to reduce anxiety during occupational engagement. Physical change strategies could include engaging the person in strength, balance, or endurance training to meet the demands of the desired occupations. Changes addressing the mediators may involve meaning transformation, reinforcement strategies to increase motivation, or graded success experiences to increase self-efficacy.

Enabling change in the occupation

Change in an occupation can be effected most simply by enabling abandonment of an existing occupation or by adding a new occupation. One alternative is to adapt specific aspects of the occupation or associated tools, in order to alter the occupation's demands so they are more consistent with persons' capacities and mediators. For example, handles on a utensil could be padded to accommodate for a limited grip, new tools could be designed and built to support performance and engagement, or occupations could be analyzed, simplified, or intensified to meet client interests in a mental health or seniors facility.

Enabling change in the environment

Enabling change in the physical, social, cultural, and institutional elements of the environment can affect fit and reduce challenges. For example, physical built and natural environments can be changed by designing and building ramps, adding grab bars to bathrooms, or placing benches as rest places along nature paths. Eliciting changes to the social environment may involve educating family, communities, or organizations to provide effective social networks, policies, funding mechanisms, and other supports for an individual, group, or population. Local change in the social environment may involve such options as having a neighbour drop in daily to visit an elderly person, or pairing a child with a community mentor or educational assistant. In eliciting changes in the cultural environment, an occupational therapist may advocate with and for a client. The occupational therapist may coordinate a meeting where individuals or groups discuss occupational challenges, abilities, strengths, resources, or other assets. Goals could be set to enable an individual or group to participate more fully in the community. Advocating for change in an individual's workplace may occur through education sessions or meetings to effect change in organizational cultures. Changes to the institutional environment may be achieved through coordinating efforts and advocating for funding for programs. Occupational therapy partners may include municipal, provincial, federal, or international levels of government. Enabling change in the environment may be as complex as developing research proposals to test occupation-based community development in Canada or internationally. Enabling environmental change could be as straightforward as coaching others to use community resources available to them — such as equipment suppliers and home delivery services offered by local grocers, drug stores, and restaurants.

Enabling change in combination: Change interactions

As the CMOP-E indicates, person, occupation, and environmental elements continuously interact: a change in one element is likely to effect change in the others. The interconnectedness of change was shown in Connor Schisler's (1996) work with the Burundian refugees (Connor Schisler & Polatajko, 2002) and is demonstrated in case 8.2 about Suhail.

Effecting change in occupational patterns

At times, the change clients want or need is not related to the performance of specific occupations, but rather to their occupational patterns — their routines, habits, or repertoires. Changes may be in the amount of time spent doing certain occupations, the time of day, patterns of occupational engagement, or the abandonment or addition of certain occupations. Client preferences will guide priorities for change to aid with the management and fulfillment of daily occupational needs and desires. Individuals may find that their daily routines, habits, or occupational patterns need to change to allow for continued participation in their predominant and most important occupations. However, changing occupational repertoires can be difficult since occupational patterns and routines are based on values, interests, perception of one's identity, and previous occupational performance and engagement (Royeen, 2003). Bontje et al. (2004) found that it was very important for many older adults with physical disabilities to maintain their daily routines in order to engage in fulfilling occupations.

Occupational therapists work with clients to restructure their occupational routines, habits, and repertoire to allow for their continued engagement in meaningful and purposeful occupations. Occupational therapists may do this by advocating with and for clients. For instance, advocacy may be directed at a work setting to create opportunities for part-time or supportive employment. Collaboration with clients is necessary to determine the best restructuring to maintain key occupations. Walker (2001) discusses the restructuring attempts undertaken by shift workers to allow them to maintain their involvement in some key occupations, while at the same time getting enough sleep to sustain them. Walker's study points to the difficulties in restructuring occupational routines. In some cases, continuous occupational restructuring may be needed, as was discovered in a study of nurses (Gallew & Mu 2004). Both studies illustrate the interconnectedness of occupational patterns and routines: changes with one person will influence the patterns and routines of others. Therefore, enabling change in routines will require mediation and negotiation by the occupational therapist and client to achieve acknowledgement and acceptance by everyone involved (see case 8.3).

Effecting change in occupational life–course narrative trajectories

Often clients experience changes in life circumstances that result in large-scale, dramatic changes to their occupations. For instance, a natural disaster, a severe injury or illness, or a life altering event may result in the inability to continue with established and familiar occupational patterns. In such cases, it is important to enable clients to reframe and reconstruct their occupational lives to recreate and

CASE 8.3 Mary's move to a nursing home

Mary is a 74-year-old widow who, until four months ago, lived on her own on the main floor of a seniors' apartment complex in a small Canadian city. Before she moved to the apartment, Mary and her husband ran a dairy farm. Mary had raised three children and had worked as a high school secretary from the time her children were grown till the age of 65.

Mary has glaucoma, insulin dependent diabetes mellitus, peripheral vascular disease, high blood pressure, and wears a below-knee prosthesis on her left leg. Mary managed well for five years after being fitted with the prosthesis; she could move around safely with a walker, look after herself, and drive her car. She was active in her church, a seniors' association, book club, and bridge club. She visited her daughter and grandchildren for weekly Sunday dinners. After a second amputation four months ago, Mary reluctantly agreed to move into Maple Valley Nursing Home. At the home, she uses a rented manual wheelchair and gets help with bathing, some dressing, transfers, and with taking her multiple medications. Mary told Jane, the consulting occupational therapist working two days per week with the home, that "four months ago the sky kind of fell in on me" when she learned that she needed an amputation to her right leg below the knee. Her doctor did not recommend a second prosthesis, given Mary's age.

Mary's daughter and family, who had been Mary's main source of support, moved four hours away because of her husband's job promotion. Mary began to feel discouraged and depressed, that her life was empty, and the days started dragging terribly. She felt too unmotivated to stick with a physiotherapy exercise program. She missed her family, apartment, friends, and previous activities and felt trapped in the new facility. Jane was asked to assess Mary and to make recommendations to facilitate her integration into the nursing home. What Mary wanted was to leave the home and recapture her former occupations. Jane undertook the negotiations and advocacy necessary to enable Mary to begin to meet her goal.

— By Wendy Pentland

rebuild a new occupational life-course. In such cases it is not sufficient to focus on the performance of specific occupations. Changes of this scale require the visualization of an ideal, yet realistic future based on assets and potential, and careful work towards meeting the occupational performance and engagement goals associated with that future. Occupational reframing will likely involve enabling a change in the client's view of the occupational self because the self-identity is constructed through occupation and social location within a particular context. Occupational reconstruction starts by considering tangible changes in the occupational life course repertoire through abandoning, altering, and adding certain occupations.

Occupational therapists start to enable such large scale changes by listening to a client's life course narrative and trying to understand and predict the impact of the change of events on the expected occupational life-course trajectory. Client narratives about their past and current situation can be used to provide information, to plot a new occupational trajectory, and to understand the necessary changes in performance, engagement, and identity.

> When people experience loss and change, the continuity of their lives is disrupted. Identity is the great integrator of life experience. We interpret events that happen to us in terms of their meaning for our life stories. This gives life a sense of coherence (Christiansen, 1999, p. 554).

In her qualitative study with people with traumatic brain injury, Klinger (2005) found that the participants focused firstly on reframing their sense of self and identity. She stated that participants needed to reframe their sense of self and reconstruct a vision of their future prior to making changes in their occupational routines. Reframing and re-visioning were key to personal transformation in their life course narrative. Change was required in progressive sequences of life events, a process that Christiansen (1999) believes is essential to bringing new meaning to one's life. Coaching or collaborating with clients to develop the narratives of their desired future occupational lives sets the stage to develop occupational goals to reframe and reconstruct an occupational life course trajectory. Klinger (2005) demonstrated that individuals who had difficulty with communication were able to use pictures and other means of communication. Creative forms of enablement are a hallmark of occupational therapy in guiding individuals to illustrate their life story—past, present and future. Thus, the focus of occupational enablement at this level is to provide people with a way to reconstruct and reframe their lives into meaningful occupational experiences through reflection and analysis (see case 8.4).

Effecting change at the level of society: Enabling occupational justice

Enabling occupational justice through social change is interwoven with enabling change in occupations with persons. With an eye to social change, occupational therapists target the environment with awareness of the influence of the environment on individual experiences (see text box 8.2). As discussed in chapter 6 on community development, organizational development, and population health, an occupational therapy approach to social change may be from the top down or from the bottom up.

Occupational therapy involvement in social change is unique in its focus on occupation and on the environmental forces — such as, the social determinants of healthy occupational engagement — beyond factors of the person. Occupational therapists typically ask these questions about effecting change at the level of society: What are individuals or those involved in a family, group, community, organization, or population actually doing in their everyday occupations? What environmental forces support and/or limit engagement in occupations for health, well-being, inclusion, and justice?

CASE 8.4 Growing up in Iran and immigrating to Canada

I (Parvin) grew up in post-reform Iran where only two per cent of women in my age group had post secondary education and worked outside of the home. I was a midwife with a private practice and also worked with the World Health Organization to implement primary health care. My job allowed me limited independence from the strict traditional role for women, but it did not give me the freedom of which I dreamed.

Even today, long after I have left Iran, I feel as though I lost important opportunities to participate in meaningful occupations from the time of my childhood until the day I left Iran. I would have liked to go camping, to spend time with my peers, to learn arts and music, or to work at a part-time job in my teenage years. Participating in activities outside of my home was strictly monitored by government regulations. Even to go shopping, I had to adhere to government restrictions regarding dress (being completely covered with a long, loose coat and wearing a hijab). There were extreme repercussions if these rules were not followed.

I especially longed for communication with my peers, with my community, and with the world. I longed to participate in leisure activities with others; and to have open friendships with both genders. Instead, I had to maintain downcast eyes when communicating with a man in the workplace and cultivate friendships with the few women I trusted.

On the only two government-regulated TV channels, the Iran-Iraq war dominated the news, which was sad and depressing. The Internet was not accessible in Iran at that time; satellite dishes were, and still are, forbidden. The political situation created a lack of trust; one could only discuss problems with immediate family and create close relationships with a few trusted friends.

Moving to Canada allowed me to participate in long awaited occupations; however, these new opportunities had their own consequences. Even though I have lived in Canada for over 11 years, I still feel uprooted. I miss my social network, as small as it was. I miss participating in family gatherings, making Persian food and speaking the mainstream language fluently. Most importantly, I miss my role as a daughter, a sister, an aunt, and as an accepted member of the core social group.

— By Parvin Eftekhar

Reflections on social place and occupational choice

As was seen in Parvin's story, gender roles in Iran clearly affected her occupational choices. Reflect for a moment, though, on gender roles in Canada and their effect on girls and boys. How many boys would love to take ballet classes, but dare not to lest they be teased unmercifully or have their sexual orientation questioned? How many girls give up their dreams of being athletes when they reach adolescence and their friends assure them that an interest in make-up, dieting, and boys is more appropriate? How many girls develop eating disorders, partly to fit in or to create an image of desirability? How many boys use steroids to become bigger, more masculine?

— By Brenda Beagan

Occupational therapists interested in health determinants will want to be consistently aware and self-reflective about their own abilities, age, culture, gender values, and experiences. By knowing herself, the occupational therapist working with Parvin from Iran may learn to understand Parvin's occupational dreams. Together, they might consider her occupational challenges with reference to the determinants of health. The therapist might consult studies, such as the one by Frankish et al. (2007), to examine the progress in Canada on non-medical determinants of health (NMDH) that gained global attention in the World Health Organization's (1986) landmark publication, the *Ottawa Charter for Health Promotion.*

In a multimethod study (2003–2005), Frankish et al. (2007) surveyed regional health authorities in Canada's 10 provinces regarding 10 non-medical determinants: income and social status, social support networks, education, employment and working conditions, social environment, physical environment, personal health practices, healthy child development, culture, and gender. They found that non-medical determinants are not clearly funded beyond health services. However, some regional health authorities are slowly stretching their mandate to address them. Issues of culture and gender may be of particular interest in Parvin's case.

An occupational therapist might offer support for her and other clients who feel that they missed out on early childhood occupations. Possible occupational solutions would be to enable Parvin to develop a new social support network (possibly a women's group), to go camping, to spend time with her peers, or to learn arts and music if such occupations are now available to her in Canada. Alternately, enablement may require consultation, prompting, and the framing of creative solutions with Parvin. She may need to consult with some people in her existing social support network to hold onto important cultural customs at the same time as she seeks outlets for her occupational dreams.

To be a self-aware practitioner with Parvin or as a researcher hearing her story, an occupational therapist who had grown up in Canada and was not female or of Iranian descent, would critically reflect on the values, beliefs, and assumptions of her or his upbringing, and of the occupational therapy profession in this country.

Occupational therapists may want to become involved in culturally oriented projects. Matuk and Ruggirello (2007) describe their Cultural Connection Project in Ontario elementary schools that focused on multiculturalism, using drama education. Multicultural projects could also be extended to examine how lifespan development and ability are taken into account. With interests in cross-cultural practices with communities, as in the cases of working with Bintu, and with Peter and Lucy in Sierra Leone (chapter 6), occupational therapists would contribute occupational and enablement perspectives to assess everyday experiences, develop creative programs, and evaluate the process and outcomes of the project or occupational therapy involvement. Enablement through program design and evaluation could be aligned with community interests in holistic education (Cavanagh, 2005) or transformative teaching (Matthews, 2005).

A familiar approach for occupational therapists in social change may be to extend the approaches for occupational restructuring suggested by Bontje et al. (2004). Beyond working with individual older adults with physical disabilities, an occupational therapist could partner with a local seniors organization, students, and local council members to investigate housing and support options as Letts and her students did in Toronto (2003a) (see chapter 6).

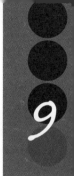

Chapter 9

Introducing the Canadian Practice Process Framework (CPPF): Amplifying the context

Janet Craik
Jane Davis
Helene J. Polatajko

CASE 9.1 Jim's negotiated return to work

Jim is a 37-year-old sheet metal worker who injured his back ten years ago. The injury left him off work for 12 months. When he returned to work he sustained a fall. He was also withdrawn from co-workers, had difficulty engaging with family, and lost interest in occupations outside work. Since the initial injury, Jim has been off work intermittently with repeated episodes of acute low back pain. He finds his job difficult due to this ongoing pain. His work relationships have eroded with rumors that he faked his injury. Jim's marriage has now broken down.

Jim recently re-injured his lower back when lifting a large sheet of metal. Eight weeks later, Sean, an occupational therapist, began working with Jim. The new injury was being treated with a range of pain medications and a daily stretching regimen, but Jim spent most of his time lying in bed. Jim was concerned that the new injury would affect his already strained work relationships. He confided to Sean that he was anxious about returning to work.

After speaking with Jim about his concerns regarding return to work, Sean visited the work site with Jim and performed a standardized functional evaluation of Jim at his job. Sean noted both the physical demands of the job and the social context. The physical demands included frequent, awkward, heavy lifting of objects between 40 and 80 lbs and prolonged standing. A fit analysis indicated that Jim's functional capacity was inadequate for a full return to work just yet; as he was only able to lift 40 lbs, could only stand up for one hour continuously, and could only work for up to four hours at one time. From a social perspective, Sean noted that Jim's co-workers avoided interacting with him and that Jim seemed awkward and nervous.

Sean spoke with Jim's immediate supervisor,who agreed to accommodate a gradual return to work for Jim. Sean recommended that they focus on working with Jim to manage his pain and to increase his physical work tolerance. Although both Jim and the supervisor agreed with these recommendations, the Workplace Safety Insurance Board (WSIB) adjudicator did not; he pressed for a full return to work. Sean set up a meeting with the WSIB adjudicator to negotiate a gradual return plan, and invited Jim and his immediate supervisor along.

At the meeting, Sean will review the evaluation findings and the return to work recommendations, specifically highlighting the poor fit between Jim's current physical capacity and the job demands, and Jim's anxiety regarding his return to work. Sean will propose a plan with a structured outline of Jim's hours and work duties, how these will be graded as Jim's capacity improves, and a routine for strategic pain management.

— *by Catherine Donnelly and Terry Krupa*

Occupation-based enablement

9.1 Introduction

Constructing a practice that includes the five essential elements of occupational enablement (chapter 8) requires careful consideration of the nature of occupational change. The discussion of human occupation in section I and of the processes of change in section II, make it clear that occupational change can be very complex, necessitating a carefully constructed process. Occupational therapy is not method driven (i.e., defined by tasks or procedures) but rather theory and process driven; that is to say defined by a vision that is theoretically grounded and a systematic series of actions directed towards enabling occupation.

The collaborative interaction of client and therapist in occupational therapy are essential to the occupational change process. This interaction is guided by abductive reasoning process to identify and solve occupational challenges. Given the idiosyncrasy and complexity of occupational performance and engagement portrayed in the CMOP-E (see figure 1.3b), each client-therapist interaction is unique with individual, family, group, community, organization, or population clients. The process of occupational enablement is a context sensitive, dynamic process. With individuals, families, and groups, the process incorporates the client's and the therapist's hopes, dreams, beliefs, and values embedded in their contexts. With communities, organizations, and populations, the hopes, dreams, beliefs, and values will be representative of a communal view, or an organizationally mandated position.

In Canada, Fearing and colleagues (Fearing, Law, & Clark, 1997) published an Occupational Performance Process Model (OPPM) in 1997. The OPPM was also published in 1997 in *Enabling Occupation* (CAOT, 1997a), and in 2002 in *Individuals in Context* (Fearing & Clark, 2000). The OPPM provided a comprehensive description of an occupational enablement process for working with individual clients. It was designed to help occupational therapists structure practice that is focused on a client's needs, based on sound theory, aimed at occupational performance, and subject to continual evaluation of the outcomes. Drawing on the core concepts of occupational performance and client-centred practice, the OPPM describes seven stages in a process of practice:
1. Name, validate, and prioritize occupational performance issues;
2. Select theoretical approaches;
3. Identify occupational performance components and environmental conditions;
4. Identify strengths and resources;
5. Negotiate targeted outcomes, develop action plans;
6. Implement plans through occupation;
7. Evaluate occupational performance outcomes (CAOT, 1997a, 2002, pp. 58-77).

The OPPM has been praised in the literature for demonstrating how core concepts of occupational performance and client-centred practice can be applied with individuals and groups (Simó-Algado, Mehta, Kronenberg, Cockburn, & Kirsh, 2002; Whiteford & Fossey, 2002). It has also been suggested that the OPPM can be used as a guide to implement evidence-based, client-centred decision making with individual clients (Egan, Dubouloz, von Zweck, & Vallerand, 1998; Egan, Hobson, & Fearing, 2006). Further, practitioners have reported that they find the OPPM useful to guide individualized practice (Craik & Rappolt, 2003). However, it has been suggested that the OPPM may not be equally useful in all situations; certain practice structures and environments make implementing the OPPM challenging (Harrison, 2000); and, aspects of the OPPM may be problematic. In particular, the selection of theoretical approaches occurs only at stage 2; occupational analysis is not named as a specific component of analysis; and, it is designed for working with individual clients, not with community, organization, or population clients.

An American counterpart to the OPPM was introduced in 2002 as part of the Framework Process of Service Delivery within the Occupational Therapy Practice Framework (OTPF) of the American Occupational Therapy Association (American Occupational Therapy Association [AOTA], 2002). The two processes have some important differences that raise questions about the Canadian OPPM:

- The OPPM provides a structured, explicit process for practitioners to follow, whereas the OTPF and the Framework Collaborative Process Model (AOTA, 2002) state what is to be done.
- The OPPM and OTPF both name key action points in practice: assessment, intervention, and evaluation of outcomes.
- The OPPM implies that the seven stages should be conducted in a linear loop, which can be repeated as often as desired in partial or full loops as necessary, whereas the OTPF specifies that the stages are not expected to be performed in a linear manner.
- The OPPM requires the selection of one or more theoretical approaches at the second stage, whereas, in the OTPF, various theories, frameworks, and approaches can be adopted throughout the process.
- The OPPM makes context — societal and practice — explicit as background information although context is not made explicit at each stage of the loop, whereas the OTPF emphasizes the significance of context throughout the process.
- Both the OPPM and OTPF are frameworks for working with individuals, whereas the application of these frameworks with community, organization, and population clients requires considerable ingenuity and abstract analysis.

Differences in comparison with the OTPF spark questions for using the OPPM: How do you incorporate a therapist's values, beliefs, and personal practice theories into the OPPM process? How does the practice context influence the process? What happens if the therapist wants to repeat process stages, particularly to do further assessment? What if the chosen theoretical framework only applies to part of the occupational challenges faced? What issues need attention at the start and conclusion of the process? What if clients are families, groups, communities, organizations, or populations?

Chapter 9 will present a new framework designed to respond to such questions: the Canadian Practice Process Framework (CPPF). The framework will be described with particular emphasis on the importance of responsiveness to context.

9.2 The Canadian Practice Process Framework

The Canadian Practice Process Framework (CPPF) for occupational therapy (see figure 9.1) is a process framework for evidence-based, client-centred occupational enablement. A generic framework that allows for application in diverse practice contexts, the CPPF is goal driven and generic, and can be used with individual, family, group, community, organization, and population clients. The CPPF is congruent with the Canadian Model of Occupational Performance and Engagement (CMOP-E) (see figure 1.3b) and the Canadian Model of Client-Centred Enablement (CMCE) (see figure 4.3), and incorporates the common aspects of assessment, intervention, and evaluation of outcomes found in any health profession process model. The CPPF is a process structure that illustrates eight action points in the occupational therapy process and provides for alternate pathways for practice.

The CPPF graphically illustrates the dynamic interchange between client and occupational therapist with continuous reflection on action within specific contexts. It is intended to be a tool for occupational therapists to work with a range of clients. Applying an occupational perspective and enablement skills, the therapist is encour-

Figure 9.1   Canadian Practice Process Framework (CPPF)

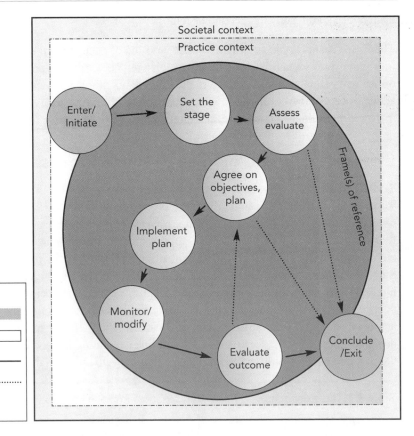

Polatajko, H. J., Craik, J., Davis, J., & Townsend, E. A. (2007). Canadian Practice Process Framework (CPPF). In E. A. Townsend & H. J. Polatajko, *Enabling Occupation II: Advancing an Occupational Therapy Vision of Health, Well-being, & Justice through Occupation* (p. 233). Ottawa, ON: CAOT Publications ACE.

aged to enable clients to realize occupational dreams, hopes, and expectations. The CPPF guides the therapist through a process of occupation-based, evidence-based, and client-centred practice, which is directed towards enabling change in occupational performance and engagement. By utilizing the CPPF, an occupational therapist would identify eight key actions in enabling any type of client to reach occupational goals.

The two principal agents in the CPPF process are the occupational therapist and the client — whether individuals or groups — who each fulfill specific responsibilities as active, engaged participants. Both are influenced by a particular set of personal and environmental factors. Because clients are experts regarding their own occupational engagement, they must be engaged in determining and implementing the process to the greatest extent possible. The therapist and client will determine acceptable solutions to occupational issues through a collaborative decision-making process. The occupational therapist enables action, from start to exit points in the client-therapist relationship, to enable the client to pursue occupational performance or engagement goals.

The desired outcome of the CPPF process is the client's goal attainment or successful enhancement of occupational performance and engagement. This outcome will be achieved by effective application of the CMOP-E, focused on occupation and using key enablement skills: adapt, advocate, coach, collaborate, consult, coordinate, design/build, educate, engage, and specialize.

The CPPF is applicable across the practice mosaic of occupational engagement including and beyond impairment reduction (see chapter 7), with any type of client. It draws on the five essential elements that are the trademarks of occupational enablement: address occupational challenges, seek occupational solutions, focus on client goals, use multidisciplinary knowledge, and employ abductive reasoning (see chapter 8).

Elements of the Canadian Practice Process Framework

The CPPF depicts the practice process as being comprised of four distinct elements. Three of the elements are contextual: the broad *societal context* (the outer box), the *practice context*, (the inner box) and the *frame(s) of reference* (the large circle). The fourth element is process based and is represented by the eight action points (the eight small circles) that guide the process of occupational enablement (see table 9.1). Since the societal context is pervasive, it is represented by the large, all-encompassing outer box and subsumes the practice context, a specific aspect of the societal context. The practice context, represented by the inner box, includes the personal and environmental factors that influence the client and therapist relationship as depicted in the CMCE (see figure 4.3). The line separating the societal context from the practice context is dotted to emphasize that the two are embedded within one

---

Table 9.1 The eight action points of the Canadian Practice Process Framework (CPPF)

1. Enter/initiate	5. Implement plan
2. Set the stage	6. Monitor/modify
3. Assess/evaluate	7. Evaluate outcome
4. Agree – objectives and plan	8. Conclude/exit

Occupation-based enablement

another and have mutual influence. The frame(s) of reference — a key part of the practice context — permeate the practice process at every action point; frame(s) of reference will change with the demands of the client-therapist interaction and practice process.

The CPPF eight action points are so named because each point requires an action to be completed. The CPPF action points not only include the processes of assessment, intervention, and outcome evaluation found in the OPPM and the OTPF, they also specify aspects of the practice process that are often not made explicit: enter/initiate, set the stage, agree on the plan, monitor and modify and conclude/exit. Depending on client need and the practice context some or all of these action points may be necessary to produce the desired outcome. Accordingly, the CPPF is designed to offer flexibility. A flexible process is achieved by using both solid and dotted action lines. The solid line shows a full linear pathway. Given that practice is rarely linear, the occupational therapist may consider the dotted lines, which indicate variations, called alternate pathways.

The shading of each context and action point holds specific meaning. The graded shading, found within the practice context, and six of the action points, represents the client and therapist collaboration within a practice relationship. The uniform shading of the societal context signals that the therapist and client engage independently in occupations outside the practice context — thus no interaction is taking place between them. Similarly, the uniform shading of the large Frame(s) of Reference circle indicates the professional knowledge the therapist brings to the process. The darker shading of the outer two actions points, enter/initiate and conclude/exit, represents the beginning and end to the practice process when the collaboration starts or concludes.

Discussion of the eight action points with case examples continues in more detail in chapter 10.

9.3 Amplifying the contexts of practice

It is clear that occupation and practice occur in context (Whiteford & Wright St-Clair, 2005). The CPPF identifies three distinct process contexts. As is frequently discussed within health services, recognition of the three contexts is key to transparent, reflective, and effective client-centred practice. The three contexts identified in the CPPF are the societal context, the practice context, and frame(s) of reference (see table 9.2). The fourth element is the eight action points in the process.

The societal context

The therapist and client are both situated within a broad societal context comprised of cultural, institutional, physical, and social environmental elements (see figure 1.3b and table 9.3).

The practice context

The client-therapist relationship begins when the occupational therapist receives the client request or referral and the two parties enter into the practice process (see

Table 9.2   Four key elements of the Canadian Process Practice Framework (CPPF)

Element	Location	Representation(s)
Contextual elements		
Societal context	Outer box with uniform shading	• Where, prior to entrance into the practice context and initiation of the therapeutic relationship, client and therapist perform and engage in various occupations within diverse environments as distinct individuals • As engaged citizens within the societal context, each holds diverse beliefs, attitudes, values, and abilities • The uniform shading depicts that the therapeutic relationship has not yet been established
Practice context	Inner box marked by a dotted line, with graded shading	• Where client and therapist meet and enter into a relationship • The initiation of this relationship between client and therapist brings together their personal and environmental factors, along with the professional's code of conduct and ethics, and the client's perceptions of his or her role within the occupational therapy process
Frame(s) of reference	Large circle with uniform shading	• The theories, models, and practice lenses that the therapist uses within the therapeutic process • The frame(s) of reference may change depending on the practice context, process, and/or relationship
Process element		
Eight action points and pathways	Eight small circles with graded and uniform shading, and bold and dotted arrows	• The action points identify the process • The pathways indicate the possible actions that may be taken at different times, and within different practice contexts and different frames of reference • All pathways will include the action points of *Enter/initiate, Set the stage, Assess/evaluate, and conclude/exit*

figures 4.3 and 9.1). Since the practice context is embedded within the broad societal context, the therapist and client relationship is influenced by personal and environmental factors. In fact, the occupational therapist cannot optimally engage clients in the practice process without closely examining personal and environmental factors. The therapist must also evaluate the specifics of the practice context, which become known once the therapist and client initiate their relationship (see table 9.4).

Personal factors

When entering into the practice context with individual, family, and groups clients, the therapist and the client each bring to every interaction their own personal resources, knowledge, abilities, skills, habits, values, beliefs, and attitudes (see table 9.5). The occupational experiences of both parties will be carried into the practice context, will influence the process and content of the relationship, and will continue to influence their lives following the conclusion of the client-therapist relationship. Although personal factors are listed under contextual factors in the ICF, the World Health Organization (2001) does not classify them because of their large social and cultural variances. However, in the Fit Chart for use with individual, family, or group clients, the personal aspects are classified as capacities composed of cogni-

Table 9.3   Societal context and the Canadian Practice Process Framework (CPPF)

Societal context: Examples	
Physical	• Natural environments: mountains, rivers, resources • Built environments: buildings, cities, transportation • Technology • Changes to the physical nature of the world over time • Physical accessibility
Social	• Social networks: family and peer support • Professional networks and associations • Workplace support • Community resources • Changes in dominant social ideologies over time • Occurrence of societal events at certain points in time
Cultural	• Ethnicity, race, gender, age • Habits and rituals based on cultural group • Cultural occupational expectations • Profession and workplace culture • Changes in cultural context over time
Institutional	• Judicial, economic, political contexts • Health care system, and governmental funding and policies • Institutional structures: schools, nursing homes, corporate • Workplace, schools: policies and procedures

tive, affective and physical ability; skill and knowledge; and the mediators of motivation/interest, meaning and self-efficacy. Personal factors for family and group clients would be a collective grouping of experiences, such as the connectedness of a group or the personalities of family members. Examples of the personal factors of community, organization, and population clients would be the collective personality of a community, or the educational level of a population.

Table 9.4   Practice context embedded in the societal context

Societal context: Examples		The practice context: Examples
Physical	• Natural enviro • Built environm • Technology • Changes to the • Physical access	**Physical** • Facility, home, or community structures • Treatment rooms • Treatment technology • Equipment
Social	• Social network • Professional ne • Workplace sup • Community res • Changes in do • Occurrence of	**Social** • Other health professionals, teams, members • Other clients • Social nature of the facility or community
Cultural	• Ethnicity, race, • Habits and ritu • Cultural occup • Profession and • Changes in cu	**Cultural** • Facility or community culture, vision, and mission • Health profession's culture, values, and beliefs • Models of practice, theories
Institutional	• Judicial, econo • Health care sys • Institutional str • Workplace, sch	**Institutional** • Facility policies and procedures • Health professional code of ethics, scope of practice • Third-party payer or insurer's regulations • Models of service delivery • Allowable number of sessions, time per session, wait-lists

Table 9.5   Personal factors: Examples

Personal factors: Examples

Personal nature and temporal aspects	• Health • Age, developmental level • Fitness, lifestyle • Gender, race, ethnicity • Emotional state of health
Knowledge, skills, and abilities	• Educational knowledge and skills • Professional knowledge, expertise, and skills • Occupational experiences • Coping and learning skills, and styles • Language • Habits
Perspectives – past, present, and future	• Values, beliefs, religion • Preconceived ideas about gender, age, ethnicity, etc. • Self, cultural, and occupational identities • Vision of future possibilities • Motivation, hopes, dreams, aspirations

Judy and Emily's story (case 9.2) illustrates the importance of reflecting on the views, values, beliefs, and experiences that individual clients hold within the broader societal context and the practice context. Reflection supports transparent, client-centred, ethical practice.

Case 9.2 about Judy and Emily highlights the impact of diverse views (in this case regarding smoking) that may be held by an individual client and an individual occupational therapist. In this situation, the occupational therapist chose to refer her client to another therapist. She made the decision because she felt that the conflict between her values, and the values and needs of her client would make it difficult to

CASE 9.2 Judy and Emily's story

Judy, an occupational therapist, received a referral for Emily, who needed an adaptive device to enable her to smoke. Although Judy was completely against smoking, she performed an assessment of Emily's occupational issues. However, Judy and Emily were unable to agree upon objectives and a plan for intervention. Although Judy identified other potential occupational issues during her assessment, Emily only wanted help with re-engaging in smoking. Judy refused to design and build a cigarette holder for Emily — who has diabetes, bi-lateral lower extremity below knee amputations, and has lost fingers on both hands because of gangrene from circulatory insufficiency — because this was incongruent with her value system. Judy and Emily terminated their relationship, and Judy recommended other service providers to Emily. Emily consulted with a different occupational therapist who agreed to implement a plan to build the required adaptive device.

— By Janet Craik and Jane Davis

practice in a client-centred manner and maintain a good client-therapist relationship. If Judy had reflected on her values and ethical beliefs about smoking upon receiving the referral and before initiating a client relationship, she might have avoided this conflict. She might have immediately referred Emily to another therapist. It is important to consider what Judy might have done if there had not been another therapist to meet Emily's needs. It is also important to consider whether Judy did indeed have the right to let her own beliefs take precedence over her client's needs.

With any client, at the first action point of enter/initiate, the client and therapist begin to interact in each others' occupational life course narrative, including personal, cultural and spiritual values, beliefs and interests. With community, organization, and population clients, the occupational therapist would typically develop a relationship with a few representatives, or a focus group. The therapist and representatives or spokespersons for the client would begin to interact at the enter/initiate action point.

An interesting point is that all professions use theoretical frameworks to organize the knowledge of the profession (Magnani, 2001). Occupational therapy is no exception. Thus the occupational therapist also brings to the relationship the ideas, values, beliefs and theories of the profession. The professional resources include professional ethics and code of conduct, competency requirements, the occupational therapy scope of practice, and the practice frame(s) of reference. Therapists enter the practice context with preconceived practice frameworks, an accumulation of professional knowledge, as it has evolved through practice experiences, and reflections on professional and personal experiences (Craik & Rappolt, 2003).

The individual client brings knowledge of her or his occupational life course narrative, including abilities, skills, experiences, and knowledge of health and occupational issues. Clients are experts on their own occupational lives. Clients hold personal values, beliefs and attitudes, and pre-conceived ideas and assumptions about their role as client and the role of the therapist. Such personal factors will influence the client's life during and following conclusion of the practice relationship. Organization and community clients bring historical knowledge of past developments and changes to their structure and culture.

Environmental factors

The World Health Organization defines environmental factors as "all aspects of the external or extrinsic world that forms the context of an individual's life" (World Health Organization, 2001, p. 193). WHO classifies the context as physical, social, and attitudinal. Within the CMOP-E (see figure 1.3b) the environmental aspects are classified as cultural, institutional, physical, and social. Environmental press is "the tendency or 'potency'" of a situation or factor within the environment to have a "facilitating or obstructing" effect on an individual (Murray, 1947). This is akin to the environmental demands and mediators identified in the Fit Chart in chapter 8. Environmental factors are dynamic and constantly changing, holding important implications for occupational therapy practice (Sumsion, 1997).

Both the client and occupational therapist are influenced by environmental factors in the societal and practice contexts (see tables 9.3 and 9.4). Since the practice context is embedded within the broad societal context, all environmental factors that were present in the societal context will also be true within the practice context. For both therapist and client, influencing factors may include transportation issues, social supports, workplace and family demands, and commonly held cultural expectations. As well, for the occupational therapist, the profession's culture and policies demand certain actions outlined by the regulatory bodies and associations. Within the practice context, the therapist's workplace context also provides a certain structure, makes additional demands on time, and holds specific performance expectations. The places where the therapeutic interaction occurs will greatly affect the process and outcomes of practice.

All environmental factors will influence the client-therapist relationship as it develops within the societal and practice contexts and throughout the process of practice, with variations associated with individual, family, group, community, organization, or population clients. In the process of occupational enablement, an occupational therapist would reflect upon the aspects of the environment that may influence the therapist and client actions. Societal and practice contexts are the background for the client-therapist collaboration. Time and place will also influence the relationship, the process of practice, and the outcomes (see text box 9.1).

Text box 9.1

Temporal influences on personal and environmental factors

Temporal factors can be viewed as part of both personal and environmental influences. Personal temporal factors can include a person's age or physical developmental stage, which is reflected within the person's life course pathway and future aspirations. Environmental factors can include historical or cultural occurrences; for example, world events, changes in policies over time, or availability of technology.

The story of Lynette and Harika (case 9.3) highlights both personal and environmental influences in the practice context, which is embedded in the societal context.

In case 9.3, Harika, the occupational therapist, entered into the practice context with Lynette, her client, knowing that Lynette has just been discharged following three months in the hospital. Harika was aware that Lynette's doctor did not think that she would be able to be cared for by her daughter-in-law, Kathy, in the family home. Harika was aware that Lynette was discharged from the hospital and required assistance with everything, and she needed the help of two people to help her safely out of bed. Harika brought to the practice context, years of experience working with older adults in the community. Her experience has included both highly effective enablement of occupational re-engagement, and minimal to ineffective enablement with her clients (see Enablement continuum, figures 4.4 and 4.5). Harika has also been an informal caregiver for her parents because they required greater levels of assistance. Harika knew that she needed to enter into this practice relationship with realistic expectations about Lynette's potential for occupational engagement, given that this would influence the outcome of the intervention.

During the first visit, Harika learned that Lynette had a strong will and was determined to get better. Lynette had been a schoolteacher for close to 40 years and had managed to juggle raising children of different ages with various occupational issues. On discovering that Lynette valued hard work, Harika realized that she would strive towards her occupational goals as an active participant. Harika planned to work equally as hard because she believed that occupational engagement is a crucial aspect of life, health, well-being, and a just and inclusive society. Harika was able to get a good understanding of the environmental factors influencing their practice relationship during that first visit. However she was aware that these influences could change throughout the process and would change as Lynette accomplished various objectives within their occupational therapy plan.

CASE 9.3 Lynette and Harika's story

Lynette is a 78-year-old woman who has six children, 14 grandchildren, and six great grandchildren. She taught school for nearly 40 years, most of that within a one-room schoolhouse in a small rural town. After her retirement at 65, she spent a great deal of time with her grandchildren, helping them with their homework, and taking them to school and extracurricular activities.

Two years ago Lynette began to experience shortness of breath and wheezing when she was doing chores and going for walks. Her doctor diagnosed her with Chronic Obstructive Pulmonary Disease (COPD) and advised her that she should use portable oxygen when doing more strenuous activities. Her son and daughter-in-law, who lived in the closest city, suggested that she move in with them so that she didn't have to worry about taking care of her home and all the chores that came with it. Lynette was hesitant to do this as she valued her independence. Her son and older grandchildren agreed to help her, to the extent that she was able to remain in her home for another 21 months.

Harika, an occupational therapist, has been practicing for 32 years, working her entire career with older adults in the community, predominantly in nursing homes. She is married with two grown children, and two grandchildren. Her parents live together in a nursing home and she visits them at least once a week. She believes that engaging older individuals in daily occupations is crucial to their health and well-being. Harika loves being an occupational therapist, and believes that with hard work by both the therapist and client in the right context, everyone can engage in significant and valued occupations.

Harika has just received a referral for Lynette, who has just arrived home after a three-month stay at the local general hospital. Lynette had developed a

Continued ...

Case continued ...

cold and pneumonia, which had been resistant to treatment. Although her doctor finally managed to get rid of the pneumonia, the three months in the hospital and the pulmonary deterioration from the pneumonia have left Lynette extremely weak and unable to even roll over in bed without help. Her doctor and social worker felt that Lynette needed to be transferred to a nursing home. However her daughter-in-law, Kathy, insisted that she come to live with her.

Harika arrived at Kathy's family's home for her initial visit with Lynette. She found Lynette sleeping in a medical bed. Kathy told her that she wasn't able to get Lynette out of bed by herself but could help her change positions in bed. The bed was in the family room while construction was underway for a new room for Lynette. At that time, Lynette could at least interact with her family because she was sleeping in the family room. Kathy was at home during the day so she could be with Lynette whenever she needed her, but also had to cook and clean. Kathy was worried that once Lynette was in her own bedroom that she would feel isolated if she couldn't move around on her own to some extent.

Harika was amazed that Kathy had decided to bring Lynette to her home given that Lynette required a lot of assistance. Because Harika saw Lynette in Kathy's home environment she had to think about how best to enable not only Lynette's occupations but also Kathy's. Within a nursing home environment, Harika would have typically provided consultation to staff on how best to position her client in bed to decrease likelihood of tissue breakdown and to allow for participation in various daily occupations. She also would have demonstrated with staff how to enable the client to build her strength and engagement in other required occupations such as bathing and toileting. Within this home environment, Harika needed to engage Lynette, as well as Kathy, to determine and prioritize the occupational goals.

— *By Jane Davis*

9.4 Frame(s) of reference as context: Models of practice, theories, and service delivery

After the enter/initiate action point, the therapist and client start to set the stage. The client and therapist begin to exchange information to clarify their views and perspectives. Occupational therapists might describe the profession's beliefs in the fact that humans are occupational beings, and that all have the need and right to perform and engage in occupations that are meaningful and significant for the client (see text box 9.2). The beliefs about occupation, enablement, client-centred practice, and inclusion (see table Intro.1) will likely continue. They are compatible with the CMOP-E and other occupation-focused models of practice.

In addition to the beliefs held by members of this profession, occupational therapists are guided in practice by frames of reference. A frame of reference is the viewpoint, context, or set of assumptions within which a person's perception and thinking occur, and which constrain selectively the course and outcome of action (Atherton,

Reflections on clients' frames of reference

As both client and occupational therapist bring themselves to the practice setting, it is important to consider how to understand the impact of clients' frames of reference. What might these include? Perhaps clients have their own theoretical understanding of illness causation? Or they may have developed a concept of the roles of health professionals such as occupational therapists and their roles as patient/client? Maybe they have a conceptual understanding of disability and the place of disabled people in society? What might be their understanding of the meaning of aging?

— *By Brenda Beagan*

2002). Occupational therapy frames of reference are sets of interrelated theories, constructs, and concepts that determine how specific occupational challenges will be perceived, understood and approached (Mosey, 1986), and that guide occupational therapists' decision making through the practice process.

Occupational therapists may use diverse theories to frame their practice (see frames of reference in text boxes 7.2 and 7.3). Most of these theories were created by other disciplines or professions, thus few are a perfect fit for the profession of occupational therapy. As the client-therapist relationship progresses, the occupational therapist may decide to employ a number of theories. In doing this, the compatibility of theories needs to be considered, reflected upon, and confirmed prior to using multiple theories simultaneously. The therapist may also decide to abandon one theory in favor of another, if the client is not progressing or goals are not being met.

Another feature of occupational therapy is the model of service delivery. Models are often specific to practice settings, although some settings now offer multiple models, such as consultation combined with direct care. In reality, occupational therapists reconcile models of practice, occupational therapy theories, and models of service delivery in decisions about what to actually do with their clients.

Case 9.4 about Benjamin and Sara highlights the reconciliation of these multiple frameworks in everyday practice. Sara, the occupational therapist, was a private-practice occupational therapist, who worked from a consultative model of service delivery and was building her practice. Sara typically embraced occupation-based, sensorimotor approaches, and wondered what theoretical approach she would use due to the beliefs and values held by the school, and by Benjamin's parents. She relied on abductive reasoning to be open to the all possible approaches within Benjamin's school environment. Sarah decided to combine her approach with the behavioural approaches favoured by the school and Benjamin's parents.

CASE 9.4 Benjamin and Sara's story

Sara, an occupational therapist with 25 years of experience, provides private occupational therapy services in the suburbs of a major metropolitan area. Benjamin is an 8-year-old boy who has been diagnosed with pervasive developmental disorder (PDD) and mild cerebral palsy. He lives with his parents and a younger sister. Currently, Ben attends a private school where intensive behavioural approaches are provided on an individual basis for the full school day. His parents have received some funding assistance from the provincial government to help cover the costs but are still responsible for much of the school fee.

Ben's parents initially approached Sara, an occupational therapist, five years ago, because they were aware that occupational therapists work with children with PDD and they wanted to make sure they had considered all approaches. They also wanted an occupational therapist to consult with the private school.

Sara has been providing consultant services to Ben and his family for the past five years. In her practice, she uses a sensorimotor approach focused on the specific occupational goals identified by the child and family.

Working with a systematic approach to address occupational challenges, Sara needed to choose a theoretical framework. The school used a formal, intensive behavioural approach, which was fully supported by the family and school staff. Sara needed to decide if her sensorimotor, occupation-based approach could be used in combination with the intensive behavioural approach. When she decided she could work in this environment, Sara and the school agreed to the consultation. Her consultation was highly successful in that she:

- Introduced a chew toy to work on increasing chewing of Benjamin's food, implemented as a program at school prior to lunch; Benjamin is now able to manage more foods (apples, pizza);

- Used a triangular cushion to improve posture while sitting;

- Introduced a keyboarding program to work on typing;

- Suggested developmentally appropriate activities for gross motor skills to be used at recess and playtime.

— By Deborah Cameron

9.5 Moving through the contexts

Entering the practice context: Professional knowledge, reasoning, and reflection

Freidson, a medical sociologist, identified one of the essential traits of a profession as specialized knowledge (Freidson, 1986). A profession is distinguished by the use of specialized, abstract, and technical knowledge applied to specific cases. The abstract knowledge of the occupational therapist includes beliefs, values, assumptions, theories, models, and a process of practice. The occupational therapist's technical knowledge may include a range of qualitative and quantitative evidence, including critical analysis of occupations, and the personal and environmental influences that shape them.

Professional reasoning is the process of reflective thought in which occupational therapists engage to determine action (Magnani, 2001). In occupational therapy, professional reasoning encompasses occupational and enablement reasoning, and is subjected to abductive reasoning as discussed in chapter 8. Reflection is the act of thinking and doing through which the occupational therapist becomes more skillful (Schön, 1983). Professional reasoning and reflection encourages the therapist to be self-questioning, to challenge accepted beliefs and practice, and take on new beliefs that may lead to more informed practices.

In their Client-Centred Strategies Framework, Restall et al. (2003) described how reflection can facilitate a better understanding of how personal factors shape practice. They described how "clarifying values assists the clinician to understand their reaction to, and resistance of behaviours when a client's values are different than their own" (p. 105). Restall and colleagues further explain:

> When a situation arises where values seem to be in conflict, clarifying and articulating values helps illuminate an appropriate course of action that allows the clinician to remain true to his or her own values while supporting the client in the enablement of chosen occupations (p. 105).

The therapist is continually questioning how personal values, beliefs, and preconceived ideas may affect practice, and is exploring how to address potential conflicts. To reduce the likelihood of conflict, clients need to understand the scope of practice and knowledge of the therapist (Wressle & Samuelsson, 2004) so that they can realize the full potential of the collaboration. Working within this framework will also provide the occupational therapist the opportunity to expand his or her personal practice framework and to expand practice repertoire, as in the case with Sara and Benjamin.

To close this chapter, let us continue with Jim's story in case 9.1.

CASE 9.5 Jim's story in context
(continued from case 9.1)

Returning to Jim's story in case 9.1, we can see how the different contexts come together. We understand that the societal context in which Jim lives views unobservable chronic pain with skepticism. His co-workers have not been supportive, and he has become increasingly withdrawn and anxious about returning to work. The case scenario doesn't provide us with information about Sean's personal and environmental influences; however, we can assume that each individual brings aspects of their own personal values and beliefs into the

Continued ...

Case continued ...

practice relationship. They possess knowledge of their own occupational and emotional lives: Jim holds the knowledge of his own experiences and brings with him certain abilities and strengths, and Sean, the occupational therapist, holds values and beliefs of his own. Some of these may be rooted in Sean's professional experience, while others will be derived from his personal experiences outside of the profession, his own unique occupational experiences.

Within the practice context, it appears that Sean and Jim have established a practice relationship based on trust and transparency. Their interactions occur in Sean's office (for planning meetings) and at Jim's workplace (for assessment and intervention). When Sean enters the practice context, he immediately explores the personal and environmental factors that may influence his practice relationship with Jim. Jim confides in Sean about his feelings of anxiety about returning to work. Sean demonstrates his belief in and support of Jim by advocating on his behalf with the WSIB adjudicator and the disability management company for gradual return to work. Within the practice context, Sean uses various perspectives and approaches to frame his practice throughout the practice process. Sean uses a consultation model of service delivery to assess Jim's capacity and motivation for return to work, and his occupational issues. Sean performs functional evaluations with a focus on biomechanics, as well as a psychosocial perspective to understand Jim's fit with the job site, especially his anxiety and pain levels. His plan uses a gradual return to work framework to enable Jim to re-engage in his previous job. This framework is congruent with the understanding that active participation will enable occupational competence and development when barriers are minimized and supports are increased.

Although Sean's practice is focused on physical injury and its outcomes, he is keenly aware that many psychosocial issues can and do arise with individuals dealing with chronic pain issues and an inability to return to work. He must utilize clinical reasoning skills, reflection and abduction to open up to all of the possibilities for interventions — both biomechanical and psychosocial — to enable Jim's return to work.

— *By Catherine Donnelly and Terry Krupa*

Chapter 10

Using the Canadian Process Practice Framework: Amplifying the process

Jane Davis
Janet Craik
Helene J. Polatajko

CASE 10.1 Margaret's non-retirement

Danielle, an occupational therapist, works as an outreach worker for a regional branch of a non-profit agency that provides services to people with low vision and other visual impairments. She works with clients in their home, school, or work environments to optimize their occupational engagement. Danielle believes that all individuals have the right to engage in meaningful and signifi-cant occupations. As an occupational therapist, her role is to enable her clients' engagement in occupations. Danielle uses the Canadian Model of Occupational Performance and Engagement (CMOP-E) to organize the information that she gathers from and with her clients.

Margaret, a 68-year-old widow, who lives alone in a two-storey home in a small rural town, was referred to the non-profit agency by her daughter who thought that her mother might benefit from devices to assist her with reading. Margaret had been having difficulty with her vision for a few years; however, up until this point it hadn't stopped her from doing what she wanted and needed to do, including her part-time job as a cook in a retirement home. Margaret was diagnosed with age-related macular degeneration (dry type) five years ago and had cataract surgery on her left eye six years ago. Results from a recent ophthalmology report indicated that Margaret was in the early stages of central vision loss but remained legally able to drive an automobile.

Based on results from the *Canadian Occupational Performance Measure (COPM)* (Law et al., 2005), and the *Visual Function Questionnaire – 25 (VFQ-25)* (Mangione et al., 2001), Danielle and Margaret, devised a plan to enhance her reading performance. They negotiated with Margaret's employer to modify her work and workplace environment to enhance her competence so that she could maintain her current job. Danielle provided Margaret with various technologies and information from the Ontario Human Rights Commission, which advocates that age should not be a factor in hiring, promotion, or retirement (Ontario Human Rights Commission, 2006).

Margaret informed her employer that she did not plan to retire. Danielle met with the employer and Margaret to discuss the employer's beliefs that low vision would limit her energy for the job. Both Margaret and the employer agreed to support low-cost occupational and environmental adaptations, such as new labeling systems for ingredients and larger print on dietary restriction information sheets. Over the next two sessions, Danielle worked with Margaret to implement the plan, and to monitor and modify it as needed.

Danielle completed a final visit with Margaret. They reviewed her goals and her progress to date, recorded an updated narrative of her experience, and re-administered the *COPM* and *VFQ-25*. Danielle and Margaret deter-mined that Margaret had met her goals. Danielle supplied Margaret with infor-mation about relevant community services as well as the contact information for the non-profit agency for which she worked, should Margaret require further services. Danielle completed her discharge report, provided a copy to Margaret, and bid her farewell.

— *By Debbie Laliberte Rudman*

Occupation-based enablement

10.1 Introduction

The CPPF, introduced in chapter 9, is a framework designed to guide practice. The framework, grounded in enablement, upholds principles of client-centred, evidence-based and occupation-based practice, and is comprised of context and process elements. As discussed in chapter 9, the three context elements are societal, practice, and frames of reference. The eight process elements are called action points (see table 9.1) that can be used in their entirety or in some combination with individual, family, group, community, organization, and population clients across the mosaic of practice.

Over the past decade there have been considerable shifts in service delivery within occupational therapy, including a greater emphasis on interprofessional, interdisciplinary, and transdisciplinary structures, consultative models, and clients who may be individuals families, groups, communities, organizations, or populations. The CPPF accommodates the multitude of service delivery models in the mosaic of practice. The language of the CPPF enables its use within various collaborative teams. The solid line in figure 9.1 shows a potential full practice pathway. Given the practice mosaic the occupational therapist would consider the dotted lines, which indicate variants on a theme, called alternate pathways.

Chapter 10 describes and illustrates each of the eight action points. The action points are discussed using abductive reasoning about occupational, personal and environmental factors, and enablement skills applied to Margaret's situation in case 10.1. To demonstrate an integration of the five essential elements of occupational enablement (see chapter 8), case 10.1 presents occupational challenges and possible solutions, client-centred goal setting, multidisciplinary knowledge, and abductive reasoning. Text box 10.1 on ageism prompts reflection on the implicit, value-laden ideas that need explicit attention in order to achieve effective enablement in Margaret's situation.

10.2 The Canadian Practice Process Framework: Eight action points

The eight action points of the CPPF, summarized in table 10.1, are: enter/initiate, set the stage, assess/evaluate, agree on objectives and plan, implement the plan, monitor and modify, evaluate the outcome, and conclude/exit.

The CPPF includes the aspects of assessment, intervention[1] and evaluating outcomes found in the Canadian OPPM and the American OTPF. The CPPF expands on these to name five central action points: assess/evaluate, agree on objectives and plan, implement the plan, monitor and modify, evaluate the outcome.

Three action points have been added: enter/initiate, set the stage, and conclude/exit.

---

[1] Although the term *intervention* is common language in occupational therapy and other health professions, the term *implementation* is used in this text to avoid using language that means to do something to or for people (to intervene), whereas occupational therapy enablement works through collaboration on all eight action points, including action to implement the plan with people.

Reflections on ageism

Ageism can be defined as "an attitude that makes assumptions about older persons and their abilities and puts labels on them. Ageism is also a tendency to view and design society on the basis that everyone is young. Age discrimination is a consequence of ageist attitudes" (Ontario Human Rights Commission, 2006). When age or attitudes about age are used to exclude aging persons from occupations they need and want to do, this can be interpreted as a form of occupational injustice. Attitudes about aging, combined with disability, can create situations of occupational injustice for aging persons wanting to remain in the workforce past what is seen socially as the standard or normative age of retirement. Despite the repeal of mandatory retirement policies in many Canadian provinces and an increase in the expressed desire of persons nearing age 65 to remain in the workforce in some capacity, systematic discrimination against older workers in hiring, training, and downsizing practices remains. Some occupational therapists are enabling occupational engagement through empowerment-directed processes to decrease real or potential occupational injustice (Townsend & Wilcock, 2004a; Townsend & Wilcock, 2004b).

— By Debbie Laliberte Rudman

The implication is that clients are engaged with the therapist in decisions about initiating, setting the stage and concluding services. In these three action points, occupational therapists can engage clients to frame the relationship for reflective, transparent, ethical, client-centred practice, and a respect for diversity of beliefs, values, and interests. These points need to be explicit to recognize the importance of building client-centred relationships, mediating power relations, and decision-making mechanisms. These are points to develop, explore options and preferences for client participation, consider potential occupational change strategies, and determine stakeholders. The final action point recognizes the essential process of explicitly concluding or re-defining relationships, clarifying understandings of what transpired during therapy, making outcomes explicit, and more. By collaborating to make these three action points explicit, clients and therapists understand the values and expectations of the relationship. The action points to start/initiate and conclude/exit are congruent with the intersections of the arrows on the CMCE (see figure 4.3), representing entry and exit from the client-professional relationship.

10.3 The process in its entirety: The full pathway

The practice process that is detailed below occurs within three contexts (see table 10.2): the societal context, practice context, and frames of reference (see chapter 9).

Table 10.1 The Canadian Practice Process Framework (CPPF): Eight action points at a glance

Action points	Key enablement skills and actions (CMCE, Figure 4.3)
Enter/initiate	• Call to action: Advocate for the client and occupational therapy to create positive first point of contact with client based on a referral, contract request, or the occupational therapists' recognition of real or potential occupational challenges with individual, family, group, community, organization, or population clients • Consult to decide whether to continue or not with practice process • Educate and collaborate to establish and document consent
Set the stage	• Engage client to clarify values, beliefs, assumptions, expectations, desires • Collaborate to mediate/negotiate common ground or agree not to continue • Adapt ground rules to the situation, build rapport, foster client readiness to proceed • Explicate mutual expectations and document the "stage" set • Collaborate to identify priority occupational issues (OIs) and possible occupational goals (OGs)
Assess/evaluate	With client participation and power-sharing as much as possible or desired • Assess (sometimes called evaluate) occupational status, dreams, and potential for change • Consult with the client and others, use specialized skills to assess/evaluate and analyze spirituality, person, and environmental influences on occupations • Coordinate analysis of data and consider all perspectives to interpret findings • Formulate and document possible recommendations based on best explanations
Agree on objectives and plan	With client participation and power-sharing as much as possible or desired • Collaborate to identify priority occupational issues for the agreement in light of assessment/evaluation • Design/build plan, negotiate agreement on occupational goal, objectives, and plan within time, space and resource boundaries, and within contexts, using requisite elements
Implement the plan	With client participation and power-sharing as much as possible or desired • Engage client through occupation to implement and document progress • Specialize in program frame of reference as appropriate to effect or prevent change
Monitor and modify	With client participation and power-sharing as much as possible or desired • Consult, collaborate, advocate, educate, and engage client and others to enable success • Adapt or redesign plan as needed in monitoring progress through formative evaluation
Evaluate outcome	With client participation and power-sharing as much as possible or desired • Re-assess/evaluate occupational challenges and compare with initial findings • Document and disseminate findings and recommendations for next steps
Conclude/exit	With client participation and power-sharing as much as possible or desired • Communicate conclusion of interaction between client and therapist • Document conclusion/exit and disseminate information for coordinated transfer or re-entry

Frame(s) of reference are defined within the local practice and daily living context, which is embedded in the larger societal context. The implication is that the frame(s) of reference and practice context are shaped by societal characteristics. Although Margaret lives in a small rural town, provincial and federal legislation on retirement age and pension regulations will determine her retirement options. Accommodation

Table 10.2 Three CPPF contexts for Margaret's non-retirement

Three CPPF contexts for Margaret's non-retirement (see case 10.1)

Societal context
- Ageism exists in Western society: historical retirement laws have produced views that older adults should not be working or are less capable than younger adults
- The case is set in a small rural town

For Margaret:
- Workplace provides her with many benefits and socialization opportunities
- Employer wants her to retire
- Lives alone in a two-storey home; has the support of her daughter
- Has had many life experiences both personal and occupational
- Has relatives and friends in Europe whom she enjoys visiting yearly
- Believes that age does not indicate an inability or lack of desire to maintain a job

For Danielle:
- Occupational therapist licensed to practice by her College
- Outreach worker for a non-profit agency that provides services to people with visual impairments
- Believes all individuals are occupational beings with the right to engage in significant occupations

Practice context
- Danielle meets with Margaret in her home and at her workplace
- Danielle is able to provide 10 sessions including follow-up with each client; to provide additional sessions, she must demonstrate a justified client need, including likelihood of an improved occupational outcome
- Danielle's role with Margaret is to enable her engagement in occupations

Frames of reference (may change throughout process)
- Danielle uses the Canadian Model of Occupational Performance (CMOP-E) to organize the information she collects from her client and through assessments
- Danielle will use a direct service model of delivery
- Danielle will use an occupational justice perspective

requirements for persons with low vision are not yet provincially mandated, and would thus be subject to company policy and her employer's attitudes.

Enter/initiate

The enter/initiate action point is the occupational therapist's call to action, or first point of contact with the client as illustrated in table 10.3. This is the point to establish collaborative enablement, and to engage Margaret as an ally in developing her occupational therapy plan and her advocacy with her employer. This may be initiated by the client or result from a referral from a health care practitioner or some other agent aware of the needs of the client and the potential for occupational therapy to make a difference. Occupational therapists may increasingly seek out contracts based on occupational perspectives on situations raised in the community or media, such as the closure of a town factory, or the need for developmental programs for children with learning disabilities or obesity.

As part of entry, the occupational therapist and client identify occupational challenges. The initial contact may review occupational challenges and consider potential or actual occupational issues. Enter/initiate is the first encounter between the therapist and client who enter into a specific practice relationship within a specific practice context, which is located within a broader societal context. Both enter with the intention of identifying and working toward the client's goals. Both parties bring with them specific personal beliefs, values and experiences, and environmental influences. The client may enter with preconceived beliefs about what will happen during this process based on previous experiences with other health care professionals, including (perhaps) other occupational therapists. Similarly, the therapist may enter with preconceived ideas drawn from information known from texts or other cases, as well as information about the client prior to entry — be it from a referral or an initial phone contact. In Margaret's case, Danielle decides that her experience is suitable to work on the case.

At entry, the client is identified as an individual, family, group, organization, community, or population. The reasons for a referral, contract, or other arrangement would be immediately identified and any conflicts of interest or ethical issues determined, including issues involving third-party payment. Also at entry, prior to obtaining any personal information from the client, the occupational therapist would ensure that the client understands that the therapist must have the client's expressed and documented consent before disclosing any client information to any individuals, groups, or organizations (CAOT, 2007). The therapist would state the necessity of reporting any situations of suspected abuse, neglect, or potential harm divulged by the client to the relevant authorities. With community, organization, and population clients, ethical guidelines would be applied to the clarification of consent on the documentation, access guidelines, and handling of information.

The model of service delivery, such as direct care or consultation, as well as the occupational therapy profile role may be determined at this point; however, ongoing changes in the practice context and frames of reference, and the process may influence changes in the model of service delivery and profile role throughout the relation-

---

Table 10.3 Enter/initiate

Enter/initiate: Margaret's non-retirement (see case 10.1)

Enablement skills
- **Collaborate** with Margaret to clarify referral and scope of occupational therapy
- **Engage** Margaret in a discussion about her occupational life course and needs, hopes

Actions and reasoning
- Initial call to action when Margaret's daughter refers her to occupational therapy services
- Client is identified: individual; 68-year-old woman
- Stakeholders identified: daughter; others not yet known
  * Danielle notes that since Margaret lives alone in a rural community, Danielle needs to explore other current or potential stakeholders during her interview with Margaret and discussions with Margaret's daughter
- Danielle consults with Margaret about her difficulty reading and listens to her occupational narrative about trying to work with low vision
- Parameters of referral are established, and Margaret, her daughter and physician are educated about the possibilities for working with Danielle
- Margaret states that she understands about informed consent and the reporting of suspected abuse; consent is documented, with a copy to Margaret as well as to the referring agent
- Danielle reflects on her experience from working in the community and determines that she has the knowledge and skills to take on the referral
- Danielle explains that she can provide direct care

---

ship. Throughout the initial contact, the occupational therapist would consider her/his professional competencies and experience to work with the client on the perceived occupational challenges. In some situations, the therapist may decide not to continue and refer the client to another professional or service. Alternately the client may decide not to continue and request to withdraw from the referral or contract.

Set the stage

Following entry into the relationship and the decision to continue, the occupational therapist and the client need to set the stage for their interaction. This action point involves determining how the occupational therapist and client will work together, and it includes rapport building, establishing ground rules, fostering client readiness to proceed, and expressing mutual expectations. At this action point, the therapist engages individual or family clients for the first time in a discussion of the occupational life course narrative. Community, organization and other clients would be engaged in narrating or otherwise documenting the relevant occupational history. Developing rapport is a critical point for discussing different perspectives, beliefs, and values between any client and the occupational therapist (see text box 10.2 and table 10.4).

Directed interviews, using tools such as the COPM (Law et al., 2005), may be useful for an initial screening of possible occupational issues and goals. Community screening tools, organization mapping, or population health data may be appropriate with clients other than individuals. When the client is a community, organization, or population, the occupational therapist would engage the client in a discussion of occupational challenges, and the history and culture for handling such challenges to date. Ground rules would be adopted, rapport built with representatives, and mutual expectations clarified and documented.

The therapist reflects on past experiences, knowledge, and possible theoretical frameworks to initiate the assessment process. The client would be invited to discuss what frames of reference fit with values and beliefs that will shape the client response to the therapist's approaches. There will likely be important points for mediation or negotiation, with the therapist advocating approaches that seem most appropriate given the therapist's professional opinion, expertise, and experience.

Text box 10.2

Reflections on developing rapport with clients

Part of the processes of entry and setting the stage is developing a rapport or connection with the client. How might differences between a therapist and client matter at this stage? What would happen, for instance, between a male therapist and female client, particularly if the two were of different ages? What about other differences? What might the occupational therapist and client talk about to examine assumptions and perceptions concerning aging?

— By Brenda Beagan

Table 10.4 Set the stage

Set the stage: Margaret's non-retirement (see case 10.1)

Enablement skills
- **Collaborate** with Margaret to set the rules and responsibilities of the practice relationship, and to determine her occupational issues and goals for performance and engagement
- **Educate** Margaret about occupational therapy and about the possibilities of workplace accommodations for working with low vision
- **Engage** Margaret in a discussion about her occupational life course and needs, hopes and dreams

Actions and reasoning
- Danielle engages Margaret by asking her about her own values and beliefs about working despite her visual difficulties
- Danielle explains her position as an outreach worker for the non-profit agency and as an occupational therapist, and discusses the frequency and duration of visits; she reviews her practice "ground rules" of occupational enablement, and discusses her expectations of herself and Margaret to be open and honest about Margaret's progress
- Danielle reflects upon her ethical and legal obligations to attain informed consent, and determines that she must explain the nature and expected benefits of the services to be provided, indicate any possible risks, identify alternate courses of action, and explain consequences of not participating in the therapy-related activities
- Margaret provides informed consent for participation in occupational therapy and for the disclosure of any information about her situation to her daughter
- Danielle suggests that they proceed with an assessment to gather more specific information before a plan can be developed and agreed upon
- Danielle and Margaret discuss her occupational experiences, including an occupational life course narrative, a directed interview, and the completion of the COPM
- Danielle makes notes on Margaret's occupational experiences, her hopes and dreams, and her conflict with her employer
- Danielle and Margaret exchange contact information, including e-mail addresses (Danielle provides a work e-mail address rather than her personal one), and decide upon telephone communication as their principal means of contact

Potential occupational issues (OIs)
- Difficulty reading fine print required for food and medication labels
- Workplace policies and attitudes that do include supportive employment or accommodations
- Uncertainty of being able to return to her job as a part-time cook in a local retirement home

Frames of reference
- Occupational perspective — using the CMOP-E to organize information
- Direct care model of service delivery

A client typically comes into contact with an occupational therapist when occupational challenges are complex or beyond commonly known enabling strategies (see table 7.1). Through the action points of set the stage, assess/evaluate, and agree on objectives and plan, the client and therapist work through a process of discussion and action from the identification of perceived or potential occupational issues (OIs) and occupational goals (OGs). The client and therapist may prioritize OIs and OGs which differ from those identified in the initial contact or referral. Part of the art of occupational therapy is to uncover a client's true occupational challenges and to engage the client in prioritizing occupational issues to assess/evaluate. Margaret identified three potential OIs related to difficulty reading fine print, workplace policies, and uncertainty about her future.

Once the initial occupational challenges and issues are identified and understood by both client and therapist, the occupational therapist may review her or his experience, expertise, skills and abilities, and how they may relate to the occupational issues. The scope and parameters of service should be clarified, including possible discussions of institutional policies. In a health setting, relevant policies might be the allotted number of visits, length of stay, time per session, and potential funding for services or resources. With community, organization, and population clients outside a health setting, relevant policies might be about access to information, routines and schedules for meeting with representatives, and funding options for new initiatives. It is important with any type of client to disclose any potential resource limitations such as a limited number of funded visits under funding constraints.

As part of setting the stage, the roles and responsibilities of the client, stakeholder(s), and the occupational therapist may be negotiated. Informed consent would be obtained before commencing to ask anyone for information for assessment or evaluation. The occupational therapist has ethical and legal[2] obligations for obtaining consent to proceed with services. Informed consent is not just to protect client privacy in releasing information to other stakeholders. Consent promotes client autonomy and fosters communication between the therapist and client. Consent is also a process through which the nature of collaboration and power sharing can be clarified by reviewing how information will be documented and handled.

An occupational therapist would respect the client's right to know the specific nature of the services being provided both initially and on an ongoing basis, and a therapist would respect the client's right to refuse to consent to participate in therapy-related activities. The therapist is responsible for providing enough information for the client to make an informed decision. It is also the responsibility of the therapist to assess if the client is capable of making these decisions. An occupational therapist must comply with appropriate provincial Freedom of Information and Protection of Privacy (FOIPOP) legislation, an example being the *Government of Nova Scotia Act* (1999). Within occupational therapy there are professional guidelines concerning ethics and consent, with additional guidelines that require attention in many settings, particularly in the health sector. The action point to set the stage (see table 10.4) is crucial in establishing communication systems, promoting the transparency of practice, and meeting legal obligations of attaining informed client consent.

Assess/evaluate

After occupational issues are identified and confirmed with the client, an in-depth assessment or evaluation would identify the personal, environmental, and occupational factors that underlie the client's occupational issues (see table 10.5). Occupational therapists would draw on their frame(s) of reference (theory, model of practice, model of service, and paradigm), past experience, expertise, and research knowledge to ascertain plausible explanations for their clients' occupational challenges. Reflection on the societal and practice contexts, and on frames of reference would guide the occupational therapist to determine what assessment(s) are most relevant and practical in the situation, from individualized standardized tests, creative

---

[2] For example, in the Province of British Columbia all health care practitioners are governed under the *Health Care (Consent) and Care Facility (Admission) Act*, 1996; in Ontario, by the *Health Care Consent Act, 1996*; in Prince Edward Island, by the *Consent to Treatment and Health Care Directive Act, 1996*.

Occupation-based enablement

Table 10.5 Assess/evaluate

Assess/evaluate: Margaret's non-retirement (see case 10.1)

Enablement skills
- **Specialize** in assessment and interpretation of occupational issues with low vision
- **Collaborate** with Margaret to determine her perceptions of how her vision loss has affected her occupational performance, through assessment
- **Educate** Margaret about the findings and their implications
- **Coach** Margaret to use self-evaluation and self-monitoring techniques
- **Coordinate** with Margaret and the team to document the assessment findings with attention to transfer knowledge in one format so that Margaret can track her progress, and in the official format for the team and institutional management of health records

Actions and reasoning
- Danielle selects the VFQ-25 as an assessment tool of best practice keeping in line with her selected frames of reference: she needs to validate Margaret's reading problems and gain a deeper understanding of her perception of her vision loss on her well-being and occupational performance, in particular, which occupations are disrupted by the visual loss and in what context these occupations are performed
- Danielle determines that she needs to assess Margaret's meal preparation capacity on site, however this will require further planning
- Danielle discusses her interpretation of the assessment findings and her recommendations with Margaret so that they can develop objectives and a plan for action
- Identify and/or confirm occupational issues
- Determine plausible explanations for issues
- Perform assessments focused on plausible explanations for issue: consider fit among personal capacity, and occupational and environmental demands, and the potential for engagement based on noted mediators (see Fit Chart in chapter 8 and analysis of fit below)
- Analyze and interpret findings
- Select most plausible explanation for issue based on best evidence (includes fit analysis, assessment results, research evidence, client knowledge, etc.)
- Discuss recommendations for possible solutions based on plausible explanation of issue, identified targets for change, and other assessment findings

Confirmed and prioritized occupational issues (OIs)
- Difficulty reading fine print on food and medication labels, books, newspapers, and sewing patterns
- Uncertainty of being able to return to her job as a part-time cook in a local retirement home

Frames of reference
- Occupational perspective — using the CMOP-E and VFQ-25 to organize information
- Direct care model of service delivery
- Measurement theories

media, and professional observation to the use of group or community assessment methods, such as focus groups, surveys, participant observation, and document review. A review of literature and local knowledge would be used to determine which assessments are viewed as best practice and most feasible with the particular client and context. The occupational therapist would discuss the choice of assessments and engage in mutual decision making with the client and stakeholder(s).

Following completion of the assessment(s), the occupational therapist would analyze and interpret the findings to determine a plausible explanation for each of the client's occupational issues. Findings and recommendations would be shared, and possibly developed, with the client. Table 10.5 provides a framework for the abductive professional reasoning that occupational therapists may follow during the assessment/evaluation action point. Reasoning would consider how best to identify, validate, and prioritize the client's OIs and OGs. It is duly noted that at this stage (and at all action points) the occupational therapist would maintain appropriate documentation and sufficient information to keep client and stakeholder(s) informed throughout the process. Clients may establish their own parallel documentation as part of their self-management in a client-centred practice.

After reviewing assessment/evaluation findings and recommendations with the client, one of two pathways may be taken: the therapist and client may go on to construct and agree upon objectives and a plan (presented here); or, the practice relationship may end (see abbreviated pathway "A" later in this chapter). Throughout the assessment/evaluation, active enablement would include collaboration with all involved, specialized enablement in the use of assessment/evaluation methods, and education, coordination and coaching to involve Margaret, and manage the team work with Margaret, the employer, representatives from the Canadian National Institute for the Blind — which provides low vision equipment — and others. Complex abductive reasoning would consider all possible assessment methods. Analysis would explore all potential explanations for Margaret's occupational issues, beyond the obvious body function impairment related to her macular degeneration. Her issues may, for instance, be more related to the employer's attitudes toward aging than low vision, or to a mandate from his boss to reduce the number of older workers who will draw from the pension fund. Possibly it will save the company funds if Margaret accesses a disability pension and leaves the company.

Agree on objectives and plan

This action point involves reflecting upon the client's occupational challenges, the priority occupational issues, and assessment/evaluation findings, including data on occupations and the personal and environmental factors influencing occupational engagement. With the client and relevant stakeholders, the occupational therapist would establish the occupational goals for the client (see table 10.6). Complex enablement is required to set objectives and plan, actions that require occupational therapy expertise. Support personnel may contribute but would not be responsible to set objectives and plans in place. Enablement would continue in collaboration, education, and coaching to reach agreement on objectives and other aspects of the plan.

This is a point where enablement to adapt, design, and build program plans is essential. Based on abductive reasoning, the occupational therapist would determine with the client the optimal objectives based on the most plausible explanation of occupational issues. The plan would follow the agreed upon possible solution to reach occupational goals based on best evidence.

Occupational therapists have an opportunity at this time to help clients extend their dreams and goals by opening up a world of realistic possibilities. Enablement would focus on engaging clients in discussions and actions. Possibilities for engagement include a review of future occupational life course narratives or future narratives about the potential for individual change, community or organizational development, or population changes. Negotiation to agree on objectives may become complex

Table 10.6   Agree on objectives and plan

Agree on objectives and plan: Margaret's non-retirement (see case 10.1)

Enablement skills
- **Adapt** the plan with Margaret as the practice process unfolds
- **Collaborate** with Margaret to determine her occupational performance and engagement goals
- **Design** and build a program plan design with Margaret, based on her personal and environmental strengths with awareness of her challenges

Actions and reasoning
- Danielle and Margaret establish and agree upon occupational goals (see above)
- Danielle and Margaret determine and agree upon objectives and plan
- Reflect on and discuss with client the fit between client's personal, occupational, and environmental factors, targets for change, and recommendations of possible solutions based on assessment findings
- Reflect on and discuss societal and practice contexts, which may delimit solutions
- Identify and confirm occupational goals with the client based on discussion of possible solutions
- Agree with the client on which solution will be implemented to reach occupational goals
- Determine objectives based on most plausible explanation of occupational issues and the agreed on possible solution to reach occupational goals based on best evidence
- Establish and finalize plan with client

Confirmed occupational performance goal
- Margaret will be able to read the fine print on labels and instructions
- Workplace accommodations will enable her employers to retain her

Frames of reference
- Occupational perspective — using the CMOP-E and VFQ-25 to organize information
- Direct care model of service delivery

with diverse stakeholders whose interests must be coordinated with a community, organization, or population client. Such complexity may be there in mediating agreement with families and groups when issues such as whether a family member can live at home, or not, are on the table.

Enablement, actions, and reasoning likely extend the collaboration, engagement, and other enablement during enter/initiate, set the stage, and assess/evaluate. Occupational goals will provide the basis for subsequent actions, such as refinement of the frame(s) of reference. The aim is to facilitate clients to name goals that are achievable and realistic, although part of enablement may be to engage the client in pilot testing what is realistic. New occupational goals that emerge after the plan has been accepted may require adjustments in the plan, or in some cases a new referral or contract.

This is a critical action point, which may require the occupational therapist to mediate or actively negotiate with clients to arrive at the best objectives and plan in light of client interests, time and space conditions, values and expertise by the client and occupational therapist. Diverse perspectives on priority objectives and plans would ideally be something that has been explicit since the client-therapist relationship was initiated.

Subsumed under general occupational goals are specific action-based objectives to facilitate goal attainment. Objectives are derived from an analysis of assessment findings. Findings would provide the most likely explanation of the source of occupational issues and point to possible solutions. Typically a number of objectives are required to attain a client's OGs, thus the completion of one objective will not necessarily lead to the end of the practice relationship.

The objectives should be clearly mapped out and linked with the plan or course of action. Plans usually include, beside objectives, an outline of the background, assessment findings that support proposed actions, a timeline, resource requirements (locations, equipment, supplies, costs), stakeholder involvement, and evaluation methods. With community or organization clients, the plan may even include revenue generation to cover costs, such as selling products, putting on workshops, or finding sponsors. The occupational therapist may utilize a variety of frames of reference and enablement skills. Collaboration would abide by client-centred enablement foundations, including client participation and power-sharing. Client voice and choice would be considered along with client rights and responsibilities for risk taking. The approaches used within the plan may range from direct hands-on approaches, as in bio-occupational splinting, to advocacy for policy change.

The plan would be documented and would include a description of the approaches to be used and who is to implement the plan. The plan would also identify what resources are available, where services will take place, and how the client and stakeholders will participate. Parties may include the client or family, employer, the occupational therapist, or assigned personnel; for example, an occupational therapy assistant or other health worker. The occupational therapist would consider suitable referrals to other health professionals as needed, discuss how the plan will be monitored and modified as required, and explain evaluation mechanisms.

Implement the plan

This action point is to implement the plan as agreed upon (see table 10.7). Collaboration is a key enablement skill to continue to engage the client in implementing the plan. The plan may, in fact, draw on a huge range of enablement skills. In Margaret's case, Danielle implemented the plan by coaching Margaret, advocating with and for her with the employer, adapting her workplace, and coordinating the documentation for the case. Danielle reasons that the best possible solution is to follow Margaret's instincts to stay on the job with accommodations, and to advocate for this with the employer. They work toward the occupational goals of Margaret being able to read labels and retain her job. Four frames of reference guide the implementation, and are used in various ways throughout the practice process: an occupational perspective on Margaret's life course and transitions, a direct service model, environmental adaptation and modification, and an occupational justice perspective to prevent occupational deprivation.

Monitor and modify

The action point to monitor and modify involves ongoing, formative evaluation to determine whether current enablement strategies are meeting the established objectives and whether the plan is being followed (see table 10.8). For the duration of the plan's implementation, the occupational therapist constantly reviews and monitors

Table 10.7   Implement the plan

Implement the plan: Margaret's non-retirement (see case 10.1)

Enablement skills
- **Coach** Margaret, using role play and encouragement to approach her employer, and advocate on her own behalf about maintaining her job (in this situation, Danielle is enabling Margaret to use her own enablement skills)
- **Enable** Margaret through encouragement to advocate on her own behalf with her employer
- **Collaborate** with Margaret and her employer to perform an on-site assessment
- **Educate** Margaret's employer about age-related macular degeneration and the benefits of employing older, long-time employees
- **Adapt** Margaret's occupation and workplace to meet her vision needs
- **Advocate** with and for Margaret with her employer and with the CNIB
- **Coordinate** and manage documentation with Margaret, the employer, and other stakeholders

Actions and reasoning
- Danielle provides information to Margaret and coaches her to develop the skills needed to approach her employer and advocate for her job
- Margaret speaks with her employer to let him know that she has no plans on retiring and feels confident that she can do her job
- Danielle educates Margaret's employer about Margaret's situation
- Danielle reasons that the best possible solution is to follow Margaret's instincts to stay on the job with accommodations, and to advocate for this with the employer
- Danielle modifies Margaret's work and workplace environment to enhance her occupational competence

Confirmed occupational goals (OGs)
- Margaret will be able to read the labels and instructions
- Margaret will remain in her job with her employer's support

Frames of reference
- Occupational perspective — using the CMOP-E and VFQ-25 to organize information
- Direct care model of service delivery
- Environmental modification and adaptation
- Occupational justice perspective

client progress towards the objective(s) and goals. Formative evaluation monitors a client's progress and provides guidance on the process of practice throughout the implementation phase. Enablement involves coordination to monitor the continuous collection of data and information on the client's progress toward desired occupational goal(s). This type of evaluation can lead to subtle changes in the objectives or plan, such as increasing the grade of difficulty and complexity of an occupation. Possibly new stakeholders will be identified, for instance, social justice or seniors groups interested in advocating for workplace accommodations for older workers. Formative evaluation could indicate the need for a more in-depth evaluation of outcomes to determine if the occupational goals have been met. New occupational issues may emerge and may require a new plan. With community, organization, or population clients, the process is the same — monitor progress toward objectives, collaborate with stakeholders to modify the plan, and confirm next steps.

Modifications to the plan are made when new issues arise, when person, occupation, or environment situations change during the course of the implementation, or when the response to the plan does not meet expectations. At this point, the therapist may need to reassess. In Margaret's case, Danielle meets twice with Margaret following the implementation of the plan to undergo an informal formative evaluation of her

Table 10.8   Monitor and modify

Monitor and modify: Margaret's non-retirement (see case 10.1)

Enablement skills
- **Coach** Margaret about how to discuss her issues with her employer and fellow employees
- **Engage** Margaret through encouragement to continue with her competence development
- **Collaborate** with Margaret to determine if plan modifications are needed
- **Adapt** Margaret's occupation and workplace to meet her vision needs

Actions and reasoning
- Danielle meets twice with Margaret following the implementation of the plan to undergo an informal formative evaluation of her occupational performance and engagement
- Danielle, in collaboration with Margaret, determines that some minor modifications are needed and makes some further adaptations
- Danielle reasons that the employer may support Margaret's employment if she has a positive attitude about requests for accommodation

Confirmed occupational goals (OGs)
- Margaret will be able to read labels and instructions
- Margaret will remain in her job with her employer's support

Frame(s) of reference
- Occupational perspective — using the CMOP-E and VFQ-25 to organize information
- Direct care model of service delivery
- Environmental modification and adaptation
- Occupational justice perspective

occupational performance and engagement. Danielle and Margaret could change the plan to improve progress, although they would both need to agree to modify the plan (see repeated pathways below). Given success with the plan, they proceed to evaluate the outcome.

Evaluate the outcome

While designing the objectives and plan, the therapist would incorporate a summative evaluation to evaluate the overall outcome of the plan (see table 10.9). A summative evaluation examines attainment of the occupational goals. If the goal or objectives have not been met, evaluation may provide useful information to guide further action. At this point in the process, at least three possibilities might occur:

1. All the agreed upon occupational goals have been met and the client has no further occupational issues, so the therapist and client conclude their practice relationship (as in Margaret's situation);
2. All the current occupational goals have been met, but the client has further occupational issues that need addressing. The practice context allows for extended occupational therapy involvement, and the therapist and client re-engage to identify further occupational goals, objectives, and a plan; or
3. The goals have not been met, and the therapist and client agree to consider next steps, which could be to reset the objectives and plan, or to conclude the professional relationship.

With community, organization, and population clients, outcomes will be evaluated according to the plan, using methods appropriate to the situation. One of the key

Table 10.9   Evaluate outcome

Evaluate outcome: Margaret's non-retirement (see case 10.1)

Enablement skills
- **Collaborate** with Margaret to determine if goals have been met and if Margaret has any other occupational issues
- **Coach** and **educate** Margaret and her employer to evaluate the strengths and gains and to document the work and other conditions that support or limit Margaret's ability to continue in her job

Actions and reasoning
- Danielle re-administers the VFQ-25 and the COPM
- Danielle interprets the reassessments and determines, with Margaret's collaboration, that the occupational goals have been met
- Margaret determines that she has no other occupational issues at this time

Confirmed occupational goals (OGs)
- Margaret will be able to read labels and instructions
- Margaret will remain in her job with her employer's support

Frames of reference
- Occupational perspective — using the CMOP-E and VFQ-25 to organize information
- Direct care model of service delivery

actions for Danielle to evaluate the outcome is to gather data for comparison with the assessment/evaluation stage. Danielle arranges with Margaret to re-administer the COPM and VFQ-25. Danielle also re-confirms with Margaret and the employer that the workplace accommodations are satisfactory from all points of view. Danielle interprets the reassessments and determines, with Margaret's collaboration, that the occupational goals have been met. Margaret can read labels with low vision technology and workplace adjustments to make large print signs. Most importantly, Margaret's employer is very satisfied and has agreed that she continue on the job.

Conclude/exit

Once outcomes have been evaluated and it is determined that occupational goals have been met or not, decisions are needed whether to pursue other objectives or conclude. If the decision is to conclude, the client and therapist arrange to end the practice relationship (see table 10.10). Although successful achievement of occupational goals is the desired outcome, there will also be occasions where the practice relationship will conclude without successful achievement of the client's goals. In this case it is important that the relationship be carefully concluded to ensure that both parties understand the reasons for ending it. At the conclusion of the practice relationship, it is important for the therapist to inform the client of the possibility of re-entry to a new practice process. Clients may receive a copy of the discharge or exit summary. With community, organization and population clients, the end point is likely a report summarizing recommendations for ongoing action. As part of the conclusion, the occupational therapist may provide a referral to another service, or information on community resources. In the end, Margaret recognized that her macular degeneration will continue to reduce her eyesight. The complexities of future occupational transitions may indeed warrant another contact with occupational therapy.

Table 10.10 Conclude/exit

Conclude/exit: Margaret's non-retirement (see case 10.1)

Enablement skills
- **Educate** Margaret about options for re-entry, as necessary
- **Engage** Margaret in the process of concluding their relationship

Actions and reasoning
- Danielle and Margaret end their relationship as her OGs have been met and no new ones have been identified
- Danielle provides Margaret with a summary of her progress and provides information for accessing occupational therapy services in the future if they are required (she acknowledges that her condition is degenerative and she may require occupational therapy services as her vision declines)

Completed occupational goals (OGs)
- Margaret can read labels and instructions
- Margaret is working in her previous position and has the full support of her employer

Frames of reference
- Occupational perspective — using the CMOP-E and VFQ-25 to organize information
- Direct care model of service delivery

10.4 Alternate pathways: The repeated pathway From evaluate outcome to agree on objectives and plan

For some practice processes, one cycle through the full pathway is not enough to address all occupational issues. A repeated pathway might follow the full route until the evaluate outcomes action point. Instead of concluding the practice relationship, the therapist and client may decide to return to the action point of agree on objectives and plan. There are three possible situations for this occurrence, assuming that funding is available to continue with a revised plan:

1. It has become apparent through monitoring and modifying the agreed upon objectives and plan that a summative evaluation is needed to guide a major modification of the overall plan to reach the occupational objectives;
2. It has become apparent through monitoring and modifying the agreed upon objectives and plan that the client's current occupational goals are not reachable with the plan; however, the client has other occupational issues or goals; or
3. The client has reached the agreed upon objectives, wants to pursue further occupational issues or goals, and funding continues to support occupational therapy involvement. Case 10.2 demonstrates this pathway.

In case 10.2, Harika, the occupational therapist, Lynette, the client, and Kathy, a stakeholder and Lynette's caregiver, worked together on two self-care goals. Upon evaluating the outcomes of the initial plan, Harika noted that not only had Lynette met her occupational goals, but she also demonstrated the physical capacity and the motivation to continue the practice relationship with new occupational goals. Funding was still available, and policies supported continuation as long as Lynette

CASE 10.2 Lynette and Harika's story (continued from case 9.3)

Lynette, who has Chronic Obstructive Pulmonary Disease (COPD), had been discharged from hospital following a three-month stay due to pneumonia, and has caregiving support from her daughter-in-law, Kathy.

It has been two weeks since Harika, an occupational therapist, began working with Lynette. Lynette's initial occupational goals were: 1) Lynette will transfer to the bedside commode with assistance from one person; 2) Lynette will engage in a sponge bath with the help of her daughter-in-law at the bedside. These two goals were important to Lynette because maintaining her own basic self-care is a priority for her. Harika felt that Lynette would be able to reach these goals within the amount of time allowed by the community health care provider; however, Lynette met these goals earlier than Harika expected.

Harika evaluated Lynette's occupational performance and found that Lynette demonstrated the capacity and motivation for increased occupational engagement in her self-care occupations. Harika discussed with Lynette and Kathy the possibility of continuing the practice relationship through the determination of new occupational goals based on Lynette's continued self-care issues. Lynette and Kathy decided that they would like to maintain the relationship and determine new occupational goals, objectives, and a plan. Based on her evaluations of Lynette's occupational performance, personal factors, and environments, Harika believed that Lynette should be able to perform her self-care occupations in the privacy of the washroom, using the standard toilet with a raised toilet seat, and bathing in the tub using a bath seat. Lynette, Kathy, and Harika collaborated to develop two new occupational goals for Lynette, with related objectives and a plan. Harika implemented this plan with Lynette and Kathy, and continued with the practice relationship until Lynette met her two new goals. The relationship was then concluded.

— By Jane Davis

was motivated. Thus, Lynette, Kathy, and Harika worked together to determine new self-care goals for Lynette, and agreed upon objectives and a new plan. On the second pathway, the plan was implemented and monitored, outcomes were evaluated, and they agreed to conclude/exit from the relationship.

10.5 Alternate pathways: Two abbreviated pathways

As noted in chapter 7, the mosaic of occupational therapy practice is extremely diverse. To provide for the unique nature of client-therapist interactions within the diversity of occupational therapy practice, the CPPF presents abbreviated pathways. Two abbreviated pathways are illustrated with dotted lines in figure 9.1. Abbreviated pathway "A" may occur subsequent to the action point of assess/evaluate if a decision is made to conclude/exit occupational therapy services with assessment recommendations but no plan. Abbreviated pathway "B" may occur after the action point of agree on objectives and plan if a decision is made to develop objectives and a plan, but there is no funding, opportunity, or interest in implementing the plan. In all cases, funding, mandate, availability of services, and service models in particular settings may influence decisions about abbreviated pathways.

Abbreviated pathway A: From assess/evaluate to conclude/exit

Abbreviated pathway "A" follows the full pathway until the action point of assess/evaluate. Following assessment, evaluation, and information gathering, services will be concluded for one or more of the following reasons: no occupational issues and/or goals are confirmed; the referral was for assessment and recommendations only; or there is a conflict in values that leads to a breakdown in determining the objectives and plan, and the therapist or client decide to end the relationship. Other reasons for this abbreviation may be reliance on an assessment consultation model, or workloads that limit time available with each client. This pathway is illustrated briefly in cases 10.A1, 10.A2, and 10.A3.

In case 10.A1, Beth, the occupational therapist, received a referral for Zayan. There was limited information describing his occupational issues. To assess his needs, Beth interviewed both his teacher and teaching assistant. The teaching assistant brought forward concerns related to Zayan's occupational engagement within his home and community environment. Upon further discussion with Zayan's mother, Beth realized that Zayan's cultural environment played a large part in his current occupational repertoire, perceived development of his occupational competence, and his social

---

Text box 10.3

Reflections on respecting cultural differences

Some other possible reflections on Zayan's story: Given Zayan's South Asian heritage, Beth might have thought about whether experience of racism was a possible explanation for Zayan's lack of play with other children. Zayan's story also highlights the complexity of respecting cultural differences while challenging the status quo in the name of justice. Beth urged Zayan's mother to involve him in lunch-making, though she had been told it was deemed culturally inappropriate for a mother to do this for her son. If Beth considers it unjust for women to be required to do all the food-related occupations in a family, she may have used this opportunity to challenge the status quo. On the other hand, she is imposing a particular cultural view on this mother. How would you handle this conflict?

— By Brenda Beagan

       Occupation-based enablement

CASE 10.A1 Beth and Zayan

Beth is an occupational therapist who graduated from university two years ago. She works in the school system and is contracted through the local home care program to provide occupational therapy services for children. Beth has just begun to work with Zayan, a 10-year-old boy with spina bifida who attends his local school. He is integrated into a regular classroom, and has a teaching assistant who helps him with schoolwork and toileting routines. As part of her assessment, Beth completes an interview with Zayan's teacher, Mr. Wright, and the teaching assistant. Mr. Wright reports that Zayan is doing well at school and that he has no major concerns. The teaching assistant reports that she is concerned that he does not play with other children while at home, and that Zayan's mother still packs his lunch and organizes his backpack. Beth agrees that the teaching assistant's concerns could be occupational issues for a 10-year-old child. However she is aware that Zayan's engagement in these occupations may be influenced by the family's cultural expectations.

When Beth speaks with Zayan's family to gain an understanding of their perspective on Zayan's occupational engagement, she discovers that the family moved to Canada within the last year from India. When asked about Zayan's social skills at home, his family reveals that in their culture, children spend most of their free time with their families. Zayan has relatives who live close by and he spends a lot of time with his cousins. According to his family, Zayan demonstrates good social skills with his relatives, yet they agree that he doesn't socialize very much with the neighbourhood children because that is not the way of their culture. In terms of packing his lunch and organizing his backpack, his mother indicates that she has always done this for Zayan and for her other children. She feels he is capable of doing these things himself, but that is not part of their culture.

Based on this information, Beth decides that at this time there are no issues with Zayan's social participation (see text box 10.3). In terms of his participation in packing his lunch and backpack, Beth decides to mention to Zayan's mother that at some point she might begin to have him engage in aspects of these occupations to enable his occupational development.

Following her discussion with Zayan's mother, Beth concludes her involvement with Zayan.

— By Debra Cameron

participation. Once this was highlighted it became apparent to Beth that Zayan had no occupational issues that required her help at this time.

Following a brief discussion with Zayan's mother about his future occupational development, Beth concluded the practice relationship with Zayan and his family.

Jacquie, the occupational therapist in case 10.A2, was asked to provide a consultation service by making recommendations based on the findings of her interviews and assessments of the women and children's occupational needs. She is not funded or mandated to continue beyond assessment. After presenting her recommendations and responding to any questions, she concluded the relationship. Therefore, no objectives or plan for intervention were developed or agreed upon with her clients, as per their request.

Case 10.A3 illustrates an abbreviated pathway from assess/evaluate to conclude/exist because Judy, the occupational therapist, chose to refer her client to another therapist.

Ethically, Judy felt that the best option was to refer Emily to another therapist. Thus, no agreement on objectives and a plan was established because of differing therapist and client values. Following the assessment, the practice relationship was concluded.

Abbreviated pathway B: From agree on objectives and plan to conclude/exit

Abbreviated pathway "B" is the route most often used by an occupational therapist acting as a consultant, whereby the interaction and engagement of the therapist occurs from assess/evaluate up to and including agree on objectives and plan before concluding the relationship. In this abbreviated pathway the client and therapist have interacted and agreed upon the objectives and plan; however, the client-therapist relationship will not be carried through to implementation. Pathway "B" is illustrated briefly in cases 10.B1 and 10.B2. There are two common possible situations for this abbreviated pathway:

1. Through the process of establishing objectives and a plan, the client decides that the professional enablement of an occupational therapist is no longer needed; or
2. The referral or contract specifies consulting services to establish a plan based on assessment.

In each of these situations, someone other than the occupational therapist will implement, monitor, and evaluate the outcome of the plan. Although the relationship is concluded prior to knowing the outcome of the plan, the client may always re-enter into the relationship if occupational issues are not resolved.

In case 10.B1, Michael's enablement involved listening and observing Isabella as she engaged in household chores. This level of involvement elicited an adaptive

CASE 10.B1   Isabella and Michael

Michael, an occupational therapist, worked with Isabella, a client in the community with degenerative disc disease. She was receiving physical therapy services when contacted by Michael. She reported by telephone that her main problem was with vacuuming. Isabella wanted to keep up with housekeeping chores, but found it painful, and her old vacuum cleaner had stopped working. She wanted to consult with an occupational therapist before purchasing a new one. When Michael made a home visit, they discussed her condition and strategies such as joint protection and proper body mechanics. Isabella came to realize that what she needed was a lightweight vacuum system to reduce bending and twisting. She was actively involved in establishing her objectives and plan when she realized that she was able to carry it forward herself. She was going to evaluate two different vacuum systems: a built-in vacuum and a lightweight, more maneuverable vacuum. Isabella contacted Michael to let him know that she chose the lighter vacuum.

— By Janet Craik and Jane Davis

CASE 10.B2 Nursing home consultation

The scope of occupational therapy consultancy in nursing homes can take on many forms. The occupational therapist may consult about particular persons — resident(s), staff, families, volunteers — within the nursing home. The therapist may also assist people in selecting a nursing home. Enablement might be to consult with the nursing home on their milieu or their sociocultural, emotional, and physical environment. A consultant occupational therapist would always gather information from as many sources as possible to understand the occupational challenges, specific occupational issues (OIs), and occupational goals (OG's) of each stakeholder.

Sometimes the consultation may be to work with someone labeled a difficult resident. The occupational therapist would seek information on difficulties from the perspective of the resident as well as from family and staff.

Franklin is an 80-year-old man who is a new resident in a nursing home in a mid-sized city. He has become increasingly agitated over the past two days following the move from his home of 47 years. At home, his wife had cared for him following his diagnosis with Alzheimer's disease three years ago. Keiko, an occupational therapist who consults with families and nursing home staff to enable successful transition of new residents, has been hired privately by the family. They hope that Keiko can enable the nursing home staff to create a supportive and safe environment for Franklin, and to decrease his agitation. Keiko works with Franklin, his family, and the staff to gain a broad understanding of Franklin's occupational issues and goals. She assesses Franklin's capacity, current and past home environment, and current level of occupational engagement. Keiko then holds a meeting with Franklin, the family, and staff to present her findings and make recommendations.

Together, they work out objectives and a plan for Franklin to engage in nursing home occupations with staff support as needed when he becomes confused. One of the key objectives of the plan is to decorate Franklin's room in a way that provides him with as sense of continuity with the environment from his home. The suggested design will highlight his life experience as an architect by putting his university degree on the wall, and photos from his work. The staff agree to re-arrange furniture in his room to make space for the desk that he loves to sit at with some drawing equipment. The changes to his room build respect, understanding, empathy, and attention from staff. Following agreement on the plan, Keiko provides her summary report and concludes her relationship with Franklin, his family, and the staff of the nursing home.

— By Anne Connor-Schisler, adapted by Jane Davis

response from Isabella. Isabella used her own strengths as a problem solver to find a solution to meet her desired occupational goal without further enablement from Michael. Through Michael's enablement to coach, collaborate, consult, and educate Isabella, they discovered that Isabella had the skills and resources to complete her plan without further professional help. At this point, Michael concluded occupational therapy services.

Keiko, an occupational therapist, has been hired in case 10.B2 to design an action plan to support Franklin's occupational transition. Keiko will design the plan within the safe, supportive, and enabling environment of the nursing home. The implementation is left to Franklin's family and staff; thus Keiko concludes the relationship and will not provide follow-up. Keiko educates Franklin's family and staff to implement the plan. Family members are aware that they are always welcome to re-enter into the relationship by providing Keiko with another referral.

10.6 Summation

The choice of alternate pathways is based on professional reasoning about the occupational issues illustrated in case 10.1 through the eight action points in the full pathway (see tables 10.3 to 10.10). One structure to organize professional reasoning is the CMOP-E (see figure 1.3b). Using a chart of the CMOP-E components, one can clarify and confirm what information is known and what information gaps in understanding occupational performance and engagement exist. One might also organize professional reasoning using a chart based on the Taxonomic Code of Occupational Performance (TCOP) (see figure 1.1). A chart based on the TCOP would be useful to document occupational issues and distinguish them from movement or activity issues in the hierarchy. A third option to chart professional reasoning would be to use the ICF (see figure 1.4) to organize information on impairments, activity limitations, and participation restrictions. The CMOP-E, TCOP, and the ICF are all tools for occupation-based enablement. They are particularly useful for five of the action points in the CPPF: assess/evaluate, agree on objectives and plan, implement the plan, monitor and modify, and evaluate outcome. The occupational therapist would use these charts in an iterative fashion to guide the process of practice, record reasoning to monitor the process, and modify actions as needed.

Using charts based on these three tools, one could reason whether or not further assessments or other data collection are required. Analysis would ideally result from discussions with the client and others. The therapist would use theoretical suppositions to guide the discussion and to gain an understanding of potential occupational engagement limitations and mediators. During all action points in the process, the occupational therapist would monitor and document change related to the person, occupation, and environment constructs and their interactions. Attention would be given to temporal aspects to understand past, present, and future occupational issues.

It is best practice for occupational therapists to qualify and document ALL statements of analyses on clients' abilities, skills, knowledge and environmental context. Best practice would qualify statements of analyses especially when the origin of the data may not be apparent or is out of the ordinary, for example, with clients who are non-communicative. All conclusions would be validated by providing the sources of data or information and the methods used to obtain it. Data may be from client reports or stakeholder reports. Data may also be from the occupational therapist's assessments or observations, research evidence, and theoretical suppositions. Data may be obtained by hearing, seeing, using hands-on assessment, knowing, or by other means. Statements such as "as reported by client caregiver," or "as observed by the occupational therapist" are key elements to the "conscientious, explicit and judicious use of current best evidence in making decisions" (Sacket, Rosenberg, Gray, Haynes & Richardson, 1996, p. 71).

SECTION IV
Positioning occupational therapy for leadership

Introduction

> *When I was in active medical practice, I thought of occupational therapy as a*
> *therapeutic tool in the biomedical model, which was to be used to increase a*
> *patient's function. I thought the therapeutic process was more important than*
> *the outcome. I gave little thought to occupation as a health benefit …*
> Enabling Occupation *opened my eyes to a new understanding about the*
> *mission of occupational therapy.*
>
> (S. Jennings, personal communication, January 2007)

When Shawn Jennings, a physician, former occupational therapy client, and reviewer
for this book, reflected on his medical practice and experience, he noted that occupational therapy is typically perceived in health services as a biomedical, therapeutic tool
to address specific functional components. Reading a draft of *Enabling Occupation II*
"opened my eyes" to "occupation as a health benefit" and "the mission of occupational
therapy," he proclaimed. Randy Dickinson, a policy analyst, former member of the
Board of Directors of the Canadian Association of Occupational Therapists, member
of the Advisory Panel for this book, and a person living with a disability, knows about
occupational therapy from the inside. He urges us to address more than biomedical
dysfunction, and be a stronger force to reduce systemic barriers, and educate people to
"fully participate as they are able in society" (see text box p. 276).

Section IV proposes four leadership strategies to guide the profession in becoming a
stronger force in both practice settings and society overall. Chapter 11 illustrates the use
of the Canadian Practice Process Framework (see chapters 9 and 10) to better integrate
scholarship and evidence on enabling occupation, using qualitative as well as quantitative
data, including client experience. Chapter 12 discusses issues and proposes solutions for
occupational therapists to demonstrate greater accountability for the effectiveness and
cost-benefits of occupational enablement. With scholarship, evidence, and accountability
strategies in hand, chapter 13 describes how occupational therapists can improve client
access to the profession by using existing and new funding, policy, and legislation opportunities in health and other sectors. Also addressing client access, chapter 14 looks at
workforce planning and a multi-stakeholder strategy. The strategy addresses the recruitment, retention, and broader utilization of occupational therapists across rural and urban
Canada. Section IV positions the profession to envision a future, and to proactively plan
to exert leadership by developing political skills (Duncan, Buchanan, & Lorenzo, 2005;
Kronenberg & Pollard, 2005; O'Shea, 1979). It proposes action for *all* occupational
therapists, with the aid of identified leaders, partners, and stakeholders to advance an
occupational therapy vision of health, well-being, and justice through occupation in
Canada and around the world.

Vision

To position Canadian occupational therapists as world leaders in advancing an occupational therapy vision of health, well-being, and justice through occupation.

Purpose

To advance the vision by escalating scholarship in practice, discovering how to frame accountability, increasing financial and policy support, and drastically expanding the occupational therapy workforce.

Objectives

- To escalate participation in scholarly practice for occupational enablement;
- To discover accountability opportunities that render an occupational perspective and occupational enablement more explicit;
- To improve public and private access to the profession by:
  - Probing current and new funding, policy and legislative opportunities for occupational enablement;
  - Accelerating occupational therapy workforce planning and stakeholder alliances in order to increase the supply and utilization of occupational therapists.
- To envision an expansive future for occupational therapy and occupational science, and to proactively plan for it.

Practice Implications

Section IV will energize you with strategic ideas for making enabling occupation and an occupational perspective of health, well-being, and justice through occupation more visible and better supported in systems and society. The section invites readers to champion an occupational perspective in society, and to facilitate opportunities for society to benefit from occupational enablement. The section's underlying message is that occupational therapists hold beliefs, values, knowledge, and skills to make important contributions in occupational enablement with Canadians and others around the world. A key strategy is to expand funding sources and lobby for support in policy, legislation, and the media. The section invites you to immerse yourself in leadership strategies and consider potential allies in occupational enablement to benefit society through clinical services, consulting, management, education, research, and policy development in both the public and private sectors.

Randy Dickinson's message to occupational therapists

There is an old parable that suggests that if you give a person a fish you may feed them for a day, but if you teach them how to fish then they will be able to feed themselves for a lifetime. Occupational therapists must be ready to do more than just assess the needs of their clients, and prescribe technical aids and other solutions that they believe will enable persons to carry out basic activities of daily living. The theory of good practice must be combined with an understanding of practical realities.

Persons with disabilities and others will present themselves with a tremendous variety of situations. Not all will have the benefit of an education or appropriate social experiences. Some will need to develop communication skills and self-confidence to be able to fully present the issues that they would like to see addressed in their lives. Others will need to learn how an occupational therapist can best help them and others.

While most occupational therapists work to enable individual change, systemic barriers in the real world outside of the clinical setting will determine what can be accomplished. Key challenges will be to work with insufficient financial resources and inadequate housing options. Affordable and accessible transportation services are scarce. The public still has poor awareness and even shows outright discrimination when it comes to inclusive employment. Personal care supports such as attendant care or homemaker services are expensive and difficult to find. Public facilities and programs that are available to the general public are often not available to those with special needs. Foremost among the challenges is the impact of poverty.

Occupational therapists can provide resource information and links to established community advocates to break down these systemic barriers. Occupational therapists can also enable people to communicate their own needs and to advocate for themselves long after the client-professional relationship has ended. Collaboration and partnership are the way to develop the knowledge base and confidence required for people with special needs to fully participate in society. A good rehabilitation plan is useless unless there are resources for its implementation.

Effective partnerships with those in need will not only enhance the lives of those persons whom occupational therapists would like to help, but also will enhance the satisfaction levels of occupational therapists and the social value attached to the profession. Clients and occupational therapists working together is a win-win scenario. Together, we are stronger!

— By Randy Dickinson, a strong advocate for and with persons with disabilities, former Board Member, Canadian Association of Occupational Therapists, and a member of the Enabling Occupation II *National Advisory Panel*

Chapter 11

Escalating participation in scholarly practice for enabling occupation

Elizabeth A. Townsend
Mary Egan
Mary Law
Mary Manojlovich
Brenda Head

CASE 11 Marjorie and Joe: Building evidence-based practice

At a local professional meeting, occupational therapists, Marjorie and Joe discuss the challenges of staying current with research and actually practising evidence-based occupational therapy. One challenge is minimal employer support to search for evidence, and to gather and analyze data on their practices. Marjorie is a recent occupational therapy graduate working in her first job providing provincial, home care services in a small community of 35,000 people. Although her caseload is diverse, the majority of her clients are over 65 years old, with occupational performance challenges and insufficient community supports to live in their own homes. In fact, Marjorie has no Internet access at her home care office. In the same small community, Joe has provided occupational therapy services for 10 years. He works two part-time jobs: one at the local hospital and one in a private occupational therapy company. Both have large caseloads and little time or support to read the literature or evaluate services.

Marjorie and Joe decide to meet at the local hospital where Joe has Internet access. They negotiate with their managers to take two hours once a month, for a three-month trial period, to discuss research and evidence during work time. Their managers will review their caseload statistics before extending the trial period. First, they read about Critically Appraised Topics (CATs) in the Canadian Association of Occupational Therapists' practice magazine, *Occupational Therapy Now*. The process framework they choose includes the typical steps to define a question, search the literature, and appraise articles to answer the question. Second they explore Web sites containing CATs that are related to occupational therapy practice. They agree on the following question: What factors support the community re-integration of seniors after a hip fracture? An approach to search for appraised information on the Internet and to complete their own CAT appealed to them. Over the next six months, Marjorie and Joe finish one CAT and invite four interested colleagues to join them in developing another one. They decide to investigate the following question: What environmental forces restrict participation in community occupations by those over 75 years of age who have experienced a hip fracture?

— *By Mary Law*

11.1 Introduction

Chapter 11 reminds us that occupational therapy's best practice is based on well-rounded evidence that has been subjected to appropriate, thoughtful, scholarly inquiry, which has not been limited to randomized controlled trials. This chapter, written for occupational therapists like Marjorie and Joe, proposes to use the Canadian Practice Process Framework (CPPF) to escalate participation by occupational therapists as scholarly practitioners, a competency role named in the new *Profile of Occupational Therapy Practice in Canada* (CAOT, 2007). It does not, however, suggest that all occupational therapists must be researchers.

In proposing greater participation in scholarly practice, we encourage occupational therapists (as Whiteford [2005] does) to raise critical perspectives on scholarship and evidence in occupational therapy. Whiteford reminds us to be wary of "levels or hierarchy of evidence" (Whiteford, 2005, p. 38). She points to the potential for us to follow old ways of thinking that devalue experiential or qualitative evidence in favour of quantitative evidence. We may "reinforce a historic and ideologic tradition of the supposed superiority of empiricism and scientific evidence" (Whiteford, 2005, p. 38). She urges us to raise critical questions about evidence-based practice, to be reflective, thoughtful, and confident — drawing on our professional knowledge and client experience — and not to respond too readily to demands for quantitative evidence.

From a cultural perspective, Iwama (2003) reinforces the need to raise critical perspectives on scholarship and evidence. Occupational therapists will want to understand how cultural influences attribute value to different types of knowledge. Iwama (2003; 2006b) has spoken forcefully about occupational therapy ontology: What is knowledge, what can be known? Like Yerxa (1991b), he has made us more aware of occupational therapy epistemology: What is valued as knowledge? How are values about knowledge known? What is a relevant and realistic way of knowing for occupational therapy? His and Yerxa's words reinforce those of Kuhn (1970) and others who recognized that ontology and epistemology are viewed differently in different contexts. It follows that different forms of scholarship and evidence will be valued differently across sociocultural contexts (Iwama, 2006a).

Iwama points to our strong tendency in the West to privilege the ontology and epistemology of Western empirical, positivist science. As a Japanese Canadian who has worked as an occupational therapist in both field and academic settings in Canada and Japan, he reminds us in the West to respect contradictory world views and to recognize what counts as evidence in Eastern philosophy. Development of the Kawa Model (see chapter 1) by Iwama (2006a, 2006b) is a direct challenge to the implicit, assumed universality and dominance of the occupational models developed in the Western world. He challenges us in the West not to claim entitlement to decide what occupational therapists will know and how the profession will be practiced. We need to include and value the voices and perspectives of occupational therapists around the world.

11.2 Escalating participation in scholarship on occupation and enablement

A good first step to escalate participation in scholarship for enabling occupation is to clarify questions about occupation and enablement, with awareness of critical perspectives on evidence and culture. For example, Marjorie and Joe would remind themselves at the outset, that scholarship is not limited to quantitative science. Rather, scholarship refers to organized inquiry that helps to produce theory and multiple forms of research evidence. Each form is recognized and valued in a particular context. Marjorie and Joe would consider their cultural context, and our tendency in the West to privilege the ontology and epistemology of Western, empirical, positivist science. Finally, Marjorie and Joe would know that occupational therapy practice is guided by scholarship — specifically, by a synthesis of knowledge of the client and the client's context, up-to-date, theoretical knowledge, and ample research evidence from multiple research paradigms.

A foremost question for scholarly practice in enabling occupation is: What theory and research evidence is most relevant at each point in the practice process? Another important question is: How might occupational therapists better integrate our growing interests in scholarship, especially for evidence-based practice, into the routines of everyday practice? We know that the prudent use of theory and research evidence is essential for a strong profession (Freidson, 1986), with growing scholarship to inform professional reasoning (see text box 11.1).

Text box 11.1

Professional reasoning in occupational therapy

Mattingly, a medical anthropologist, and Flemming, an occupational therapist popularized the term *clinical reasoning* in occupational therapy (Mattingly & Flemming, 1994). Mattingly contracted with the American Association of Occupational Therapists to study clinical reasoning in occupational therapy with reference to the work of Schön (1983), particularly drawing on his 1987 landmark publication, *Educating the Reflective Practitioner: Toward a New Design for Teaching and Learning in the Professions*.

Mattingly & Flemming (1994) proposed that occupational therapy is based on three forms of reasoning: narrative reasoning around client and other stories; empirical reasoning around medical and other quantitative data; and conditional reasoning around the socio-cultural conditions of practice and of clients' and therapists' lives. It is noteworthy that the three forms of reasoning reflect the major research paradigms in the Western world.

The broader term *professional reasoning* encompasses clinical reasoning (narrative, empirical/positivist, conditional) without being limited to clinical practice, given that occupational therapists also practice as managers, consultants, educators, policy analysts, and researchers in non-clinical as well as clinical contexts. The focus of occupational therapy professional reasoning is occupational reasoning (see Section I) and enablement reasoning (see Section II). Abductive reasoning (see chapter 8) invites examination of possible explanations and solutions.

— By Elizabeth Townsend

A cultural critique is particularly important to consider, especially in light of the value of different research paradigms in Eastern and Western global contexts, and in different systems within Canada. The global value of occupational therapy knowledge (see text box 11.2) lies in critically appraising the cultural and professional construction of knowledge and its use as evidence, particularly related to the complex concepts of occupation and enablement.

Reflections on the global value of occupational therapy knowledge

The social value of occupational therapy knowledge is extremely high, although still largely undeveloped, underestimated, implicit, and taken for granted as common sense.

Occupational therapy *common* sense knowledge is a synthesis of positivist biomedical sciences, positivist organizational or management sciences, phenomenological and interpretive sciences of the world of everyday experience and meaning, and critical sciences about power relations and structures that determine what people and societies do. The synthesis of this multi-faced knowledge base touches on many concepts, ideas, values, beliefs, assumptions, and information focused within the core domain of occupation and the core competency of enabling/enablement, as captured in the seemingly simple description of occupational therapy as *enabling occupation*.

The global value of this complex, dynamic, evolving knowledge is emerging. An occupational perspective of health, well-being, and justice is emerging as research shows that occupation is necessary for human survival: thus knowledge, evidence, and scholarship about what humans do and how occupation influences human health, well-being, and justice is essential not only for individuals or communities, but also for global survival. Research on enablement, which seeks to involve citizens in shaping their lives and the structures of societies, is showing the importance and effects of professional collaboration and partnerships, which in turn, enable choice and meaning to be valued in decision making.

Beyond the treatment of disease, scholarship and evidence on enabling occupation appear to be essential to promote individual, family, group, community, organizational, and population health, well-being and justice. By extension, scholarship and evidence on enabling occupation attend to questions about health, wellness, and (in)equitable inclusion or other injustice in everyday situations for those whose lives are disrupted, alienated, imbalanced, marginalized, or oppressed by chronic illness, disability, aging, or disempowering social conditions.

— By Elizabeth Townsend

Research on wound care and daily life is an example which illustrates a multi-method approach to integrate positivist, phenomenological, and critical social sciences for use in health services. Occupational therapists are recognized for their expertise in the prevention and resolution of pressure sores in daily routines (Registered Nurses Association of Ontario, 2005). When working with individuals or groups of clients whose occupations are affected by pressure sores, multiple forms of evidence are useful, including evidence from the client. Quantitative research based on the positivist paradigm, is extremely helpful to raise questions about, or find evidence on, the amount of pressure, shear, heat, and moisture that cause a pressure sore, ideally with reference to the occupations of client concern, and which types of cushions and mattresses are most effective in preventing or healing a pressure sore.

Narrative evidence from a qualitative (interpretive, phenomenological) paradigm of inquiry (Holstein & Gubrium, 2000) is also extremely helpful. We might raise questions or find evidence about what clients understand regarding the origins of pressure sores, and about their preferences for different types of cushions, mattresses, and positioning for engagement in various occupations.

Analyses of health systems and social structures based on critical inquiry (Bourdieu & Johnson, 1998; Grenfell & James, 1998), are also important in scholarship and evidence-based practice. Critical inquiry informs us how power and social structures work to shape performance, engagement, routines, and the meanings we attribute to occupations. We gain insights and become conscious of the policies, funding, and regulatory conditions that support and limit transformative learning, client participation, empowerment, inclusion, and justice for our clients (and our profession). With reference to wound care, we need critical analyses of health policies and funding priorities to understand why there has been a failure to mobilize the material and human resources to limit the burden of pressure sores. This failure to act seems to disregard considerable knowledge related to the prevention and treatment of pressure sores that not only interfere with body function but also restrict social participation in occupations. Given that knowledge seems insufficient to change behaviour, we need to determine what helps or hinders family members from implementing the recommendations of occupational therapists and other health professionals, e.g., recommendations regarding positioning and use of mattress overlays.

In summary, questions about the effectiveness of wound care and other rehabilitation programs in promoting social participation – a core construct in the ICF – might combine the use of a positivist rehabilitation research paradigm with an interactionist perspective. Consequently, one would inquire about multiple interacting factors (body structure and function, activity, and participation) in the context of personal and environmental factors (Bartlett et al., 2006).

The following suggestions to escalate participation in scholarly practice (see table 11.1) are linked to the Canadian Practice Process Framework (CPPF) first introduced in chapters 9 and 10. Given that scholarship refers broadly to organized inquiry and is not limited to formal research, we invite readers to reflect on the suggestions and to add their own questions. We acknowledge that the time and mandate for scholarly inquiry in everyday practice will be negotiated differently in different contexts.

Throughout the action points, a client-centred occupational therapist would engage the client to participate in scholarship and the search for evidence, according to the ability and wishes of the client, whether the client is an individual or an organization. Collaborative power-sharing would be in the forefront, with respect, awareness, and explicit ground rules for participating from different power bases: professionals in the field, researchers, and clients.

Enter/initiate and set the stage for scholarship

To initiate scholarship in enabling occupation, key enablement skills will include collaborating and consulting with both the client and team members. Within the

Table 11.1   Integrating scholarship in practice

Enter/initiate scholarship
Determine client readiness and interests in organized inquiry to escalate participation in scholarly practice

↓

Set the stage for scholarship
Start to collaborate and consult with the client to identify what knowledge exists and what needs to be known to work with various clients in diverse setting

↓

Assess/evaluate scholarship options
Based on existing research, select occupation-based, client-centred tools to assess/evaluate occupation and influencing factors in persons and the environment using flexible methods to elicit client participation where possible and desired

↓

Agree on objectives and plan for scholarship
Collaborate to use both client and professional knowledge to name valued and feasible occupational objectives, and organize plans

↓

Implement the scholarship plan
Based on the plan, use a dynamic process of moving between what is known about a specific situation and generalized theories regarding the complex process of engaging or re-engaging in valued occupations and emerging knowledge

↓

Monitor/modify scholarship
Monitor and modify the dynamic process by being explicit about what is being done through practice, the theories driving practice, and the ongoing processes of testing practice assumptions

↓

Evaluate outcome of scholarship
Re-apply the same tools and processes that were used to assess/evaluate and compare data before and after implementation of the plan

↓

Conclude/exit
Conclude/exit services and monitor what happens after conclusion of occupational therapy, raising questions such as: Are supplementary services (i.e., analogous to a "booster" shot for health protection) needed to retain gains in occupational performance? How might re-assessment at critical points after services are concluded determine the need for follow-up services?

Adapted from Egan et al. (1998), Head (2005), and Manojlovich (2006).

context of a referral or contract, an occupational therapist would use scholarship as the starting point of practice. The therapist would start by determining client readiness and consent to participate with the occupational therapist and others; together they would raise questions about their occupational issues and possible solutions. Some clients may feel discomfort if they perceive that inquiry implies that the occupational therapist lacks professional expertise. The occupational therapist would determine, with the client if possible, what is already known and what further knowledge is needed. Ideally, the occupational therapist would collaborate with the client through occupation, such as searching the Internet or library, organizing a file or database to store evidence collected, or documenting conversations with key people.

With children, adults, or seniors who are hesitant or not accustomed to communicating their experiences to others, enablement would use skills to adapt communication, coach others in communication options, design communication technologies, or educate others about scholarship. Enablement would foster non-judgmental collaboration, openness to listening to diverse perspectives, and use the arts, technology or other creative communication. In team or collaborative, interprofessional practice, and with caregivers or other stakeholders, the occupational therapist would discuss ground rules and encourage and support client participation, particularly when clients may not be able or wish to express their views verbally.

Using enablement skills, objectives for the occupational therapist at this point are to build trust in the client-professional relationship, determine client readiness to proceed, clarify values and beliefs about different forms of knowledge and expertise, mediate differences in cultural expectations for appraising local and research knowledge, mediate power to clarify how decisions will be made, and support clients to identify their priority occupational issues based on their own and other evidence. Decisions and ground rules to pursue scholarship in practice would be documented for all involved, possibly using multiple strategies such as writing a brief guideline, uploading notes to the Internet, or making copies of meeting results.

Assess/evaluate options, and agree on objectives and plan for scholarship

When clients name and prioritize performance, satisfaction, engagement, choices, or other occupational issues, the occupational therapist and client would continue to collaborate to assess/evaluate the supporting and limiting factors for the issues identified.

The *Canadian Occupational Performance Measure* (COPM) (Law et al., 2005) continues to be a research milestone to assess/evaluate, and prioritize occupational objectives and plans. We know that the *COPM* seems to work best when administered with individuals who are able to communicate their goals with occupational therapists (Warren, 2002). Methods for eliciting valued occupations from individuals who may have difficulty identifying and/or communicating their occupational aspirations, due to depression or aphasia for example, continue to be tested in practice.

We are learning that occupational narratives (Kirsh, 1996) and visual cues (Mandich et al., 2004) are promising methods to assist clients who may have difficulty using the *COPM*. Such methods warrant further investigation.

In developing tools and methods to assess/evaluate, research is needed to describe and critique how enablement works and what enablement skills are paramount with diverse clients in varied contexts. There is tremendous scope for research to develop and test other individualized, client-centred tools and methods, both qualitative and quantitative, including tools and methods to assess/evaluate the occupational environment for community, organization, and population clients.

To review assessment/evaluation data, the occupational therapist and client would agree on occupational objectives and a plan. The next step is to conduct scholarship research in order to identify occupation and enablement factors for client-centred assessment/evaluation (Law et al., 2005). The following examples, along with previous chapters in this book, present current knowledge on occupation, person, and environment factors.

Although a new field of research, the use of activity analysis (Perlman, Weston, & Gisel, 2005) (see Chapter 1, A Taxonomic Code for Occupation for the link between activity and occupation) and dynamic performance analysis (Polatajko, Mandich, & Martini, 2000), has greatly enhanced knowledge about *occupational factors* as well as how occupations can be analyzed and adapted to better fit the resources of the individual. The question of how occupation-related factors affect occupational performance and engagement, has not yet received much attention in occupational therapy, although the growing body of scholarship in occupational science (see chapter 3) will help to answer this question.

On the other hand, knowledge about *person factors* that affect occupational performance is extensive within and outside the profession (see for example, Desrosiers' [2005] discussion of person factors that affect occupational performance following a stroke).

Canadian occupational therapy scholars have been pioneers in the study of *environment factors* critical to occupational performance. Research is growing on the influence of the environment on physical occupational performance factors (Cooper & Day, 2003; Ringaert, 2003), social (Letts, 2003a; McColl, 2003), cultural (Baptiste, 2003), and institutional (Dyck & Jongbloed, 2000; Jongbloed, 1996, 2003; Letts, 2003a; Raponi & Kirsh, 2004; Rebeiro, 2001; Townsend, 1998).

Implement the plan, monitor/modify scholarship

After agreeing with a client on objectives and a plan for scholarly inquiry as part of practice, the occupational therapist would document the plan and disseminate it in various forms to all parties involved. The next step is to participate with the client in implementing the plan. Combining scholarship with practice requires a dynamic process that can integrate: (a) knowledge of a specific situation; (b) generalized theories regarding the complex process of engaging or re-engaging people in valued occupations; (c) emerging knowledge about what can be changed; and (d) how the client wishes to change or minimize change. Our understanding of this complicated process remains largely implicit, residing in the minds and hearts of occupational therapists who do this work. Perhaps the greatest challenge to occupational therapy scholarship at this time is for front-line and academic occupational therapists to find time, resources, communication systems, and strategies to work together. In occupational therapy, we are all challenged — whether as academic researchers or front-line practitioners — to be more explicit about occupational therapy, to elucidate the general theories driving it, and to test its assumptions.

A dilemma for occupational therapists is the extent of potential directions for scholarship related to enabling occupation. A broad-based profession like occupational therapy must maintain its focus and identity in the face of all of the interesting lines of inquiry that relate to practice. An examination of the daily work of occupational therapy will reveal the broad topics of occupational therapy research that are most important. Research is needed, for instance, on basic questions about occupation and enablement. We need to know more about how to assess/evaluate the issues that are crucial for clients to move toward their occupational goals by engaging or re-engaging in valued occupations.

To illustrate how scholarship can inform practice and how practice can inform scholarship, consider a few brief research examples on transformative learning, client-centred practice, and spiritual issues in practice. As noted in chapters 5 and 8, the educational theory of transformative learning is helping occupational therapists to understand the concept, processes, and power relations of enablement. Therapists are learning to design client programs with a critical awareness of the profound personal and social changes attached to the meaning of self and occupation.

Transformative learning seems necessary for client re-engagement in valued occupation in light of a major life change such as may occur following a stroke (Dubouloz, et al., 2004). We are learning that the opportunity to experiment through *doing* occupations with changed abilities in a safe environment — a key aspect of occupational therapy — appears to play a large role in client re-engagement in productive occupations (Petrella, McColl, Krupa, & Johnston, 2005). Research on the client-therapist relationship is guiding occupational therapists to recognize issues such as choice, responsibility, and power in client-centred practice (Law, 1998; Sumsion, 2005). Studies of spirituality that are informing aspects of occupational therapy that address the spirit and spirituality, for instance, in guiding clients to identify their most valued, meaningful occupations (McColl, 2003). Research in these three areas alone shows that attending to suffering, enabling choice, and supporting hope appear to be essential aspects of enabling occupation (Egan & Swedersky, 2003).

Friedland (2001) describes what we now call *enabling occupation* from a historical perspective:

> As in war time, when the spirit can so readily be broken, much of our work today requires us to help mend broken spirits. It is here that we use our interpersonal skills to understand our client's view of the world, and to enter into an alliance with them; it is here that we draw upon our own sense of compassion (p. 67).

Today, we can heed Frank's (2001) warning not to increase the alienation of our clients through attempts to fit their experience into predetermined frameworks. At the same time, occupational therapy scholars will likely continue to describe and examine successful ways to address suffering, enable choice, and support hope with individuals, families, groups and other clients, in order to help make their occupational goals a reality.

Evaluate outcome of scholarship and conclude/exit

Ideally, methods such as the COPM, which have been used to assess occupational performance, are repeated for comparison of findings before and after the implementation of a plan. A scholarly approach in this final action point is to conclude/exit services and to monitor what happens after occupational therapy is concluded. For example, we would investigate the following questions: What strategies are effective to ensure that an occupation-based program is a point on a trajectory of increasing satisfaction with occupational performance? Are gains made during occupational therapy maintained at a later date, or is some form of supplementary service — like a booster for immunization — needed to maximize the effect over time? What kinds of innovative programs and policies may be needed to allow clients to re-access their occupational performance at critical points in time?

Two recent scholarship developments are of tremendous assistance to describe, analyze, and test occupation-based enablement. First, as noted throughout this book, the worldwide adoption of the ICF (WHO, 2001) ensures that questions about engagement in valued occupations – which the ICF calls participation – will be viewed as important in health-related research. Similarities between the Canadian Model of Occupational Performance and Engagement (CMOP-E) and the ICF (see figure 1.4) may encourage occupational therapists to use this international, interdisciplinary language to communicate their practice and research questions. The ICF language offers a strategy to approach funding agencies and researchers from other fields (Stewart, 2002).

Second, the development of post-professional graduate, doctoral, and post-doctoral studies is preparing a new generation of occupational therapy and occupational science scholars. Occupational therapy is such a broad profession that master's, doctoral, and post-doctoral studies may encompass numerous fields, such as occupational therapy, occupational science, architecture, engineering, the humanities, rehabilitation science, and many others. With few post-professional degrees available that are specifically designated as occupational therapy or occupational science in Canada, the question of how best to build the profession's knowledge base is still being debated.

In Canada, 7.4% of the CAOT membership in 2004 (CAOT, 2005b) were engaged in scholarship as part of their jobs. For many occupational therapists working directly with clients, participation in research projects can be a valued adjunct to enrich, focus, and refine practice, providing new learning and personal development. Marjorie and Joe's positive experience in developing their first Critically Appraised Topic (CAT) enticed four of their colleagues to join them in doing another CAT, thereby showing how scholarly inquiry can invigorate occupational therapists. Emerging collaborative research models (Kielhofner et al., 2006) raise the profile of scholarship in practice. Direct service providers are learning to connect with academic occupational therapists (and vice versa) to jointly develop and answer research questions. Such collaboration can maximize research validity/trustworthiness and research utilization in the field. Collaborations between clients and occupational therapy researchers may range from seeking advice to full decision-making partnerships in participatory action research (Trentham & Cockburn, 2005). This type of research — along with other collaborative research strategies — is important to test the relevance of knowledge generation and transfer with those served by our profession.

11.3 Escalating participation in evidence-based practice in enabling occupation

Marjorie and Joe, like all occupational therapists, have an ethical and moral commitment to provide their clients with the best service possible. Occupational therapists need to access, critically reflect on, and communicate what is already known about best practice (Precin, 2002).

Not surprisingly, different models of health, wellness, and justice tend to be aligned with different forms of evidence, grounded in different research paradigms. Biomedicine and rehabilitation research have drawn heavily on quantitative, biological sciences to examine evidence of body function, disease, and impairment. In a medical context, evidence-based practice has been defined as "the conscientious, explicit and judicious use of current best evidence in making decisions about the care of individual patients. Evidence-based (practice) means integrating individual clinical expertise with the best available ... evidence from systematic research" (Sackett et al., 1996, p. 71).

In occupational therapy, a Joint Position Statement published by four of Canada's national occupational therapy organizations (CAOT, ACOTUP, ACOTRO, PAC, 1999) supports evidence-based practice focused on enabling occupation. The statement takes the same position on multiple forms of evidence as Whiteford (2005) did in cautioning the profession to be wary of "levels or hierarchy of evidence" (p. 38). The Canadian position is that "the occupational therapist provides knowledge of client, environment, and occupational factors relevant to enabling occupation. Ideally, this evidence is derived from a critical review of the research literature, expert consensus and professional experience" (CAOT et al., 1999, paragraph 3). The statement emphasizes that clients, from individuals to organizations, expect that occupational therapy practice will be based on evidence, that service will be provided by competent practitioners, and that approaches will be effective. Taking a broad view of evidence-based practice, the Canadian position guides practitioners to make practice decisions based on the results of good quality research, clinical reasoning, and other evidence. Decisions based on evidence inform a plan that is enriched by the occupational therapist's knowledge of the specific client's experience, explicitly expressed client perspectives, and occupational therapy judgment. In other words, occupational therapists are strongly reminded to look for and use professional reasoning well beyond quantitative evidence.

Evidence-based practice is integral to all forms of occupational therapy practice, from clinical work to management, education, consulting, policy analysis, and research. As with the integration of scholarship in practice (see table 11.1), the Canadian Practice Process Framework (CPPF) introduced in chapters 7 and 8, provides a framework to advance the integration of evidence in practice (see table 11.2).

Table 11.2   Integrating evidence in practice

Enter/initiate evidence-based practice
Generate or respond to a referral or request for services and clarify interests in requesting occupational therapy

Set the stage for evidence-based practice
a. Define scope, role, underlying theory, desired outcomes of practice

b. Develop research question to focus the search for evidence, with client participation where possible

Assess/evaluate the evidence
a. Gather literature, client's evidence, experiential knowledge of self and colleagues, evaluation of outcomes

b. Critical appraisal, relevance to practice environment, significance of data

Agree on objectives and plan for evidence-based practice
Communicate evidence to client, team, funders, and stakeholders in ways that are meaningful and that prompt mutual planning

Implement plan for evidence-based practice
Integrate evidence into practice with ongoing communication with client

Monitor/modify approach for evidence-based practice
Continue to search, evaluate, and use evidence to adjust services with client input

Evaluate outcome of evidence-based practice
Evaluate changes in practice with client input

Conclude/exit
Use evidence on exit, follow-up, community supports to educate client about future self-management and to educate communities, systems regarding opportunities

Adapted from Craik (2003), Egan et al. (1998), Head (2005), and Manojlovich (2006).

Enter/initiate and set the stage for evidence-based practice

Evidence-based practice starts with a referral or request for services. In order for the occupational therapist and others to proceed, it is at this stage that informed client consent is recorded; this is the first piece of evidence gathered in evidence-based practice and will form the basis of quality service. The scope, role, theoretical framework, values, beliefs, and desired outcomes need to be known or negotiated before developing the practice question/or questions to focus the quest for evidence. In an opening call for evidence, the following are potential questions: Are literature searches and other work to gather evidence funded as part of the referral or request?

In a client-professional collaboration, what agreement is needed on the types of evidence that will be valued and used? Once clarification of funding and other support have been established, one of the most important tasks in setting the stage is to define and document the scope of practice — and thus the scope of evidence — in the situation.

Assess/evaluate the evidence

Once one or more questions have been agreed upon by the client and the occupational therapist, they can turn their attention on the search for evidence that answers or is related to their question(s). Different questions will lead to different types of evidence. Quantitative evidence is found in systematic reviews or randomized controlled trials, and is most likely to inform questions about intervention effectiveness. General search databases such as those found within the Cochrane Library (http://www3.interscience.wiley.com/cgi-bin/mrwhome/106568753/HOME), are excellent for providing up-to-date systematic reviews and information about randomized controlled trials. Qualitative evidence is found in narratives, ethnographic stories, critiques and reflections, and is most likely to inform questions regarding human experiences and their meaning. Critical analyses of power and social structures will address questions about how an organization works, how some theories and practices dominate while others tend to be marginalized, and how policy, funding, and legislation determine what is possible in specific sociocultural, political, institutional, and economic contexts.

Using evidence in practice involves creating a culture of questioning and investigation, with practitioners and researchers working together to assess research information (Craik & Rappolt, 2003). In an evidence-based culture, research information, professional experience, and client knowledge and desires are woven together and documented to ensure that each client — whether an individual or organization — receives the most effective and appropriate services. The Web sites listed in table 11.3 are excellent sources of information about evidence-based practice in occupational therapy (web sites were current when consulted). As well, CAOT members have access to the CAOT Information Gateway. This is a specialized web-based tool designed to provide therapists with easily accessible resources for evidence-based

---

Table 11.3   Internet sources of evidence for occupational therapy

Evidence-based occupational therapy Web portal (http://www.otevidence.info)
* This Web portal has been designed in partnership with international colleagues to provide strategies, knowledge, and resources to aid occupational therapists in finding out about and using evidence

* **Resource Guide for Evidence-Based Rehabilitation Practice**
  Contains many rehabilitation-related evidence-based practice resource links (http://www.library.ualberta.ca/subject/evidencerehab/guide/index.cfm#sources)

* **Netting the Evidence (http://www.shef.ac.uk/scharr/ir/netting/)**
  Gives access to helpful evidence-based, health care-related organizations. Contains useful learning resources, such as an evidence-based virtual library, software, and journals

— By Mary Law

---

occupational therapy. The Information Gateway can be found online at http://www.caot.ca//default.asp?pageid=281.

When searching, one can easily become overwhelmed by the amount of evidence available. A focused and methodical search will not only save time, but will also make information easier to find. Critical appraisal of the literature and other evidence will guide decisions about whether the evidence is age-, gender-, or population-specific, and if the research is reliable and trustworthy. If the studies found are sufficiently relevant to the question and their quality is adequate to produce credible results, the information should be synthesized and applied to the practice question. Conversely, the evidence found may prompt revision of the question. Useful resources are listed in table 11.4, including a self-study guide on searching for evidence called ADEPT. The occupational therapy and rehabilitation databases in table 11.4 are also good places for occupational therapists to search for evidence (web sites were current when consulted).

Not all research is conducted with the same level of rigor — research articles, grey (unpublished) literature, experience, and other evidence need to be critically

---

Table 11.4   Evidence-based search strategies

- **Centre for Evidence Based Medicine** (http://www.cebm.net/levels_of_evidence.asp)

- **ADEPT** (http://www.shef.ac.uk/scharr/ir/adept.index.htm), a self-study guide to searching for evidence

- **OT Search — American Occupational Therapy Association** (http://www.aota.org/otsearch/index.asp), OT Search is a bibliographic database of occupational therapy literature as well as related subject areas

- **OTseeker: Occupational Therapy Systematic Evaluation of Evidence** (http://www.otseeker.com/default.htm), this database contains abstracts of systematic reviews and randomized controlled trials relevant to occupational therapy. Trials have been critically appraised and rated to assist you to evaluate their validity and interpretability

- **OTDBASE:** developed by a Canadian, Marilyn Ernest Conibear; an Internet-based indexing and abstracting service (http://thebishops.org/otdbase/FMPro?-lay=List&-db=otdbase_database. fp3&-format=search.htm&-FindAll)
  Note: available to faculty and students with access to Canadian university databases and to members of the Canadian Association of Occupational Therapists

- **OT Education Finder — Canadian Association of Occupational Therapists** (http://www.caot.ca/default.asp?pageid=1296), CAOT has created a database with periodicals, position statements, and papers including those from the *Canadian Journal of Occupational Therapy* and *Occupational Therapy Now*, dating back to 1998

- **OTCATs — Occupational Therapy Critically Appraised Topics** (http://www.otcats.com/index.html), OTCATs contains a series of critically appraised topics (or CATs) produced by occupational therapy students at the University of Western Sydney in Australia. A CAT is a short summary of evidence (less rigorous than a systematic review) on a topic of interest, usually focused around a clinical question

- **Critically Appraised Topics in Rehabilitation Therapy** (http://www.rehab.queensu.ca/cats/) CATs, prepared by graduate students in the School of Rehabilitation Therapy at Queen's University in Ontario, Canada, present another source of information
                                                                        — *By Mary Law*

Table 11.5   Checklists to critically appraise evidence

- **CASP** (http://www.phru.nhs.uk/casp/critical_appraisal_tools.htm), CASP is a critical appraisal skills program developed in the United Kingdom

- **McMaster University** (http://www-fhs.mcmaster.ca/rehab/ebp), McMaster University's Occupational Therapy Evidence-Based Practice Research Group developed this site focused on best practices in occupational therapy

- **OTseeker Tutorial** (http://www.otseeker.com/tutorial.htm), the OTseeker Tutorial explains how to examine a clinical study's results to see if an intervention is effective. Results need to be clinically significant, not just statistically significant

- **The American Occupational Therapy Association's Evidence-Based Practice (EBP) Resource Directory** (http://www.aota.org/memservices/login.aspx?PLACE=/memservices/ebp/index.aspx &Stay NET=Y)
  Note: available to members of the American Occupational Therapy Association

- **The American Occupational Therapy Association's Evidence Briefs Series**
  (http://www.aota.org/memservices/login.aspx?PLACE=/members/area15/evbriefs.asp)
  Note: available to members of the American Occupational Therapy Association

- **The American Occupational Therapy Foundation: Evidence Based Practice Self Study**
  (http://www.aotf.org/html/evidence.shtml)

- **OTdirect** (http://www.otdirect.co.uk/index.html)

— By Mary Law

appraised. Table 11.5 lists key resources and checklists to establish whether a research study has reached valid conclusions.

Mediate agreement on evidence for objectives and plans, and implement plan

Typical challenges to the implementation of evidence-based practice include lack of time, limited research skills, and poor or restricted access to literature as a routine part of work (Townsend, Le-May Sheffield, Stadnyk, & Beagan, 2006). Ideally, occupational therapists decide – in partnership with the client – on how to use available evidence in setting clear, focused objectives and plans for occupational therapy. Decisions about objectives and plans will include whether to act on available evidence and whether to act without evidence if none can be found. Is the evidence at hand relevant for this client, the occupations of concern, and the particular environment? The usefulness of research evidence in a particular situation is determined by many factors. With individual clients, for instance, considerations are the client's living environment, cultural beliefs, priorities, and values. In community development, occupational therapists and community representatives consider the socio-cultural values of the community, and the knowledge and skills of those involved. Other factors are the practice setting, professional expertise, involvement of team members, and the resources available to the occupational therapist.

Monitor/modify, evaluate outcome, and conclude/exit

Much has been written about research priorities and agendas, and the various barriers encountered by practitioners engaging in evidence-based occupational therapy(Cusick & McCluskey, 2000; Rappolt, 2003). The evidence-based practitioner needs to monitor and modify the search for, and use of, evidence. As well, organizational contexts that, as with Marjorie and Joe, do not readily support occupational therapists to integrate evidence in practice must be considered (Rehabilitation Outcomes Measurement System Vendor Survey II, 1999; Bowman & Llewellyn, 2002; Dubouloz, Egan, Vallerand, & von Zweck, 1999; Humphris, Littlejohns, Victor, O'Halloran, & Peacock, 2000).

Occupational therapists recognize the importance of evaluating the outcomes of their practice. A common struggle is to find the time and resources to do so. Evidence of the inhibiting effect of workload pressures, and in some cases inadequate human resources, is repeatedly cited by occupational therapists. Pringle (1996) reported that occupational therapists are subject to organizational changes that can increase or limit freedom to structure their workload to include outcome evaluation and evidence. Evidence can be found on how the imposed demands of non-patient/non-client contact activities — such as administrative duties and the collection of routine statistics — reduce the time available for direct client work and professional reflection (Hollis & Madill, 2006; Hunter & Nicol, 2002; Townsend et al., 2006). Craik, Austin, & Schell (1999) noted that the move to community-based mental health services, has resulted in a loss of professional leadership and the fragmentation of mental health services, as occupational therapy services are often absent beyond acute care settings. Occupational therapists need to be vigilant and collaborate with managers to ensure that evidence on occupation and enablement is used to monitor and modify programs, evaluate outcomes, and plan an exit strategy with follow-up and links to relevant community supports. To address the real-life occupational issues of concern and the enablement approaches required in enabling occupation, evidence on length of hospital stay or impairment outcomes for example is woefully insufficient.

11.4 Getting involved in scholarship and evidence-based practice

Canadian occupational therapists already possess a considerable amount of information about scholarship, evidence-based practice, barriers and enablers, the process of evidence-based occupational therapy, and suggestions for increasing our use of evidence in practice (Craik & Rappolt, 2003; Manojlovich, 2006; Rappolt, 2003). Despite such knowledge, occupational therapists like Marjorie and Joe struggle to get involved in scholarship and evidence-based practice. One way of getting involved is to use the CMOP-E for self-reflection (see Figure 11.1).

Figure 11.1 The occupation of getting involved in evidence-based practice

Occupation
- Evidence integral to choice of occupation
- Promotes practice effectiveness
- Enhances accountability for practice
- Maintains standards of practice
- Provides framework for evidence
- Contributes to body of knowledge

Environment
- Time
- Access to evidence
- Supports for evaluation
- Mentoring
- Context for practice
- Culture

Person
- Belief in value of evidence-based practice, program evaluation, and research
- Skills
- Confidence
- Practice knowledge and experience

— Adapted from Mary Manojlovich (2006) & Brenda Head (2005)

The occupation of getting involved in scholarship and/or evidence-based practice

The question to ask is: How might I get involved in scholarship and/or evidence-based practice? Getting involved may begin by learning to search, critique, and synthesize literature and other sources of evidence to answer a practice question. Getting involved in scholarship may mean many things: organizing data for program evaluation, collecting client data for a researcher, or participating in or leading an externally-funded research project. In Canada, 7.4% of occupational therapists (CAOT, 2005b) who belonged to the Canadian Association of Occupational Therapists in 2004, declared that their primary work was research. For most occupational therapists who are interested in scholarly work but devote the majority of their time to direct client services, collaboration with full-time researchers is a manageable way to be involved in critical appraisal and synthesis of research evidence, program evaluation, and the testing of theory in practice.

Occupation factors which are inherent to evidence-based practice and scholarship, can facilitate or limit this occupation. In reflecting on occupation factors in scholarship and evidence-based practice, occupational therapists might consider these questions: How may engagement in scholarship and evidence-based practice expand or refine my choices about ways to practice? How may evidence be used to develop greater effectiveness and accountability in practice? How may time and space be managed to make participation in scholarship and/or evidence-based practice a more manageable component of everyday practice? What opportunities exist naturally in this occupation to use evidence, and to organize and manage data already being collected?

In terms of *person factors*, self-reflection might spark questions like these: What are the strongest motivating factors to integrate scholarship and evidence in practice? What beliefs and values will guide evidence-based inquiries or scholarship? What

Positioning occupational therapy for leadership

is the knowledge and skill base for involving clients or drawing on client/consumer knowledge? What expertise — attitudes, knowledge, and skills — will be needed to engage in scholarship and/or evidence-based practice? How might skills be developed to define practice from an occupational perspective, develop practice questions, locate and appraise the evidence, integrate evidence into practice, evaluate the outcomes, and communicate the new knowledge to the client, team, and funder? What professional reasoning will support recommended changes in patterns of practice that may involve changes for the whole team?

Self-reflection on *environment factors* might raise the following questions: What resources are needed (space, computers, information technology support services, and Internet connections without firewall restraints)? Who will make good partners (examples of partners to consider are client groups with interests in research, students with Internet and library skills, health professionals with research experience, and academic scholars)? What challenges need to be addressed if the necessary supports for scholarship and evidence-based practice are not present in the work environment? How might advocacy help to change the environment, to make time to reflect on practice, read and evaluate the literature, search the Web, network with colleagues, consider client experience, document evidence, and make changes in practice? How might library and technology resources be organized for timely access to the literature and education on the use of technology? Who else (if anyone) in the same setting is already using methods to collect and analyze data for practice evaluation? What mentoring is available to assist in making appropriate decisions about design and methodology in research? Occupational therapists are more likely to engage in scholarly and evidence-based practice in a workplace that already values, models, and supports these activities (Craik & Rappolt, 2003; Hollis, Madill, Darrah, Warren, & Rivard, 2006; Manojlovich, 2006).

Management strategies to integrate scholarship and evidence in a process of practice may be needed to create the necessary work environment. A strategy used successfully in one workplace for example, involved the introduction of practice development groups as forums for evidence-based practice discussions. Discussions identified sources of evidence appropriate to the needs of the group, and helped group members develop documents to support the transfer of knowledge into practice. Key to the success of these groups was the structure introduced by a skilled facilitator; the facilitator kept the process going and enabled therapists to overcome roadblocks, which might otherwise have discouraged them from continuing or even starting the process (Head, 2005). In this same workplace, reflection on the theory underlying practice — that is to say, adopting an occupational perspective and enablement reasoning — had previously been overlooked. This new way of approaching practice became critical to the development of questions that guided the search for evidence. The practice development group provided an environment that welcomed innovation and change. Management provided support for questioning practice, and supported therapists in being open to debate and questioning. It was an intentional process that required time and commitment, but it was successful in changing the culture of practice in this workplace.

Another strategy may be to develop reciprocal arrangements between practitioners in the field, and faculty and students in academic occupational therapy programs. A new opportunity has emerged for advancing scholarship and evidence-based practice by collaborating with students in Canada's new master's, entry-level, occupational therapy curricula. These graduate programs are rich in educational content for evidence-based practice, program evaluation, and research. In the same way, academic and fieldwork courses can be enhanced by seeking the involvement of practitioners who bring real life experiences and their own expertise to the class-room. University faculty-preceptor-student fieldwork collaborations can provide opportunities for new learning for the occupational therapist in the field, and it can greatly enhance student learning. Students can be sources of expertise about technology and Web-based resources, and can teach therapists how to use technology when it is integrated as part of fieldwork. Occupational therapy programs can create partnerships with preceptors to provide access to the university library holdings and, potentially, distance technologies for communication and networking among occupational therapists. Employers whose mission includes research, may welcome and support collaborations, particularly when they enhance occupational therapy recruitment and retention while building scholarly practice.

Occupational therapists as well as clients and stakeholders will certainly benefit from evidenced-based practice and scholarship. A key point in positioning occupational therapy for leadership is to be explicit about different values around scholarship and evidence (see text box 11.3).

Text box 11.3

Reflections on different values around scholarship and evidence

What kinds of scholarship and evidence are most valued where you work? Are there some who express different points of view about scholarship and evidence? What are their points of view, and what socio-cultural beliefs and values are they expressing? How are the dominant beliefs and values about scholarship and evidence put forward so that they are likely to prevail in decision making? What limits the credibility of alternate points of view in your work setting?

Where do you stand in your beliefs and values about scholarship and evidence? How do your views fit with what tends to be highly valued in your work setting when it comes to decision making about clients, funding, policies, or programs?

— By Brenda Beagan

Chapter 12

Accountability for enabling occupation: Discovering opportunities

Elizabeth A. Townsend
Andrew Freeman
Lili Liu
Judy Quach
Susan Rappolt
Annette Rivard

CASE 12 Esther's story of managing accountability

Esther is a registered occupational therapist who is manager of rehabilitation services in a large regional health authority. She reports to Carol White, a nurse who is the program coordinator of medicine and surgery. The end of the fiscal year is approaching, and Carol has indicated that crucial decisions regarding staff levels are required. Esther knows that two occupational therapy staff positions are on the line for cuts, because case numbers and direct contact time per case are regularly lower for occupational therapists than for physiotherapists, respiratory therapists, recreational therapists, and support personnel in rehabilitation services. Esther arranges to meet with all the rehabilitation services team leaders and follow up with the occupational therapy team leaders Gina and Martha.

The occupational therapists' primary strategy to critically review the value of their team is to prepare a report, "Accounting for Enabling Occupation," which will include the following sections: an executive summary to educate the health authority about effectiveness and efficiency of participatory approaches (client-centred enablement) with an occupational perspective on rehabilitation goals; an analysis of existing re-admissions to rehabilitation services over the last five years; satisfaction survey data; data from the Statistics Canada Web site on the costs of long-term disability; and evidence on population outcomes associated with occupational therapy from an evidence-based occupational therapy Web portal (http://www.otevidence. info). The report will also include plans for a long-term strategy to collaborate with a local social scientist, who, captivated by the field of occupational science, initiated a longitudinal study to collect "best and worst case stories of occupational disruption and transformation in a rural community." Esther must now negotiate with Carol to hold the line on the occupational therapy staff budget for six months until the "Accounting for Enabling Occupation" report is available.

— *Adapted from Andrew Freeman and Lynn Stewart*

12.1 Introduction

Those who make their occupational perspective publicly known are well positioned to be accountable for enabling occupation. Chapter 12 explores accountability for enabling occupation so as to make our contributions better known, funded, and otherwise supported within systems and society. The proposed strategy for leadership in accountability is to critically reflect on the structures and processes of power: to be aware of the influence and power of documentation in decision making; and, to use documentation strategically to evaluate and refine the quality of practice, refocusing continually on enabling occupation.

12.2 Professional autonomy issues in a biomedical context

A hallmark of professional autonomy is accountability for the effectiveness of practice (Freidson, 2001; Hall, 1968). Accountability is a powerful tool to define what *counts* (matters) (Stein, 2001; Waring, 1988). Occupational therapy team leaders, like Gina and Martha, develop their enablement skills to collaborate, consult, and coordinate while engaging with others; at the same time, they must retain their ethical and professional responsibilities for enabling useful and meaningful occupational outcomes with clients. In developing new accountability systems, Gina and Martha might want to learn more about accountability issues such as the biomedical context of practice, program evaluation, quality assurance, and professional regulation.

Defined simply, accountability refers to the responsibility to give account of, and answer for, the discharge of duties or conduct (*Oxford English Dictionary*, 1989). The traditional basis of health professionals' accountability is their special duty of fidelity to their clients by virtue of their clients' vulnerability (Pellegrino, 2002). Accountability in working with agency, organization, community, or population clients requires adaptation of this special duty of fidelity to a collective body and society instead of to individuals.

Health professionals are facing growing accountability demands (Donaldson, 2001), which are legitimized by professional decisions incurring health and other service costs (Morreim, 2001) that may not always be well justified (Wenneberg, 2004). As an occupational therapy manager, Esther navigates the paradoxical position of being accountable to others while also retaining professional autonomy. While cooperating and collaborating with others, professionals are also accountable for best practices to serve the public, based on their specific knowledge and skills. They may also be responsible for advocacy, which although positioning occupational therapy more explicitly within accountability systems, also requires attention to documentation; as a consequence, practising client-centred, evidence-based practice requires that the occupational therapist become acquainted with documentation and documentation practices.

Documentary processes are used to manage modern institutions, such as health services. Efficiency, safety, liability, cost control, personnel management, consent, codes of ethics, protection of privacy, supervision, public relations, and other processes are all managed through documents, not by direct observation or supervision (Smith, 2005). Although documentation may seem to be an innocuous and dreary part of practice, choices about what to document and how to use the data have a powerful influence in determining whether or not occupational therapy is accountable for enabling occupation.

Occupational therapists make daily choices about documentation by complying with the routine, taken-for-granted documentation of workloads, admissions, discharges, and other data. It is true that making such choices is largely automatic and unquestioned, with little time to reflect. Moreover, advocacy to reduce systematic barriers may be unthinkable for many occupational therapists if they risk losing their position and salary. It is also true, however, that becoming conscious of the power of documentation is a strategy to develop occupational therapy leadership.

The occupational therapy workforce in Canada is primarily funded by health services (see chapters 13 and 14). The implication is that occupational therapy is, for the most part, accountable to the powerful biomedical system, which operates through a medico-business paradigm. Accountability systems are organized to manage costs for impairment-based diagnoses and treatments, and emergency health management. Understandably, the primary data of interest are those that guide decisions for cost containment. Evidence collected is primarily quantitative, and the emphasis is on the effectiveness, efficiency, and cost-benefits of producing diagnostically-based outcomes in body function. The accountability data of greatest interest are direct contact time, length of hospital or clinic stay, and time and costs of diagnostic and treatment procedures for specific categories of disease. These data place occupational therapy at a disadvantage: they do not capture the full scope of enabling occupation, which goes beyond isolated acts to diagnose and treat functional limitations, which, unfortunately, cannot be accomplished as quickly (Cockerill, Scott, & Wright, 1996).

Typically, accountability data on occupational outcomes, (e.g., management of self care, return to work, or ability to live at home with a chronic illness) are viewed as worthwhile from a quality of life perspective. Furthermore, client-centred enablement, family- and patient-centred care, and collaborative health initiatives are becoming the standard expectation of Canadians who want to participate in decisions about their health and health services. However, our horizontal, collaborative occupational and enablement models (see figures 1.3 and 4.3) operate contrary to hierarchically organized biomedical structures (Townsend et al., 2003). Our concerns as a profession and the accountability data that would record the work of enabling occupation do not easily fit with current,biomedical accountability systems.

Occupational therapy is not alone in facing the challenges of making occupational outcomes and enabling processes relevant and accountable in the health sector; being at odds with the existing power relations can be overwhelming (Griffin, 2001). Alternatively, critical awareness of the difference between collaborative and hierarchical power structures, and between occupational and biomedical models of health, can be liberating. Four strategies can position occupational therapy leadership for enabling occupation with others who are concerned with the non-medical promotion of health.

The first strategy is to build alliances with others who recognize the necessity of new forms of accountability for health, well-being, and justice through occupation. We know that the biomedical model does not explain how health and disability are experienced (Engel, 1977), nor do biomedical practices adequately promote health (Epp, 1986; Lalonde, 1974; Romanow, 2002). Our occupational model aligns strongly with social models of health (Barer, Marmor, & Evans, 1994). Occupational and social models are consistent with the *Ottawa Charter for Health Promotion*'s (World Health Organization, 1986) call for health services and societies to act beyond the medical treatment of disease. A biopsychosocial view of health, which incorporates biological, psychological, and social factors (Cooper, Stevenson, & Hale, 1996), is now championed in many fields (Turner, 2000). Generally accepted accountability processes — such as functional outcome measurement — increasingly use multiple forms of evidence not limited to quantitative data. Client perspectives and professional judgment are gaining recognition (Craik & Rappolt, 2003; Pearson, Wiechula, Court, & Lockwood, 2005; Rappolt, 2003).

As emphasized throughout this book, the *International Classification of Functioning, Disability and Health*'s (ICF) (World Health Organization, 2001) view of health, has various components in common with the occupational model of health that underpins enabling occupation (Stamm et al., 2006). The ICF could be used as an accountability tool — a diagrammatic and linguistic bridge to visually connect bio-medical interests in impairments on a continuum with activity, social participation, and occupational engagement (see table 1.3 for a comparison of the CMOP-E and ICF). With like-minded partners, we can contribute the trademarks that are essential elements of occupational therapy — knowledge, skills, and attitudes — to address occupational challenges, find occupational solutions, enable client-centred priorities, draw on multidisciplinary knowledge, and apply comprehensive thinking using abductive reasoning. Occupational therapy is a profession whose time has come.

A second strategy is to build a body of knowledge to make occupational enablement more explicit (Backman, 2005; Wood, 1996). Occupational therapists can advance the profession's vision by building a body of evidence on occupational outcomes and enabling occupation (Egan et al., 1998; Whiteford, 2005). Hocking (2001) asserted that we best demonstrate our interests in occupation through evaluations of occupational performance, beyond performance components.

A third strategy is to ask critical questions: What might occupational therapy services that enable occupation actually look like? What administrative infrastruc-tures best support the enablement of occupation, beyond traditional health services structures? What would accountability look like for the increasing number of occupational therapists who work at organizational and policy levels, instead of with individual clients? Further evolution will require the development of compe-tency-based accountability frameworks that generate data on what occupational therapists actually do in enabling occupation.

A fourth strategy is to gather data on the costs, cost-effectiveness, and cost-benefits of enabling occupation. It is true that gathering, interpreting, and analyzing data make it difficult for professionals to fulfill their obligations to clients, given the administrative efforts required to monitor and control rising costs (Robins, 2001; Walker, 2001). Nevertheless, occupational therapists are starting to demonstrate their responsibility in evaluating costs while maintaining standards and being responsive to clients. Collaboration among occupational therapists, managers, and economists could produce new accountability models to raise awareness of the economic value and social capital in enabling occupation (Whiteford, 2005).

Landry and Mathews (1998) support economic evaluation as an approach to deter-mine the economic value (worth or importance) of an outcome, given the cost of a service. They describe *cost-minimization* as a comparison of two or more services to identify the least costly one; cost-effectiveness is a calculation of cost per unit of improvement in functional independence; *cost-utility* is an analysis of scenarios to decide how to allocate limited staff resources; and *cost-benefit* is a sum of costs against measurable benefits. Economic evaluation data allow comparisons of the costs and consequences of alternative programs or services; comparisons can examine the relative worth of alternatives using cost-minimization, cost-effectiveness, cost-utility, or cost-benefit calculations (Drummond, O'Brien, Stoddart, & Torrance, 1997).

To illustrate a potential use of economic evaluation in occupational therapy, consider the following. It has been established through research that economic status is the most important determinant of health (Evans, Barer, & Marmor, 1994; Public Health Agency of Canada, 2004). Low-income Canadians die earlier and experience more illnesses than Canadians with higher incomes regardless of age, sex, race, and place of residence (Raphael, 2004). It follows that cost minimization, cost-effectiveness, cost-utility, and cost-benefit calculations of enabling occupation with low- and high-income Canadians would produce useful data. Conversely, the costs of *not* including occupational therapy for enabling occupation in health services would be useful. Studies could evaluate the savings when this profession is included, for example, in hospital admission and discharge planning, or in the development of employment accommodations for those unemployed because of disability or chronic illness. As a profession, we could develop cost-minimization alternatives that address socio-economic status and income level. Low-income clients with or without disabilities may want to prioritize collective action in community and economic development occupations, to improve their socio-economic status and weekly incomes. Higher-income adults and older clients may ask that occupational therapists focus more on leisure occupations. They may also want to help others through volunteer occupations.

The challenges and opportunities in using these four strategies are worth studying as the subject of accountability is central for shaping the future of occupational therapy. With increasing bureaucratic control of standards and resources, occupational thera-pists may experience strong pressure to reduce, refine, or even increase the scope of practice, by consulting for example, rather than working through direct client contact (Freeman, McWilliam, MacKinnon, Rappolt, & DeLuca, June 2006). Resource reduc-tions may prompt a downward spiral in which occupational therapists struggle to accomplish even the most technical, narrow interpretation of practice, such as providing assistive technology without the time for a quality assessment and follow-up. Resource reductions are certainly not the only driving force that narrows practice. In Alberta, where resources are far more plentiful than in many other regions of Canada, new health funds are still directed to basic science research, and high-technology and high-profile medical procedures such as islet cell transplants. Currently, more health fund-ing in Alberta seems to produce only more of the same, as in expanding the numbers of traditionally structured, long-term care beds (Hollis et al., 2006).

An opportunity that may present itself to make enabling occupation explicit in accountability systems, is to know when to hold the line and to learn to recognize when to advocate for change when services are unable to produce desired outcomes; in other words: to know when to speak or not speak up. The message is that some-times we need to compromise. This position is pragmatic, but it comes with a warn-ing: in the pressured context of today's rising costs for medical tests and treatments, health services will understandably give priority funding to the measurable elements of health practices, with little funding to attend to the whole person and their envi-ronment (Valkenburg et al., 2003).

Another opportunity may be to seek public support to influence spending priorities in health services. Clients, regulatory bodies, and courts expect professionals to exercise autonomous, professional judgment. Occupational therapy professional judgment is to enable engagement in human occupation as necessary for survival of humankind. Occupational therapists might profile the ineffectiveness of some forms of standardization and cost restraint. For instance, cost restraint to omit occupational therapy services or to support only ineffective enablement (see figures 4.4 and 4.5) will deprive societies of a profession dedicated to health, well-being, and justice through occupation.

Occupational therapists might search for literature to explain the limitations of a health system that only offers impairment reduction. Efforts to predict health service resource allocation may emphasize standardized clinical pathways to control costs (Kravitz, Duan, & Braslow, 2004; Timmermans & Berg, 1997). Conceptual, generic practice guidelines, such as those offered in this book, tend to advance best practice (Blain & Townsend, 1993; Burgers, Grol, Klazinga, Mäkelä, & Zaat, 2003). The danger to occupational therapy lies in prescriptive guidelines, which can become a management tool to maximize the predictability of resource allocation, often based on measurable biomedical outcomes for accountability. Prescriptive guidelines may merely increase professional responsibility to account for expenditures (Armstrong et al., 2000; Degeling, Maxwell, Kennedy, & Coyle, 2003; Robins, 2001). Used in isolation from other evidence, clinical pathways and prescriptive guidelines potentially reduce professional autonomy and best practice. It follows that reduced autonomy in standardized practice can dehumanize services, as noted by Stein (2001) in her Massey Lecture *The Cult of Efficiency*. Her mother was described to Stein as an "outlier" when her needs for nursing were different from those of other patients. These and other stories that profile the narrowness of biomedicine ignoring everyday life, are essential for occupational therapists to publicize.

Overall, the idea is to develop accountability for enabling occupation with both a short- and a long-term view. Enabling occupation may not always be the least costly alternative or have measurable benefit in the short run. In some short-term situations, such as discharge planning and crisis management, *brief occupation-based enablement* may be the least costly alternative with accompanying measurable benefits. The least costly alternative and most measurable benefit may result from employing occupational therapists to enable people to stay at home or continue their work, rather than incurring the immediate and extensive costs of institutional care or lost economic productivity.

To reshape accountability, occupational therapists might present themselves as belonging to a **translational profession**: translate the ideas, language, practice, and research methods between the everyday world and the medical world. We know how the medical world works and can translate medical terms, diagnoses, and treatment expectations into possibilities for occupational engagement outside bio-medicine. Our medical knowledge is invaluable for working with individual, family, group, community, organization, and population clients. We can interpret the occupational consequences of disease, impairment, and disability. Conversely, within the medical world, we know how everyday life works: can translate the occupational demands and affordances of everyday life to clients, health professionals, community members and others. We know the influences of the environment and of persons on occupations, and the requirementsfor successful occupational engagement in employment, housing, transportation, school, and other settings. Our assessment methods are becoming increasingly sophisticated in providing data for predicting self-management, return to work, and successful community living with an impairment, chronic illness, disability, or participation restriction. This is not strictly quality of life data; for example, the information collected may also be used to predict hospital re-admissions, an area of concern in the medico-business world. Possible professional autonomy issues in a biomedical context include the development of greater occupational therapy leadership, given the essential nature of occupation for human existence.

12.3 Accountability opportunities in program evaluation and quality assurance

Occupational therapists, such as Gina and Martha, ideally seek opportunities to coordinate services for efficiency, align services with targeted service goals, and contain costs. In a biomedical context, we will want to expand accountability data beyond biomedical concerns. Our best strategies in program evaluation and quality assurance are (as noted in 12.2): to develop alliances; generate a body of evidence; raise critical questions; and analyze the cost benefits of occupation-based enablement. In balancing accountability requirements with professional autonomy, occupational therapy will need to exercise leadership in program evaluation and quality assurance.

Program evaluation is different from client evaluation; it involves collecting, analyzing, and interpreting data about a program. Program evaluation determines if program goals and objectives were met. Evaluation data can be used to inform service providers and make decisions, plan, or justify resources for stages of evaluation of outcomes for a program (Law et al., 2005, pp. 40-44). Program evaluation encompasses program planning and design as a framework for evaluation. Program evaluation can take on many different approaches, depending on the purposes of evaluation (examples include needs assessment, cost benefits, or client satisfaction evaluations). An outcome-based program evaluation examines the impacts on clients and costs, for example, of a particular intervention or program.

Quality assurance refers to "maintenance of quality (of a program or service) by constant measuring and comparison to set standards" (Jacobs, 1999, p. 121). The discussion here focuses on quality assurance as a core component in continuous quality improvement. Continuous monitoring of evaluation and other accountability data management are used to improve the quality of services beyond the evaluation of specific programs.

While program evaluations determine if program goals are met, quality assurance is broader. The Donabedian (1966, 1994) framework for quality assurance encompasses the structure, processes, and outcomes of a program or service. Guidelines, indicators, protocols, and standards are examples of quality assurance tools that are used to guide reviews for quality assurance. Audits, certification, and accreditation structures may be mandatory or voluntary. For example, the Canadian Association of Occupational Therapists' academic accreditation of university, entry-level occupational therapy programs is mandatory. Data on workload measurement, a client's length of stay in hospital or a clinic, and quality indicators on a Minimum Data Set (MDS) (Hirdes & Carpenter, 1997) are also examples of routine, mandatory data collection. The MDS tracks minimum indicators and does not replace in-depth client assessments based on profession-specific expertise.

As professionals working in inter-professional environments, occupational therapists face many challenges when introducing program evaluation and quality assurance indicators related to enabling occupation. For example, client outcomes cannot be entirely explained by the performance or time invested by any occupational therapist. Indeed, the strength of an enabling occupation framework lies in diverse and extensive collaboration, with the client at the core, while the success of an occupational therapy program depends on accountability at individual, team, community, government, and societal levels. This and other challenges raise questions about the autonomy of occupational therapists developing accountability in our own practice.

Businesses may wish to enhance their credibility and competitive edge through voluntary compliance with program evaluation and quality assurance standards set out by bodies such as the Canadian Standards Association International (CSA International) or the International Standards Organization (ISO). In health services, the Balanced Scorecard Performance System, which originated in business, is an example of a voluntary approach used in quality assurance. One can also use the five principles of successful organizations described by Kaplan and Norton (1992). These principles have been adopted by Ontario Public Health (Woodward, Manuel, & Goel, 2004) and are articulated in health services terminology: (a) strategy; (b) health determinants and status; (c) community engagement; (d) resources and services; and (e) integration and responsiveness. Occupational therapists could frame questions and indicators, and build strategic alliances so that occupation-based questions might become part of quality assurance standards.

Given the emphasis on impairments, body, and individual persons in a biomedical context, it is not surprising that measures for performance components abound and that occupational therapists often use them to guide practice and demonstrate accountability. To counter the strong trend in biomedical contexts to focus on the body and person, occupational therapists are urged to consider client evaluations of occupation and the environment, which can be collected for program evaluation as illustrated in the following examples.

Occupational therapy researchers are gradually leading the development of measures that produce empirical accountability data on occupation, including client perspectives. The accountability opportunity in using such measures is to contribute to occupational therapy's top-down, client-centred, occupation-based perspective on real life in biomedical contexts — which tend to concentrate on bottom-up components. The *COPM* (Law et al., 2005) and the *Assessment of Motor and Process Skills* (AMPS) (Nygard, Bernspang, Fisher, & Winblad, 1994) both provide occupation-based data on individuals. For program evaluation and quality assurance, data from these tools can be collected, reported, debated, and ultimately used to inform evidence-based practice and the development of practice guidelines.

International researchers are showing leadership in developing occupation-based measures that focus on the environment. The School Setting Interview (SSI) (Hemmingsson, Egilson, Hoffman, & Kielhofner, 2005) generates data on the school environment, including physical accessibility, the support provided by teacher assistants, and parental and school resources. Iwarsson and Slaug (2001) developed The Enabler and are using it in interdisciplinary research with European colleagues to examine old age participation in community environments. Fisher (1994), who works from the USA and Sweden, has challenged occupational therapists to develop and use measures that reflect our unique perspective.

Qualitative data needs to be used for accountability in program evaluation or quality assurance. Occupational therapy researchers have long recognized the importance of narrative phenomenological and interpretative data (Yerxa, 1967, 1991b). A prime example is the growing use of client stories in evaluation, such as stories of transformative learning (Ashe et al., 2005; Dubouloz et al., 2004), and stories of the value to clients of having a voice and an affirming environment (Rebeiro, 2001). Critical analyses of the context (the environment) of occupational therapy practice are scarce, and are not widely used in occupational therapy program evaluation and quality assurance as yet. However, data are starting to emerge to evaluate and monitor occupational therapy in different economic contexts (Jongbloed & Wendland, 2002). Data to evaluate and monitor the impact of the regulatory context on occupational therapy are becoming available in some jurisdictions, such as Ontario (Rappolt, Williams, Lum, Deber, Verrier, & Landry, 2004). Data to evaluate and monitor power relations and the impact of institutional governance policies, from admissions to accountability methods and budgets, are starting to emerge. One example of such data is from the critical analysis generated through an institutional ethnography (Townsend, 1998, 2003; Townsend & Wilcock, 2004a). Critical analyses raise awareness in occupational therapists and others about opportunities and limits for developing data on occupation and enablement for program evaluation and quality assurance.

Quantitative data are, of course, important in occupational therapy as well. Yet occupational therapists need to go beyond quantitative workload measurements, analyses of length of stay, and minimum data sets. In this age of information management, occupational therapists might think critically about occupation-based information and enablement information. The Canadian Institute for Health Information (CIHI) and the field of health informatics are two avenues to explore what quantitative data exist and what might be gathered to better account for enabling occupation.

Consistent with regulated practice standards, program evaluation and quality assurance are integral components of service provision. Using reports to negotiate work time and funding, as Gina and Martha (see case 12) are doing, would help to strategically position occupational therapy to become more accountable for enabling occupation.

12.4 Accountability opportunities in occupational therapy regulation

Professionals exercise autonomy through their expertise in applying abstract and technical knowledge to the cases or clients they take on (Freidson, 1970, 1994). While exercising autonomy, professionals must also demonstrate accountability. How can professionals reconcile the exercise of autonomy with demands for accountability? The paradox is managed through the mechanism of professional self-regulation. Governments delegate authority to a regulatory college to ensure that registrants of a profession carry out their practices in the interests of their clients and the public at large. Regulatory colleges have two strategies for managing the tensions between professional autonomy and accountability: quality assurance programs, including standards and guidelines to promote individual practitioners' self-regulation; and systems for investigation, remediation, and discipline.

Occupational therapists want to exercise professional autonomy in enabling occupation (CAOT, 1997a, 2002). The opportunities to become more explicitly accountable for enabling occupation are to develop data on occupation and enablement, and to strategically use the data in following guidelines and regulatory requirements for transparency, confidentiality, consent, professional boundaries, open communication, and avoidance of conflict of interest. Since occupational therapists are self-regulated professionals, we are also subject to the accountability provisions established by our regulatory colleges, who act in the public interest (Tuohy, 2003).

Three forces are converging to bring accountability to the forefront for occupational therapists: standards of practice stipulated by regulatory colleges; administrative benchmarks and limits set by managers; and escalating demands for accountability by consumers (Allsop & Saks, 2002; Degeling et al., 2003). To establish standards of practice, all 10 provincial occupational therapy regulatory colleges in Canada[1] refer to the competency framework called *Essential Competencies of Practice for Occupational Therapy in Canada* (ACOTRO, 2003). The seven units of essential competency identified by ACOTRO have been mapped with those established in the *Profile of Occupational Therapy Practice in Canada* (CAOT, 2007) (see text box 12.1). Moreover, the units of competence in the *Profile* have been mapped with the 10 enablement skills found in section II (see table 4.7 and text box 4.6). Differences between the ACOTRO *Essential Competencies*, the CAOT *Profile*, and the enablement skills, reflect the different interests of regulatory colleges, professional organizations, and professional guidelines for practice. Regulatory colleges are mandated to maintain the standards of professional practice to protect the public, while professional organizations are mandated to promote excellence in professional practice. Regulatory colleges use competency frameworks for quality assurance and to organize educational materials regarding professional accountability for self-regulation. Some colleges provide practice scenarios and other tools for individuals to monitor the quality of their practice. Professional organizations, such as CAOT,

---

[1] Canada's northern territories do not yet regulate occupational therapy.

Competency roles and skills for accountability

The Profile of Occupational Therapy Practice in Canada (CAOT, 2007) includes the following seven roles: collaborator, communicator, change agent, practice manager, scholarly practitioner, professional, and expert in enabling occupation.

Where enabling occupation is not explicit, the occupational therapist might draw on the change agent and practice manager roles to collaborate and communicate with others, and to negotiate acceptance and inclusion of new indicators and evidence. The occupational therapist might negotiate accountability indicators and evidence with other team members and managers, and advocate as a change agent in redesigning program evaluation or quality assurance for continuous quality improvement. The scholarly practitioner and professional roles might be used to accelerate the integration of scholarship and evidence as a routine part of both everyday practice and program evaluation.

The occupational therapist might actively engage some clients, who are interested and prepared to do so, as participants in documenting their own narratives, goals, and outcomes.

use practice guidelines, such as this book, and competency frameworks, such as the *Profile*, to stimulate learning, critical reflection, and professional development by members both individually and collectively.

Administrative benchmarks and escalating consumer demands for accountability could be inspired by the competency framework of the regulatory colleges and professional organizations. Occupational therapy leadership in enabling occupation will advance by developing evidence and accountability systems specific to the interests of administrators, funders, client groups, and the public.

12.5 Ethical and moral issues in being accountable

Accountability is expected by virtue of professional status and the social contract that professionals have with those they serve (Cruess et al., 2004). In other words, professional autonomy requires more than the exercise of power and expertise: professionals must uphold and adhere to specified values, and the competent, discretionary use of expert knowledge and skills.

Professional values and behaviours were defining features in claiming professional autonomy long before the establishment of professional regulatory bodies. Regulatory legislation was developed in part to inform and assure the public about the responsibilities, competency, and integrity expected of professionals. In Canada, the ethical aspect of professionalism is addressed in the codes of ethics of national and provincial professional associations. Certainly, the practice of enabling occupation is subject to workplace challenges. Codes of ethics are a guide to managing such challenges. For example, the updated CAOT Code of Ethics states that occupational therapists must engage in moral agency that is respectful of her or his own values and their influence on how practice is accomplished (CAOT, 2007). Congruent with client-centred enablement and Canada's Joint Statement on Evidence-based Practice (CAOT et al., 1999), the CAOT Code of Ethics stipulates that practice must respect the stories and lived experiences of the client, and must not cause injury nor create or foster false expectations (CAOT, 2007).

Occupational therapists also make an ethical and moral commitment to base practice decisions on scholarship, and on multiple types of evidence including client experience, program evaluation, and quality assurance to avoid unnecessary or irrelevant services that consume a client's time and energy, as well as private or public funds.

Distributive justice and the reality of finite resources demand that services be available to those for whom there is evidence of demonstrated benefit. Ever-increasing demands on limited human resources require that occupational therapists decide who they will take on as clients, who will wait for services, and who will go without occupational therapy. Decisions such as these must be ethically justifiable, not based only on cost-minimization.

Ethical and moral imperatives require that occupational therapists employ enablement skills to collaborate, consult, and coordinate with others, while applying the competency roles expected of a scholarly practitioner and professional. The occupational therapist is expected to act as a moral agent on behalf of others in everyday, ethical practice and in potentially conflicting situations. An important aim is to ensure an efficacious allocation of services and resources. Rapid change, scarce resources, the prolific emergence of new technology, and a growing emphasis on risk management affect today's health and other service fields. Occupational therapists face a triple challenge of simultaneous demands: to use new and innovative approaches to involve clients in enabling occupation in order to uphold professional autonomy; to manage a caseload, maintain safety, and be accountable; and to maintain personal job satisfaction and quality of life.

12.6 Developing accountability opportunities for enabling occupation

Occupational therapy colleges may use the phrase *conscious competence* to alert those registered that a tacit and taken-for-granted understanding of practice guidelines is no longer sufficient. The Conscious Competence framework, developed by the College of Occupational Therapists of Ontario (2002a, 2002b), is an accountability tool that prompts consideration of the subject (target audience), object (outcomes), and methods used to demonstrate accountability (see table 12.1).

To complement use of the Conscious Competence tool, occupational therapists may draw others into critical reflections on accountability (see table 12.2). We might stimulate discussions on questions such as: What data would demonstrate accountability for enabling occupation? What data would allow us to evaluate the opportunities and limits for enabling occupation in a particular context?

Table 12.1   Conscious competence as a tool to define accountability opportunities

Focus	Accountability	Reflections for conscious competence
Subject of accountability	To a client	Name the funding agent
	Individual, family, group, community, organization, population	Identify the type of client
		Determine what the subject-client wants to know for accountability (outcomes, processes, efficiencies, effectiveness, indicators of success)
Object of accountability	For occupational outcomes	What does the subject-client want to know about what people do during or at the end of services?
	Examples: occupational performance, engagement, satisfaction, importance, choice, etc.	What is *already known* about occupational outcomes to present as "accountability?"
		What *could be known* from assessment or other new data?
Methods	Through enabling	To focus on occupational outcomes, ask: • What key and related enablement skills were employed (section II)?
	Examples: narratives to illustrate foundations, skills, and competencies	• What main competency roles from the *Profile of Occupational Therapy Practice in Canada* (CAOT, 2007) were employed?
	Examples: measures of practice processes and collaboration with clients, teams, others	• What main continuing competency strategies were employed to maintain competence and enablement skills? • What supports and limits optimal enablement?

Adapted from College of Occupational Therapists of Ontario (2002), *Conscious decision-making in occupational therapy practice.*

Table 12.3 offers discussion points on personal- and systems-level strategies. The strategies to seize accountability opportunities start with personal change management and scarce resource management. Other strategies are the balance of technical proficiency and professional reasoning; safety and risk management; and professional and self-empowerment.

To seize accountability opportunities, occupational therapists may wish to audit their own practice. An Enabling Occupation Audit checklist (see table 12.4) may spark ideas for occupational therapists to develop their own checklists. The purpose of

---

Table 12.2   Accountability questions

How would you answer these four questions?

1. To whom are you accountable in your practice (clients, funders, managers, regulators, communities, etc.)?

2. What accountability data or evidence do you provide to each party?

3. How do you demonstrate accountability for enabling occupation?

4. What helps and limits you from enabling occupation?

— *By Andrew Freeman*

Positioning occupational therapy for leadership

making such lists is to raise the awareness of occupational therapists and others to opportunities to negotiate new accountability strategies with managers and funding bodies. Such an audit may help to stimulate innovation. The development of accountability for occupation and enablement processes is a precursor to triggering a different distribution of funding for health and other services to provide greater support for enabling occupation.

Critical reflections on conscious competence, accountability questions, self and systems change management, and an enabling occupation audit may not be of high priority during or at the end of a busy day. For some occupational therapists, critical reflection may seem like a luxury that is best left to educators and researchers. Moreover, if the emphasis each day is on technical procedures, it may be difficult to take time for professional reasoning about the breadth and scope of enabling occupation. Yet we know that professional autonomy and growth in today's world, requires us to participate in accountability systems. Gina and Martha in case 12 are acting on that awareness. To realize a vision of being world leaders in enabling occupation, occupational therapists will want to become more critically aware and make use of the power of documentation. The situational nature of accountability must be considered as data are only relevant to the context and to the questions that they are collected to answer (see text box 12.2). An important strategy to position occupational therapy

Table 12.3 Accountability opportunities

Opportunities	Discussion
Personal change management Motto: Change is upon us. If we do not manage change, change will manage us.	Readiness to cope with change and the demand for change depends in part on how resilient individuals are to change and how many changes they have recently undergone. Resiliency to change also depends on the person's perception as this will shape their reality and influence how they react to change (Keagan & Lahey, 2001). For some, change means distress and the need to resist. For others, the pressure to change is translated into opportunities. They will direct change and interpret the change positively. Occupational therapists are accountable for being proactive with changes in the health care system (Jones, 2006). We need to avoid becoming numb or resistant to change, and influence decisions for change that positively impact our practice.
Scarce resource management Motto: The load can be overwhelming when it is carried alone and less when shared with others.	How might occupational therapists advocate successfully for adequate resources? How might we balance accountability with effectiveness and ethical best practices? Like all professionals, occupational therapists practice with conflicting priorities and commitments. To retain control and balance, one combines the following elements: • Professional reasoning and common sense • A client-centred focus • Best judgment to practice due-diligence • Networking with others • Sharing of resources • Development of strategies to increase individual responsibility and initiative • Communication of difficulties without ignoring confidentiality • Development of a learning context to create a path for experimentation and research • Solution to the problem situation and communication of evidence-based recommendation to policy-makers (Champagne, 2002; Simonson et al., 2005).

Continued ...

Table continued ...

Table 12.3 Accountability opportunities

Opportunities	Discussion
Management to balance technical proficiency and professional reasoning Motto: If we use technology, use it correctly and use it well.	Is more always better? Under constraint for time and staffing resources, people tend to turn to technology for quick and easy solutions. With the onslaught of technology in daily occupational therapy service delivery, occupational therapists may rely on technology to do the diagnostic work. Technology is not really a quick fix and it cannot replace the professional reasoning and problem-solving skills of an occupational therapist. There is excitement when new tools assist in professional decision making, using best practice evidence to produce positive results for clients. Occupational therapists are urged to assess, enquire, appraise, and apply the technology in the right context. It is expected that professionals exercise their autonomous, professional judgment in choosing what technology to use, use it efficiently and responsibly, always allowing time to learn the technology so that we can use it comfortably. There is a balance of how much technology to use, and how we need to keep things simple and useful for our clients. The same can be said about new knowledge. Despite new technology and new research, evidence-based practice is still the exception rather than the rule (Simonson et al., 2005). In order to promote accountability and best practice for enabling occupation, occupational therapists need time to create a work environment that fosters practice reflection and information sharing. This by itself will build capacities for absorbing new learning.
Safety and risk management Motto: Competency grows with self-direction and life-long learning.	Occupational therapy has tremendous, unfulfilled potential (Townsend, 1993). The demand and financial support to expand our services depend in part on taking responsibility for safety and risk management with our clients. Safety and risk management means creating a culture of safety and quality for a sustainable health system (Cowell, 2005; Kuhn & Youngberg, 2002). Safety and risk management, and professional accountability require competency to meet standards, be accurate, and constantly develop and change.
Self and professional empowerment Motto: Occupational therapists cannot avoid risk. Instead, we can find ways to manage it.	It is easy to feel that our professional hands are tied, and to limit what we can and will do. When we give up, another profession will respond to demands for which occupational therapists may have the most effective responses, if we are confident in our knowledge and skills. At the other extreme, the real danger is to grow too fast without the necessary resources and spread ourselves too thin to make a difference. Occupational therapists are encouraged to manage their own lives, and to ask periodically: What are my hidden fears and limitations? What stops the profession from being accountable for enabling occupation? Who defines our scope of practice? We can take stock of what we do best, and retain our focus on occupation-based, client-centred enablement.

— By Judy Quach

for leadership is to develop program evaluation and quality assurance with accountability data on occupation-based enablement. Occupational therapists can then document and interpret current practice to envision and plan proactively for the future.

Table 12.4   Enabling occupation audit

- Who creates and controls documents, and when, where, and how do clients have a voice?
- How are clients categorized — as active participants or passive objects (for example, residents vs. patients, individual vs. collective category such as a community)?
- When, where, and how do services occur, and what is documented?
- When, where, how, and by whom is enablement focused on environmental change? What enablement skills are used? What is documented?
- When, where, how, and by whom is enablement focused on personal change in clients? What enablement skills are used? What is documented?
- Who controls decision making? What enablement skills are used? What makes it client-centred? How is enablement documented?
- How are occupations used? What enablement skills are used? How are occupations and an occupational perspective documented?
- What risks are associated with enabling occupation? How are shared choice, risk, and responsibility handled and documented?

Adapted from Townsend, E. A. (1999). Client-centred practice: Good intentions overruled. *Occupational Therapy Now, 1*(4), 8-10.

Text box 12.2

Reflections on the situational nature of accountability

In considering how to make your work accountable, what holds you back from presenting your case in favour of enabling occupation? How likely is it that your accountability data would resonate with clients and their families? Would you be likely to collect the same or different data if you worked in a smaller or bigger organization? Would you collect different data if your practice was in a rural vs. an urban setting, or with people from diverse ethnic backgrounds? Might you present your data on program evaluation or quality assurance differently if you are female, male, a new graduate, or an experienced practitioner?

— *By Brenda Beagan*

Chapter 13

Funding, policy, and legislative opportunities

Elizabeth A. Townsend
Lyn Jongbloed
Robin Stadnyk
Hilary Drummond

CASE 13 Paulette: A policy analyst in community services

Paulette is a registered occupational therapist with 15 years of experience and a master's degree beyond her B.Sc. (OT). She has just accepted a policy analyst position in a provincial community services department, in its services for the aged division. Although a degree in occupational therapy was not an advertised requirement for the position, Paulette decided to apply, and emphasize her occupational therapy background and experience. Intrigued to consider what they might gain from appointing an experienced occupational therapist, and with no other experienced applicants, the hiring panel selected her for the position. In a strategic planning meeting, Paulette learned that departmental staff members were divided on whether they wanted to invest in more community support services or more nursing home beds.

The nursing home model, typically used in the province in both public and private settings, is to employ a few senior nurse managers, many nursing attendants for day-to-day nursing, one consultant each in occupational therapy and physiotherapy, and a recreation therapist to run activity programs. The seniors' health promotion and primary health care programs have yet to include occupational therapy. Paulette's responsibility is to analyze the range, utilization, and costs of services for diverse cultural groups of seniors, and to recommend policy updates to improve efficiency, effectiveness, and cost containment to the department head.

— By Elizabeth Townsend

13.1 Introduction

Occupational therapy needs funding, policy, and legislative support in order to flourish as a profession that can serve the occupational needs of society. Quality client-centred occupational therapy services attract and retain funding (Fearing & Clark, 2000). The health benefits of occupation and the collaborative nature of enablement are strong features to emphasize. Occupational therapy solutions for dealing with chronic illness, disability, and old age are timely, given escalating social, health, and economic costs. With such positive potential for occupational therapists to contribute to society, chapter 13 probes the current and new funding opportunities to facilitate greater public access to the profession. It supports occupational therapists to hold on to our vision of leadership in enabling occupation. We and society have much to gain if we can resist pressures to find quick, technical solutions that minimize attention to occupational challenges. The chapter includes guidelines for getting involved in private practice.

13.2 The Canadian health system

Canada is structured as a federation in which resources and considerable decision-making power are allocated to 10 provinces and 3 territories. Federal decision-making power is exerted primarily through federal taxation, and the development of national guidelines and policies. Health services, education, natural resources (fish, land, mines, oil, etc.) and industrial development are largely under provincial/ territorial jurisdiction, and are funded through provincial/territorial taxation and federal tax distribution. What makes Canada work is the constant mediation of the taxation and decision-making powers of provinces/territories and the federal government. Canadian occupational therapy is situated in public and private initiatives, which are embedded in this interplay of federal and provincial/territorial power relations.

Canada's public health insurance was designed to be universally accessible, fuelled by strong beliefs in collectivism and the value of government intervention to build a just society (Hall, 1980). To receive full payment from the federal government for insured medical services, the provinces/territories must adhere to the five principles of the *Canada Health Act* (Government of Canada, 1984; Kirby, 2002): accessibility, universality, comprehensiveness, portability, and public administration. Hospital and physician services for all citizens have been publicly funded since the 1960s (Evans, 2000). Public insurance was designed on a biomedical paradigm of health to cover individual, medically necessary services, primarily in hospitals (Evans, 2000). Yet the *Ottawa Charter for Health Promotion* (WHO, 1986) emphasized that health is more than the absence of disease, and that social determinants, such as income, education, housing, and employment have an incredible influence on health. Clearly, universal access to comprehensive medical care is not sufficient to promote health, nor eliminate health and social inequities (Pincus, Esther, DeWalt, & Callahan, 1998).

13.3 Public-sector health funding for occupational therapy

The Canada Health Act (Government of Canada, 1984) does not require the provinces/territories to offer occupational therapy, nor can occupational therapists who set up private offices bill the public health system. Nevertheless all provinces/ territories provide some public funding for occupational therapy services. Since the publicly-funded system is largely hospital-based, publicly-funded occupational therapy services are primarily based in, and managed through, the hospital system (Jongbloed & Wendland, 2002). With considerable variation across provinces/ territories, occupational therapy is available in acute care, in- and out-patient rehabilitation, and in- and out-patient mental health services. The greatest disparities in access to occupational therapy in health services are in long-term care, home care, primary care, and community mental health services (see chapter 14). Community services, not health services, generally fund long-term care (such as nursing homes) with the emphasis placed on nursing care. Therefore, it is important that managers such as Paulette (case 13) develop new funding, policy, and legislative conditions to expand long-term services, including occupational therapy (Swedlove, 2006).

There is considerable debate about whether Canadians should have more choice in health services and in the education, housing, and other services associated with the determinants of health. Wait times for medical diagnostic and treatment procedures tend to dominate discussions about health funding in Canada. To date, public debates have not raised questions about occupational therapy services. Yet occupational therapists should be attentive to the discussions of wait times and medical procedures, because increased funding to reduce wait times for acute medical and nursing care may result in fewer publicly-funded positions for occupational therapists. Increasing private occupational therapy, however, will not resolve the problem. Greater numbers of occupational therapists will move into private practice, which differs enormously from publicly-funded practice (Jongbloed & Wendland, 2002). In essence, publicly-funded practices are more likely to work with the whole person, their occupations, and their environment. Privately-funded practices tend to be driven to demonstrate accountability for measurable, technical solutions.

13.4 Occupational therapy in rehabilitation services

Occupational therapy in Canada is typically known as a *rehabilitation profession*. Public funding for occupational therapy continues alongside a growing range of private rehabilitation services. Important opportunities for occupational therapy rehabilitation are in interprofessional collaboration and teamwork. Rehabilitation funding supports the involvement of families and community members in occupational therapy, and addresses the individual issues of self-care, employment, housing, transportation, and social support in the short-term management of physical impairment and disability beyond acute care.

Although funding, policy, and legislative support for rehabilitation services traditionally created opportunities for occupational therapy in Canada, the profession has always had an uneasy alliance with rehabilitation services (Friedland, 2003). The uneasy alliance results from occupational therapy needing to narrow practice to focus on physical, affective, or cognitive impairments, with minimal attention dedicated to the environment and on occupation as a therapeutic medium or as an outcome. Certainly, occupational therapists have much to offer in impairment-based rehabilitation, and rehabilitation services need occupational therapy. Of concern is occupational therapy's close identity with physiotherapy in rehabilitation services. The dangers arise when occupational therapy focuses too narrowly on physical dysfunction, without an occupational perspective. Minimal, missed, or even ineffective enablement (see figures 4.4 and 4.5) may result without client-centred collaboration in contexts where caseloads and workload statistics are expected to mirror those of physiotherapy. Occupational therapy's strong identity as a rehabilitation profession may, in some situations, limit opportunities to generate interest from new funders for occupational enablement. Occupational therapists whose interests lie outside physical rehabilitation, struggle to see themselves as part of the profession, despite the historic and emerging occupational therapy services in mental health, public health, population health, healthy workplace initiatives, community development, child development, corrections, schools, and other sectors where occupational therapy has untapped potential (Wilcock, 2006).

13.5 Occupational therapy in mental health services

Occupational therapy services are not very accessible to those with severe and persistent mental health disorders, even though the majority of occupational therapists likely address the mental health or psychosocial components associated with many occupational challenges. Yet between 2003 and 2005, only slightly more than 12% of CAOT members (CAOT, 2004d, 2005b, 2006) reported that their primary service was in mental health services. In the same years, slightly more than 9% of occupational therapy researchers focused on mental health issues.

With concern for the limited access of Canadians to mental health occupational therapy services, the Canadian Association of Occupational Therapists (CAOT), in collaboration with Health Canada, produced *Occupational Therapy Guidelines for Client-Centred Mental Health Practice* (CAOT, 1993). These guidelines offer broad support to include psychosocial issues in all practice areas; specific attention on the role of occupational therapy with persons diagnosed mental disorders is included. Occupational therapy aims are cited as enabling empowerment in acute care, out-patient, day programming, and psychosocial rehabilitation services designed for persons with mild, moderate, and severe and persistent mental illness. The 1993 guidelines incorporate the growing call in the 1990s, emphasized by Woodside (1991), for client-centred attention to the inclusion of a consumer voice in mental health services.

To highlight occupational therapy's history and importance in mental health services in Canada, Rebeiro (1998) traced the historic use of occupation-as-means to mental health as an early contribution by occupational therapy in mental health services. Despite the limited presence of occupational therapy in modern mental health services, important research – for instance on work accommodations, affirming environments, and quality of life for adults with schizophrenia – continues to draw out the issues and options for Canadian occupational therapy in this field (Laliberte Rudman, Yu, Scott, & Pajouhandeh, 2000; Rebeiro, 2001).

In Australia, Scaletti (1999) proposed community development approaches for working in the field of mental health. In Britain, Creek (2002) published the third edition of her text on occupational therapy in mental health services. Fieldhouse (2000) found that a focus on occupation, using occupational science, is helping to sustain occupational therapy in community mental health services in Britain. In an American example, Dressler and MacRae (1998) showed that American interest persists in the kinds of advocacy, partnerships, and client-centred practice that we champion in mental health services in Canada. There is a huge potential for enabling occupation in mental health services, including the client-centred approaches of participatory research (Townsend, Birch, Langley, & Langille, 2000). The challenge is to probe for funding, policies, legislation, and other systems-level support to sustain, introduce, and in some instances restore occupational therapy as a cornerstone of mental health services.

13.6 Private-sector health funding for occupational therapy

Private-sector access to occupational therapy exists largely because of the way in which the disability income system in Canada is structured. The employment insurance structure has also been a strong driving force to increase private-sector access to occupational therapy.

Throughout the 20th century, insurance programs were developed to help injured workers with disabilities return to work or to compensate them financially if they could not do so. The first disability programs in Canada were funded through workers' compensation insurance and nationally-funded veterans' programs (Jongbloed, 2003). Later, programs such as the Canada Pension Plan disability benefits and social assistance began to provide some financial assistance to other individuals with disabilities. In recent years, there has been growth in private, long-term disability plans and automobile insurance (Jongbloed, 2003). For example, both the British Columbia workers' compensation board and the provincial automobile insurance company are corporations that operate separately from the health care system. They employ occupational therapists in private practice to accomplish specific, individualized objectives with particular clients (Jongbloed & Wendland, 2002). The Canadian Association of Occupational Therapists' members reported (CAOT, 2005b) that private-sector access to services was principally funded by workers' compensation boards, automobile insurance, private health insurance, and lawyers.

13.7 Funding for occupational therapy beyond health services

Public and private access to occupational therapy in Canada is slowly increasing outside the health sector, although funding remains an issue. Two key policy-related factors may increase access: a focus on the social determinants of health, which include occupationally related areas such as employment, housing, and education (Public Health Agency of Canada, 2004); and a focus on social inclusion and participation as an outcome of interest for persons with chronic illness or disability, and older adults (Office for Disability Issues, Social Development Canada, 2005). The following examples illustrate existing services available outside the health services paradigm.

Private insurance-funded services

Occupational therapists are privately contracted by insurance companies and lawyers representing individual clients, primarily in the area of personal injury claims. Occupational therapists consult with these organizations to develop policies and their recommendations are often used to help determine the services, equipment, and/or financial compensation for claimants, or the development of life care plans (Kennedy, 1997; Klinger, Baptiste, & Adams, 2004). Most insurance coverage is for physical rehabilitation. Private funding for occupational therapy in mental health services is almost non-existent, unless this is part of a physical rehabilitation claim. Consequently, advocacy is needed to develop insurance for mental health services, primary health care, and other areas in which occupational therapists can contribute.

School-based services

Occupational therapy is not universally available in all of Canada's provinces/ territories in public or private schools at the pre-school, elementary, secondary, or post-secondary levels. Where it is available, health services funding is typically for elementary level, school-based, rehabilitation services that include occupational therapy. Occupational therapists work with individuals or groups of students with developmental, sensory, physical or learning impairments, or with mental health issues. Occupational therapists also facilitate the transition from school to work life or higher education. Working with teachers, teachers' aides, in-class assistants, and families, occupational therapists aim to improve students' performance in school occupations and to better integrate students into the school environment (Whalen, 2002).

Universal design and housing

Occupational therapists work privately with individuals, architects, contractors, or planners to use universal design principles in new or renovated housing and the development of public spaces (CAOT, 2003a). The occupational therapist can emphasize client-centredness to advocate for inclusive designs that enable participation by those with diverse ability, vision, hearing, or mental health. Occupational therapists are typically on contract with the builder or planner, and in some instances with an architecture firm or planning department.

Wellness and older persons

Occupational therapists are typically funded on private contract by some community organizations or housing complexes. The usual occupational therapy contribution is to encourage wellness, social participation, increased quality of life, and reduced incidence of falls (Steultjens et al., 2004). Methods may be through the provision of assistive devices (Boudreau, 2004), or through engagement in meaningful occupations and active living (CAOT, 2003a; Pranger, 2002). With increasing attention to those with Alzheimer's disease and mental disorders, new funding will be needed to increase access to occupational therapy in mental health services. Concern for older adults and safe driving (CAOT, 2005a; Millar, 1999) will require increased access to occupational therapy driving assessments and rehabilitation.

Work-related services

Work-related occupational therapy services appear to be on the increase in Canada. Assessment services include ergonomic, activity of daily living, vocational, pre-employment/post-offer assessments, and functional capacity evaluations with individual clients (Archer-Heese & Stratton Johnson, 2002; Strong, 2002).

Return-to-work services include pain management, work relationship development, work hardening, and job modifications, sometimes with employers as an organizational client (Archer-Heese & Stratton Johnson, 2002; Gowan & Strong, 2002). Prevention services include injury prevention, employee wellness, and health promotion (Archer-Heese & Stratton Johnson, 2002; Baril, Clarke, Friesen, Stock, & Cole, 2003; Pond Clements, 2002). Disability management is a comprehensive, workplace-based, collaborative approach that sometimes includes occupational therapists. Disability management includes workplace wellness, injury prevention, early intervention following onset of disability, rehabilitation services, and early return to work (CAOT, 2004a; Westmoreland, 2003). Work-related services may be funded by insurers (including workers' compensation boards) or by industries.

13.8 Emerging funding for occupational therapy

Federal initiatives in health, education, housing, employment, and other sectors are not necessarily accompanied by provincial/territorial funding, policy, and legislation; conversely, provincial/territorial policy initiatives may wither without the support of federal funding and guidelines. Possible employers/payers for new occupational therapy initiatives include Aboriginal organizations, addictions services, correctional services, departments of education, social services, mental health, and primary health care services. An effective way to launch new initiatives is through demonstration or pilot projects with public or private funding agreements. New initiatives are seldom targeted only to occupational therapists, and may not be explicit about including occupational therapy. Five areas of social policy development highlighted below are worth noting.

Aboriginal health

Aboriginal health has been a longstanding concern in Canada. The *Blueprint on Aboriginal Health*, written collaboratively by government and Aboriginal organizations (Government of Canada et al., 2005) combines traditional and Western approaches. The focus is on non-medical health determinants and areas such as mental health, addictions recovery, and services for persons with disabilities in Aboriginal communities. Occupational therapy is emerging as a service in some Aboriginal health programs for children, youth, adults with disabilities, and seniors.

Child health

A 2006 federal report on human resources and social development in Canada (Human Resources and Social Development Canada, 2007) recognized the importance of childhood experiences to lifetime development and choices. Proposed initiatives fit well with occupational therapy interests in enabling healthy occupations for children and youth by advocating a rights-based approach (CAOT, 2004b).

Anti-poverty and anti-exclusion

New federal initiatives recognize that poverty involves exclusion from many aspects of life related to employment, safe housing and neighbourhoods, and social networks (Policy Research Initiative, 2005a). Homelessness and poverty are major issues for the occupational development of children from early life throughout their school years (Humphry, 1995).

Building social capital

The concept of social capital refers to the network of friends, family members, and acquaintances that we use for support, information, or for obtaining what we need in our communities, and has been found to be a component of well-being and a resource for surviving difficult times (Policy Research Initiative, 2005b). If, as the 2005 Policy Research Initiative suggests, we consider social capital as a process, then an important outcome of social capital development may be the person's ability to engage in occupations that they need or want to pursue. Proposals by occupational therapists to collaborate with social agencies and non-governmental organizations will improve access to occupation-based services to develop social capital with individuals, families, groups, communities, organizations, or populations.

Work-life balance

Access to occupational therapy is emerging in private counselling-based practices, which focus on work-life balance and the needs of an aging workforce (Duxbury & Higgins, 2001; Hunsley, 2006). Work-life balance is an area where the evaluation of occupational routines and habits provides essential data for individual, group, or organizational clients to adjust time use, and to modify work and home environments.

13.9 Positioning new occupational therapy initiatives

Three key issues in positioning occupational therapy for new funding, policy, and legislative support are: third-party payers, professional autonomy and identity, and practice skills.

Third-party payer issues and multiple clients

Occupational therapists working in schools or workplaces are usually paid by a third party (Strong, 2002). This can create a dilemma if the payer, such as an employer, has competing interests with the person, such as an employee, whom the occupational therapist may regard as her or his primary client. As well, as Jongbloed and Wendland (2002) found, private occupational therapy services are more likely to focus on physical dysfunction and measurement as required by insurers, whereas in Canada's publicly-funded health services, occupational therapists expect funding to cover at least some time to be client-centred in listening to client issues and addressing environmental, psychosocial, and other issues.

Professional autonomy and identity

Occupational therapists work with or in competition with other health professionals who may share certain work components (CAOT, 2004c; Strong, 2002). Overlapping scopes of practice and vigorous marketing of new professions has produced role blurring (Archer-Heese & Stratton Johnson, 2002). In a competitive market, the need for efficiency and standardized reporting may outweigh the desire for occupation-based enablement. Occupational therapists may find themselves working in organizations or for employers who are not focused on occupation as a process or an outcome. The greatest challenges to occupational therapy autonomy and identity are from management accountability practices, where decisions are made based on case-load size and turnover in tight fiscal conditions rather than on occupational outcomes and client-centred enablement (Freeman et al., 2006; Jongbloed & Wendland, 2002; Rappolt et al., 2004; Townsend, 1998). Although occupational therapists in Ontario reported high levels of job satisfaction, a majority perceived future threats to their professional autonomy with the rise of commercial controls over the services they provide (Rappolt et al., 2004).

Some occupational therapists work for private rehabilitation or home care companies, where they have neither the benefits of a public-sector position (steady pay, benefits, perhaps a union) nor those of working in their own businesses (independence, potential profits). For autonomy in the private sector, occupational therapists need to educate insurers who are not aware of the health and social benefits of occupation or occupational therapy.

Practice skills

Increasingly, practice areas outside of health care require enablement skills in consultation (Mullan, 2003) or systems/policy level practice (CAOT, 2004c; 2005b; Baril et al., 2003; Westmoreland, 2002, 2003). Skills for enabling social change, that is to say at the systems/policy level, vary from competences used for enabling individual change (see chapters 5 and 6). Occupational therapists will increasingly draw on advocacy, coordination, consulting, education, and engagement enablement skills to be occupation-based and client-centred with multiple stakeholders, including policy makers and other service providers. Working in many of these areas requires sociocultural competence and collaboration with the groups requesting services (Gerlach, 2005; Urbanowski, 2005). Advocacy skills extend, not replace, important enablement skills with individuals, families, and groups.

13.10 Getting involved in private occupational therapy practice

Most areas of Canada have experienced a dramatic increase in the rate of occupational therapy self-employment with private sources of payment. The number of CAOT members in private practice rose from 3% in the early 1990s to over 22% in 2004, with over 50% of members reporting that they received some private payment for their services in 2004 (CAOT, 2005b).

Occupational therapists often choose self-employment because of the opportunity for greater autonomy (Bridle & Hawkes, 1990; McLain, McKinney, & Ralston, 1992). We place a high value on intrinsic employment factors such as the autonomy to perform job tasks (Painter, 1990). However, private practice may be the only choice for some occupational therapists when public-sector positions in their areas of interest and expertise are not available where they want to live.

The occupational therapist considering going into private practice has many decisions to make and should give careful thought before starting down this path. Not all occupational therapists have the skills required to run a business, and they may not have exercised the business skills required for owning their own practice while working as salaried employees. While there are some great advantages to being in business (e.g., flexibility and control of work time) there are also challenges: slow times with few clients, cash flow management, dealing with business issues, and constant marketing.

In the start-up checklist (table 13.1), the first step is to create a clear outline to save both time and money in the long run. Occupational therapists should clarify their vision for private practice early on and work steadily toward what they see as their ideal practice. Values should be clearly identified to create a successful business that is compatible with personal goals. It is helpful to outline areas of importance and to set specific goals in each of them. Planning will assist in determining how to best allocate time and financial resources, and will help in making decisions when life can feel overwhelming.

Table 13.1   Private practice start-up checklist

• Vision and values	• Business skills	• Potential payers
• Planning	• Knowledge of regulations	• Business partners
• Structure of the business	• Financial business plan	• Marketing

– By Hilary Drummond

Occupational therapists may want to give serious thought to whether or not they are really entrepreneurs with the personality factors to succeed in private practice. They may want to take personality or entrepreneur tests (available through business development sources) to help determine their chances of succeeding. It is helpful to know one's areas of relative strengths and weaknesses before making any commitments.

Multiple roles are available to occupational therapists in private practice, under various business structures. Occupational therapists can own their own practice and subcontract their services to other companies. They may establish a sole proprietorship — a business owned and operated by one person — or a partnership operated with another individual through a partnership agreement. Or they may form a corporation that offers the advantage of limited liability — but also the challenges of managing the regulations and obligations of a corporation. Rulings about business ownership, proprietorship, and partnerships are available on the Canada Revenue Agency Web site.

A business plan is essential for occupational therapists who will be establishing a line of credit or other lending arrangement with their financial institutions. Of utmost importance is the need to develop a personal relationship with an accountant and banker. This will facilitate business growth by ensuring that the financial demands of the business are met. An accountant can provide invaluable information and support to the new business, as can a lawyer for items such as contracts and partnership agreements.

As professionals, Canadian occupational therapists in private practice are subject to the guidelines and ethical codes of provincial regulatory organizations. Private practitioners also need to develop their own policies on important issues such as ethics, conflict of interest, consent, and access to private information. The private practitioner is subject to the accountability, policy, funding, and legislative conditions associated with local, provincial, and federal governments.

It is confusing at times to determine: Who is the client? Is it the payer for the service or the person receiving the service? From a business perspective, the client is the service payer. However, it is crucial that private practitioners clearly outline their roles and responsibilities to both the payer and those receiving services. The question about the client extends to ownership and privacy of information, both generated through service provision. Occupational therapists in private practice need to set policies around these issues.

There are endless opportunities for the occupational therapist considering retail business. For example, as the population ages in Canada, there is an increasing call for access to assistive technology to enable people to live at home and stay as active as possible. Occupational therapists will find challenges in promoting the use of assistive devices that are commonplace to the profession, but that are unfamiliar to the public or insurance payers. Maintaining an inventory of items and covering the overhead for a storefront are challenges in a retail business. Selling on-line may be a more economical way to reach a large number of consumers.

Occupational therapists in private practice may want to develop alliances with business partners. Partnerships may evolve from requests for proposals or from ongoing relationships with service payers. An important strategy is to diversify the business to avoid being overly dependent on one payer. In fact, the Canada Revenue Agency may consider that a therapist is an employee for tax purposes if there is only one payer, even if payment is on contract. There are many resources available to help with the processes for creating and developing a request for proposal or other business offer.

Occupational therapists in private practice must be prepared to continuously market themselves and their profession. Being highly visible in the community, they must act as exceptional ambassadors for the profession, both as service providers and as business persons. They must be ready to compete fairly and openly with colleagues. Private practice occupational therapists face many challenges but the benefits can be rewarding for those who have the personality, business skills, vision, and tenacity to work in the private sector.

Let us reflect on funding, policy, and legislative opportunities for Paulette (case 13) and other occupational therapists that can improve access to this profession (see text box 13.1). Public and private funding for rehabilitation health services are important core access points. Mental health services — particularly the acute, out-patient, and day program options funded through hospital services — provide some access to occupational therapy. Occupational therapists, such as Paulette, who work in community services, may bring an occupational perspective to long-term care and other sectors where access to the profession is still very limited. The ethical issues that go with privatizing occupational therapy are in fact central issues for all Canadians. The greatest opportunities to increase access to occupational therapy may be to match services to population trends. New partnerships with primary health care and other sectors concerned with the social determinants of health provide the opportunity to coordinate new initiatives. Given popular support for universal health care, Canadians will likely want to retain publicly-funded access – with supplemental private access – to the breadth of occupational therapy, which is emerging with an occupational perspective of health, well-being, and justice. To position occupational therapy for leadership, we can take a proactive stance to develop funding mechanisms and policy support for occupational enablement within and beyond health services.

Text box 13.1

Reflections on funding, policy, and legislation opportunities

How would you search for funding if you were in a well-resourced province? A resource-challenged part of Canada? How might your own experience or cultural background influence whether or not you were willing to seek funding outside health services? What kinds of assertiveness might this require? Do you see patterns in who is or is not able to be assertive in those ways? What types of occupational challenges receive the most attention in your community? What funding, policy, and legislation support programs and services are available for older adults with a severe and persistent mental illness? How might you compare programs for poor and disabled older women versus well-off and disabled young children in your community? What professions are attracting new funds? How are they the same as or different from occupational therapy?

— *By Brenda Beagan*

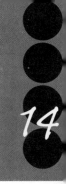

Chapter 14

Occupational therapy workforce planning

Elizabeth A. Townsend
Claudia von Zweck
Sue Baptiste
Terry Krupa
Huguette Picard
Louis Trudel

CASE 14 Eugene's dilemmas in recruitment and retention

Eugene is an occupational therapist who is registrar of a provincial, occupational therapy regulatory body. He knows from anecdotal information shared among occupational therapy regulators, professional associations, and educators that demand is increasing for occupational therapy. Yet some new graduates face unstable contracts, casual employment, and little opportunity for supervision and mentoring. Moreover, some experienced occupational therapists are letting their registrations lapse when they move to management, policy, and consulting positions without the title of occupational therapist. Others with experience are leaving the profession after 20 or so years, saying that they need a new challenge. In essence, registration of occupational therapists is only slowly increasing despite the increasing potential supply from Canadian educational programs and immigration.

While the public is seeking greater access to occupational therapy, funding for new positions is slow to come. One thing that Eugene knows is that demand will only increase given an aging population, advances in technology, and greater emphasis on quality of life. With better recognition of the value of rehabilitation, mental health services, and home care, he receives frequent calls from individuals and agencies who are looking for occupational therapists. Immigration holds promise to increase numbers and enrich the profession's socio-cultural diversity in the province. The growth of occupational therapy support personnel is also promising to raise public awareness about occupational therapy, although Eugene must monitor occupational therapists to ensure that they are supervising all support personnel.

The impacts on employment, systems costs, recruitment, retention, and career development associated with changing entry-level education requirements to the master's level are still unknown. Because the number of registered members is not sufficient to meet provincial demands, Eugene decided to participate in a national project on occupational therapy workforce planning. He familiarized himself with the project, and agreed to collaborate with the Canadian Association of Occupational Therapists and the Canadian Institute for Health Information to develop a national database to track trends in the age, education, and practice of provincially registered practitioners across Canada. He is also working with local practitioners to develop a new competency portfolio. What he really wants to know is how the new competency profile can make the profession's identity clearer to the public and how a clear identity, career path, and new funding options will help to recruit and retain the most competent and proficient practitioners in his province.

— By Claudia von Zweck

14.1 Introduction

Chapter 14 targets workforce planning as an essential strategy to increase Canadians' access to occupational therapy. The chapter presents key issues for the profession in integrated workforce planning: (a) the historical context and contemporary professional profile; (b) factors that influence supply, namely, occupational therapy education, immigration and emigration, and occupational therapy support personnel education; (c) demand and utilization; (d) Québec as a unique case; (e) retention and career development; (f) partnerships and interprofessional collaboration; and (g) implementation of an integrated, multiple stakeholder strategy to improve public and private access. Data to track the occupational therapy workforce in this country are available primarily from the membership database of the Canadian Association of Occupational Therapists (CAOT), and the emerging national occupational therapy database being developed by the Canadian Institute for Health Information (CIHI). Since 2005, CAOT has worked with CIHI and Canadian regulatory organizations in a Health Canada-funded initiative to develop a national health human resources database for occupational therapy in Canada. Beginning in 2007 this database will provide consistent, supply-based data regarding the demographics, education and practice of Canadian occupational therapists (CIHI, 2005a).

The Canadian context for occupational therapy workforce planning is an officially bilingual and multicultural federation under the *Canadian Charter of Rights and Freedoms* (Government of Canada, 1982), which was drafted to protect the rights of minority groups without discrimination based on race, national or ethnic origin, colour, religion, sex, age, or mental or physical disability (see text box 2.3). Canada's commitment to minority rights reflects an ideology that Canada is made up of distinct socio-cultural groups with equal status. In terms of race and national or ethnic origin, individuals of British and French descent constitute more than half of the people of Canada. Immigration over many years has enhanced population growth among those with Chinese, South Asian, German, and Italian backgrounds (Statistics Canada, 2005b).

Occupational therapy in Canada, by all accounts, is a very small, female-dominated profession that is little-known outside the specialized worlds of rehabilitation, mental health, and disability services. An occupational perspective is hardly recognized by anyone outside occupational therapy and occupational science. Considerable planning and vision will be needed to position occupational therapy for leadership to advance a vision of health, well-being, and justice through occupation.

We can briefly look at other health professions in order to put the size and profile of the occupational therapy workforce in Canada in perspective. Nursing is a very large, female-dominated profession with specialty areas that overlap with occupational therapy, and professions such as social work, physiotherapy, psychology, and special education, all share some component of the occupational therapy domain of practice. New fields, such as disability management, health promotion, kinesiology, recreation therapy, and vocational counselling are professionalizing rapidly, growing in numbers, becoming regulated, and extending their scope of practice to overlap with occupational therapy. In Ontario alone, there are now 13 kinesiology education programs with a total of approximately 2000 bachelor's and master's level graduates each year (Health Professions Regulatory Advisory Council, 2006), almost triple the number of annual graduates in occupational therapy for the whole country.

It is known that the value and capacity of a profession depend, to a large degree, on defining a clear demand that is not met by other professions, and on organizing education and quality practice to make a difference in society (Griffin, 2001). Professions that serve a niche demand, such as audiology and speech pathology, may thrive with a small, specialized workforce. A small, female-dominated, broad-reaching profession like occupational therapy urgently needs an integrated workforce planning strategy for growth and development in order to:

1. Increase the supply of occupational therapists throughout Canada to improve universal access to the breadth of this profession;
2. Retain experienced practitioners who can influence funding, policy, and legislative decision making to support occupational enablement for all citizens;
3. Develop a clear identity with the public about both our potential contributions, and the limited and inequitable access Canadians have to this profession and its services.

We need not be shy to present ourselves. Members of this profession offer an integrated, reasoned occupational perspective of health, well-being, and justice through occupation with a range of clients in diverse contexts, drawing on multidisciplinary knowledge and professional reasoning about occupations and enablement. Done well, occupation-based enablement is poised to attend to diversity and inclusion in enabling all people to engage in their everyday occupations, and enabling societies to become more inclusive and just. This profession is an important human resource to prevent or ameliorate the everyday consequences of chronic illness, disability, aging, or social disadvantages.

While service to others must be the core rationale for a profession, an important strength to accelerate workforce planning is that occupational therapy is interesting, meaningful, and well-paid work. The profession rightly attracts people who want to make a difference in people's lives and society, beyond treating the body (Rozier, Gilkeson, & Hamilton, 1992). It engages those who combine vision with enablement skills to influence the lives of all Canadians. One can imagine that many would want to join and remain active over a long career in such an attractive profession.

14.2 A brief history of occupational therapy in Canada: Context for workforce planning

A historical context provides important insights for Eugene and others in workforce planning. As a registrar, Eugene must not only organize policies and procedures to regulate today's practices, he and other registrars will also want to understand how the scope of practice, access to occupational therapy, and influences on workforce planning evolved in Canada.

Issues facing the Canadian occupational therapy workforce in the 21st century are influenced by both today's conditions and the profession's historic foundations in mid-19th-century mental asylums and poorhouses in England and France. The origins of occupational therapy in Canada are in the 19th-century work of occupation aides or occupation workers. They engaged people in looking after themselves to promote their health and reduce the impacts of their poverty through, for example, cooking, cleaning, farming, craftwork, and creative expression (Dickinson, 1990; Wilcock, 2006). Occupational therapy developed in Canada as opportunities were provided by actual ideas and events (Friedland, 2003), a few of which are highlighted on a timeline in figure 14.1.

Occupational therapy emerged in Canada at the beginning of the 20th century as part of rehabilitation medicine and psychiatry. Not all influences were medical, however. Early initiatives to form the profession also drew inspiration from social movements, notably the Arts and Crafts Movement, the Settlement House Movement, and the Mental Hygiene Movement (Friedland, 2003). The predominance of women in the profession of occupational therapy in Canada also has historic roots; early feminist initiatives were a social influence in opening up new opportunities to educate and employ women (Litterst, 1992).

With an educational vision of experiential learning drawn from Dewey and others (Dewey, 1900; Dewey & Bentley, 1949; Schwartz, 1992), early practitioners used handcrafts to implement century-old ideas about the therapeutic value of purposeful activity, learning through doing, and the physical and mental health benefits of

Figure 14.1 Evolving ideas in Canadian occupational therapy

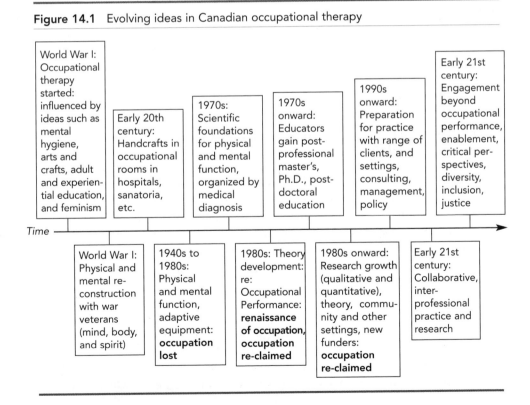

engaging in meaningful and purposeful occupations (Alaszewski, 1979; Ernest, 1972; Gritzer & Arluke, 1985; Wilcock, 2001b, 2002). Early enablement involved the engagement and education of individuals to overcome functional limitations, and the design and building of adaptive equipment (Jongbloed & Crichton, 1990). Enablement likely included collaboration and advocacy with sympathetic groups to improve conditions for living with a disability. Practitioners would have coordinated and consulted with others in the new managerial systems that brought medicine into complex hospitals (Freidson, 1986, 2001). In this context, occupational therapists learned to organize practice around men's and women's handcrafts that could be easily accomplished within the space, safety, housekeeping, labour union, and management parameters of medical institutions. Today's emphasis in workforce planning for practice in hospitals and other health settings is thus historically-based.

Today's occupational model has emerged to guide modern practice (see figure 1.5), but medical sponsorship was critical in launching the profession in the early 20th century (Maxwell & Maxwell, 1979). Some physicians recognized the lack of activity for those with mental illness or tuberculosis who were hospitalized for long periods of time. Physicians in military hospitals championed the inclusion of occupational therapists to enable wounded veterans to return to employment and off compensation as soon as possible (Friedland, 2003; Howland, 1944, 1986). Key Canadian physicians, such as Charles Kidner and Goldwin Howland, were champions for occupational therapy, recognizing the importance of engaging people in mind, body, and spirit in purposeful and meaningful activities (Friedland & Davids-Brumer, 2007). Howland's insights, which open section I, pointed to an early awareness "to remedy human dissatisfaction and mental unrest by providing daily tasks so that minds may be occupied, bodies may be healthy, and the means of sustenance may be found" (1933, p. 4). While concern for occupation gave rise to occupational therapy (Howland, 1933), awareness and publication about occupation as the core domain disappeared between 1940 and 1980 (Polatajko, 2001; Whiteford et al., 2000). Following World War II and into the 1950s and 1960s, demands for an occupational therapy workforce in rehabilitation services increased (Robinson, 1991). During this time, occupational therapy education and practice focused more on physical than mental health and psychological concerns (Madill, Cardwell, Robinson, & Britnell, 1986).

Beginning in the 1970s, the occupational therapy workforce began to introduce scientific foundations into practice, including theories about human activity and the measurement of functional limitations. A new component of the occupational therapy workforce developed: researchers began to emerge with graduate level education, and with interests in quantitative research and the development of standardized tests. Some practitioners and researchers began to express aspirations for career development (Brintnell, 1985).

The growth of theory-based practice has been a critical turning point in workforce planning from the early 1980s to today. Regulators and practitioners alike expect practitioners to apply theory in practice, and to test practice against theory. Such theoretical development has transformed awareness of the ontology and epistemology of occupational therapy, and has sparked awareness of critical perspectives on diversity in clients, communities, and the profession (ACOTRO et al., 2006). The last 25 years have been described as a period of *renaissance* when occupation was reclaimed as the profession's core domain (Whiteford et al., 2000).

14.3 Supply profile of Canada's occupational therapy workforce

Three sources of supply influence access to the profession in Canada: Canadian graduates of occupational therapy university programs; immigration and emigration of qualified occupational therapists; and, formally trained support personnel. The dominant profile of an occupational therapist in Canada is that of a young female who provides services directly to individual clients. An optimistic statistic from CAOT data (2005b) is that occupational therapy is growing faster than the population of Canada. Canada had 5887 active full- and part-time occupational therapists who retained membership with CAOT in 2004. Total membership in CAOT (including students) has grown between 2001 and 2006 by 1099 (17.2%). This is an encouraging figure, although the potential total membership increase from graduates of Canadian occupational therapy education programs would be over 3000, almost 2/3 of whom did not become CAOT members. Current available seats in occupational therapy education programs will provide an additional 3500 occupational therapists who will be eligible for full, active CAOT membership by 2010.

CAOT growth statistics for occupational therapy only reflect part of the story on access to occupational therapy. National data collected by the Canadian Institute for Health Information from provincial regulatory organizations indicate that 10,984 individuals were registered across the 10 provinces to practice occupational therapy in 2004 (CIHI, 2006). Québec has one of the highest ratios of occupational therapists per population in Canada. CAOT is a voluntary organization, and only a few provinces require CAOT membership as a criterion for provincial registration. In 1984 and 1985, almost all Canadian occupational therapists were members of CAOT (with the exception of Québec). Only a small percentage of the 3126 occupational therapists in Québec were members of CAOT in 2004. CAOT data include approximately 20 occupational therapists who are not in CIHI data because they work in Canada's three territories where practice is not regulated and, thus, not reported to CIHI.

Data on numbers of practitioners in Canada provide one view of the supply profile. However, we want to look critically at the age, gender, race, and other descriptive features of this profile if we want to uncover trends that need to be considered in planning. CAOT data from the 2004 membership indicate that the large majority (75.3%) of members were under 45 years of age (CAOT, 2005b) (see figure 14.2). The average age of occupational therapists in 2004 was 36 years (Human Resources and Skills Development Canada, 2005), younger than members of professions such as medicine and nursing, where aging of the workforce has created significant concerns for replacing workers who will retire in the coming decade. The younger age profile of occupational therapists is to some extent a reflection of increases in the number of occupational therapists graduating from Canadian university education programs over the past decade, while the number of seats in other professions such

Figure 14.2 Age categories of CAOT members in 2005

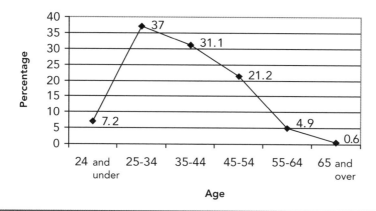

as medicine and nursing have dropped (CIHI, 2005b, 2005c). Whereas occupational therapy is growing faster than the population in the last decade, the number of family physicians has barely kept up with population growth (CIHI, 2005b). The supply of nurses has grown by 60% in the past 25 years, but large increases occurred in the 1980s, followed by workforce reductions in the next decade (CIHI, 2005c). Occupational therapy statistics are, of course, based on keeping pace with population increases, but do not, however, consider the disparities between those in need and access to occupational therapy that continue to exist in Canada.

The younger age profile of occupational therapists may also reflect the short career lifespan of occupational therapists. While the profession is growing in numbers, we know very little about the retention of occupational therapists. The largest membership losses occur when occupational therapists reach 45 years of age and again after they reach age 55. These data suggest that many experienced occupational therapists do not retain their registration and leave the profession after 20 to 30 years of practice, well before retirement age. Many members do not retain the title of occupational therapist when shifting to positions not linked to direct client care; consequently, they are not required by law to be registered to practise. The lack of "occupational therapist" senior-level positions, has been reported as a factor that limits promotion and retention in the profession (Brown, 1998; Wilkins & Rosenthal, 2001). Without experienced members, the profession is also limited from developing necessary expertise and senior-level networks in education, scholarship, consulting, management, and policy development.

Anecdotal evidence reports a worrisome trend that retention is becoming an issue for new graduates. In 2004, CAOT attracted approximately 79% of graduates of Canadian occupational therapy education programs who successfully completed the national certification examination. One wonders: Why did 21% of 2004 graduates decline to join? Why do some graduates either decline to join or let membership lapse with CAOT? To better understand the career paths of Canadian occupational therapy graduates, CAOT is investigating ways to follow new occupational therapy graduates during their first five years after graduation and throughout their careers.

Over 90% of occupational therapists in Canada are female (CAOT, 2005b; CIHI, 2006). The few studies that exist on this gender profile, point to lack of career options and salary advances, and to perceptions and reinforced that occupational therapy is caregiving, women's work (Frank, 1992; Griffin, 2001; Irvin & Graham, 1994; Litterst, 1992). This view is perpetuated and reinforced by individualized, direct contact with persons with disabilities and the profession's emphasis on self-care — an occupational area that has traditionally been associated with women. Traditional views of occupational therapy as women's work sustain the image that the profession has limited power and prestige (Maxwell & Maxwell, 1979), as well as insufficient financial compensation when compared with male-oriented roles in technology, business, and medicine (Beagan & Kumas-Tan, 2006). Male occupational therapists in Canada reported that they planned to leave the profession within 10 years because of dissatisfaction with earning potential, upward mobility, and recognition (Brown, 1998). Men are as likely as women to leave the profession after about 20 years of practice.

The race or social class profile of Canadian occupational therapists is not well known. A survey of Ontario occupational therapists indicated that those from visible minority groups were under-represented in the occupational therapy workforce, despite the culturally and racially diverse population of that province (Lum et al., 2004). Socio-economic status is known to correlate highly with academic achievement: individuals from higher income families are significantly more likely to attend university in Canada, because of influences such as parental support for education (Finnie, Lascenes, & Sweetman, 2005). As a result, some racial and social groups may be disadvantaged in attaining the qualifications to practice occupational therapy.

The lack of diversity in the age, gender, race, and, possibly, social class of practitioners likely limits workforce flexibility. Lack of diversity is also an access issue; those who might refer to or use occupational therapy may see the profession as lacking the perspectives of particular groups. The lack of diversity in occupational therapy will be an ongoing, workforce planning issue, in light of the transition to increase the entrance credentials for occupational therapy from a bachelor's to a master's degree. This higher credential requirement is part of the transformation to position the profession for leadership in enabling occupation. On the one hand, the higher entry-level credential may attract students with a greater diversity of intellectual backgrounds, such as anthropology, biology, business, engineering, kinesiology, science, and sociology. The entry-level bachelor's degree is no longer a disincentive to graduates with a bachelor's degree who are looking for a profession in which they are almost guaranteed employment (Ontario Hospital Association, 2003). On the other hand, the higher educational requirements are likely another barrier to marginalized groups who want to enter the profession. A prime example is that of Aboriginal Canadians who report overall lower rates of participation in post-secondary education (Finnie et al., 2005).

14.4 Supply of graduates from Canadian occupational therapy university programs

Over 90% (90.4) of CAOT members in 2004 had graduated from one of 12 occupational therapy university education programs[1] that were then accredited by CAOT to offer occupational therapy education in Canada (see table 14.1). Two to three additional programs are in the works in Québec within the next decade. As well, discussions have been re-initiated by CAOT and the Saskatchewan Society of Occupational Therapists regarding the need for an education program in Saskatchewan. Canadian occupational therapy programs supply approximately 700 graduates each year (ACOTUP, 2006). Enrollment and graduate data are essentially the same because the attrition rate is low — most students who enroll in occupational therapy education in Canada complete their programs.

Table 14.1   Accredited Canadian Occupational Therapy University Programs 2006

University of British Columbia (1962)	University of Ottawa (1986)
University of Alberta (1960)	Queen's University (1967)
University of Manitoba (1960)	Université de Montréal (1954)
University of Western Ontario (1970)	McGill University (1950)
McMaster University[1] (1989)	Université Laval (1968)
University of Toronto (1926)	Dalhousie University (1982)

[1] In 1974, the Ontario government decided to introduce a new three-year diploma course at Mohawk College, a new community college. Despite strong protestations from CAOT and from several individual members, the program was launched. It was several years before this issue was resolved and the course became part of the McMaster University program (Cockburn, 2001, p. 5).

In 2006, 8 of 12 programs were governed within faculties of medicine, thereby reflecting the historical, medical sponsorship of occupational therapy. The other four (University of Alberta, University of Western Ontario, University of Ottawa, and Dalhousie University) are among Canada's newer occupational therapy education programs, found in faculties other than medicine.

The evolution of occupational therapy ideas in Canada (see figure 14.1) is paralleled by the evolution of occupational therapy education, which is summarized in figure 14.3. Until recently, when immigration and support personnel added to the supply of occupational therapy personnel, university education programs were the major supply source.

The first education courses for ward aides in Canada began in Ontario after World War I. These courses laid the foundation for the creation in 1926 of a two-year diploma in occupational therapy at the University of Toronto (Friedland, 2003). In 1945, CAOT decided that the Toronto program should be extended from two to three years in length. McGill University opened the second three-year, combined program in Canada beginning in 1950. In 1954, the Université de Montréal opened the world's first university-level, occupational therapy program in French. This too was combined with a physiotherapy program.

[1] Occupational therapy education in Canada has always been offered at the university level, not at the technical collage level.

Positioning occupational therapy for leadership

Figure 14.3 Evolution of Canadian occupational therapy education

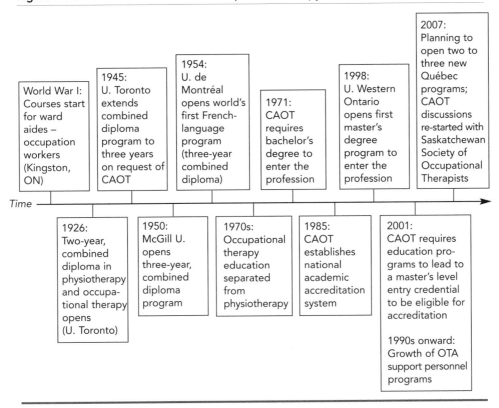

In 1953, CAOT recognized that combined occupational therapy and physiotherapy programs were a disadvantage for occupational therapy, given that, by far, the greatest numbers of graduates were choosing a career in physiotherapy (Friedland, 2003). In the 1970s, universities began to offer separate occupational therapy programs. Universities also complied with the 1971 CAOT decision to accredit only education programs that produced graduates with a bachelor's degree.

Recognizing that the supply of occupational therapists must be well qualified, CAOT began to establish national standards for education in 1975, and created a national Academic Accreditation Council in 1985. All entry-level occupational therapy programs in Canada are now accredited by CAOT. Registration with most provincial regulatory colleges requires proof of graduation from an accredited program. The CAOT academic accreditation standards are congruent with, and exceed, minimum, international standards for education set by the World Federation of Occupational Therapists (2002). Programs must demonstrate that their graduates are educated in the competency areas of the *Profile of Occupational Therapy Practice in Canada* (CAOT, 1997b, 2002, 2007) and the *Essential Competencies* (ACOTRO, 2003).

In 1998, The University of Western Ontario opened the first Canadian, entry-level, occupational therapy, master's degree program. CAOT announced in 2001 that, beginning in 2008, only entry-level programs leading to a Master's degree will be eligible for academic accreditation. A similar requirement for a post-baccalaureate degree exists in the United States. Canada continues to accept the qualifications of new Canadians whose education was from a non-Canadian program, which has been accredited by the World Federation of Occupational Therapists.

In addition to offering degree programs in occupational therapy, Canadian universities offer post-professional coursework and research master's degrees, as well as doctoral programs for occupational therapists. These were introduced to build scholarship and generate knowledge, to provide an educational ladder for career development, and to develop future academic occupational therapists. Most Canadian, post-professional master's, doctoral, and post-doctoral studies are in rehabilitation science. A few post-professional, master's degree programs are in health or related sciences. At the time of the writing of this book, there is one post-professional, master's degree program in occupational therapy and two doctoral-level opportunities to focus on occupational science within a rehabilitation science degree.

In 1982, Canada's 12 university-level, occupational therapy programs developed a national organization, the Association of Canadian Occupational Therapy University Programs (ACOTUP). ACOTUP aims to uphold standards of education, facilitate an exchange of ideas, foster research in occupational therapy, and liaise with other national and international institutions with occupational therapy education and research mandates. To strengthen the voice of occupational therapy education in Canada, ACOTUP established a permanent secretariat in 2004 and started to articulate position statements on the education of occupational therapists in this country.

The change to a master's degree requirement in entry-level education is intended to better prepare new graduates to provide evidence-based accountability for occupation-based practice, and to engage in more autonomous practice with diverse populations in diverse settings (CAOT, 2004c). CAOT is involved in the strategy which Statistics Canada (2006) is developing to examine education as a primary source of supply for health professions, such as occupational therapy, in Canada.

With a growing interest to supply practitioners who are well versed in enabling occupation, programs now educate students in qualitative as well as quantitative research, client-centred practice, and enabling occupation. Graduates learn the theory and use of occupation-based models, such as the Canadian Model of Occupational Performance and Engagement (CMOP-E). They draw evidence for practice from many sources, including the new, interdisciplinary field of occupational science (see chapter 3). With an eye for future demands and new ways to utilize occupational therapy in the workforce, today's occupational therapy education is strong on such issues as evaluation, interprofessional learning, professional autonomy, accountability, management of funding, policy and legislative requirements, and the integration of scholarship and evidence in practice. Students learn about social issues, ethics, globalization, citizen participation, inclusion, and justice. In addition to developing a workforce strongly rooted in occupational therapy knowledge and skills, students learn important competencies for interprofessional practice, including communication, collaboration, and professionalism. Research is growing to understand the broad concepts of occupation and enablement, and to advance an occupational therapy vision in practice, as this book attests.

14.5 Influences of immigration and emigration on workforce supply

In 2004, 9.6% (563) of CAOT members were educated outside Canada. Immigration and emigration are a growing influence in occupational therapy workforce planning. Regulators in Canada report that 262 occupational therapists educated outside the country, registered for practice from 2000 to 2005. Over half (136) of the international graduates settled in Ontario, with another 20% (51) moving to British Columbia. Only 5% (13) chose to live in one of the four Atlantic provinces (von Zweck, 2006). Occupational therapists educated in Canada also move to other countries to practice. From 2005 to 2006, 238 CAOT members lived outside of Canada; of these, 56.3% (134) were educated in Canada.

The supply of Canadian-educated, occupational therapists is enriched greatly by immigration. Canada is a country of immigrants and, over the past century, waves of immigration have shaped much of our country's history. From 1890 to 1920 alone, the population of Canada almost doubled. The second major influx of immigrants, from the 1940s to the late 1960s, was tailored to suit the labour market needs of the country. This wave introduced a much wider diversity of people, and reflected humanitarian concerns for the plight and chaos experienced by the citizens of many nations. The ethnocentric selection criteria that favoured European and British immigrants, slowly adapted to embrace a much more flexible approach during the later half of the 20th century. Today, there is a greater emphasis on cultural and ethnic diversity to reflect the needs for migration.

At the beginning of the 21st century, thinking has shifted and consideration is given to how immigration enhances the Canadian population. The advent of the global village, ready access to every corner of the world, and greatly enhanced communication systems have created an attitude of welcome for those who are suffering or escaping repressive regimes. The federal government's Bill C-11, the *Immigration and Refugee Protection Act* (Citizenship and Immigration Canada, 2002), declared Canada's intention to assess appropriateness for immigration based on skills and abilities rather than on credentials. Bill C-11 highlights key principles that include: respect for Canada's multicultural character; support for the development of English and French linguistic minority communities; the notion that new immigrants and Canadian society have mutual obligations; the idea that refugee protection is, in the first instance, about saving lives; and the commitment to work in cooperation with provinces/territories to secure better recognition of the foreign credentials of permanent residents and their accelerated integration into the workforce. Bill C-11 attempts to strike a balance between measures to address the security and safety of Canadians, and the legacy of welcoming immigrants and protecting refugees. This is indeed laudable, however, the Bill challenges occupational therapy and other professions to protect standards of practice, while also embodying the Canadian principles of inclusion and respect for others.

Canadian occupational therapists will want to consider the need for consonance between our profession's mandate and philosophy, and the intentions of Bill C-11. The construct of culture is an important element of the environment in the Canadian Model of Occupational Performance and Engagement (CMOP-E) and in other occupational performance models. A very real conundrum for occupational therapists in Canada is to develop a workforce that practices in concert with the profession's values, beliefs, and models. Yet Canadians want to enable our professional colleagues with diverse educational, practice, and cultural backgrounds from around the world to join our ranks.

To address this conundrum, in 2005 CAOT received funding from the Government of Canada Foreign Credential Recognition Program to conduct a review of issues that influence the ability of international graduates to work as occupational therapists. The review indicated that international graduates are marginalized in various ways and do not readily enter the occupational therapy workforce. For instance, there are complex national and provincial procedures for qualifications review. Added challenges are language difficulties, expectations of familiarity with Canadian models and terminology, and procedures in the Canadian health system or other sectors that are unfamiliar to international graduates. If occupational therapists are able to effectively implement solutions to this conundrum, it would truly be a fitting next chapter in Canada's legacy of welcoming the world while also building professional excellence.

14.6 The growing supply of occupational therapy support personnel

Formally-trained occupational therapy support personnel are a major, new, positive-supply resource in occupational therapy workforce planning as long as their positions are clearly aligned with occupational therapy. Just over 42% of CAOT members in Canada's provinces report that they assign services to support personnel (CAOT, 2005b) (see table 14.2). CAOT data (2005b)[2] indicate that 35% of associate members in 2004 were occupational therapy support personnel. The extended use of support personnel is reported by many provinces as a powerful workforce planning strategy to improve access to occupational therapy (Atkinson & Hull, 2001; New Brunswick Department of Health and Wellness, 2002; Newfoundland and Labrador Health Boards Association & Department of Health and Community Services, 2003). Congruent with this perspective, CAOT members working in provinces with lower than the national average of per-capita numbers of occupational therapists, report higher rates of support personnel, particularly in Newfoundland and Labrador, and Saskatchewan (CAOT, 2005b).

Only one program was publicly-funded in 1990 (Okanagan College in British Columbia); by the 1990s, there were 7 publicly-funded programs and 6 have opened since 2000 for a total of 16 programs in six provinces in 2006.[3] The exceptions are Québec, New Brunswick, and Nova Scotia, which are all planning programs, and Prince Edward Island. In the four years between 2002 and 2006, 835 rehabilitation-related support personnel graduated from publicly-funded programs, and more graduated from a rapidly growing number of privately-funded programs. The two largest programs, at Okanagan College in British Columbia and Mohawk College of

---

[2] The three Canadian territories are not included due to limited availability of data on support personnel.

[3] The opening dates of two programs were not available in CAOT data that was collected through contact with individual programs and with a fledgling national organization for support personnel education programs.

Table 14.2 Occupational therapists working with support personnel in Canada per province

Province	Occupational therapists per 100,000 population	Percentage of CAOT members who assign work to support personnel
Newfoundland and Labrador	28.3	60.2%
Saskatchewan	21.5	60.2
Alberta	37.0	53.2
British Columbia	32.1	48.6
Manitoba	37.6	47.4
New Brunswick	31.8	43.4
Nova Scotia	30.2	40.3
Ontario	31.1	37.3
Prince Edward Island	25.3	35.9
Québec	41.1	19.8
Canada	34.0	42.4

CAOT (2005b)

Applied Arts and Science in Ontario, graduated almost 300 of the 835 support personnel noted above. On average, 150 support personnel graduate annually. Several colleges offer a two-year diploma program that will allow graduates to upgrade to a general bachelor's degree. With a bachelor's degree, some may apply for admission to the new master's programs to enter the profession.

Occupational therapists working with support personnel in Canada per province

At present, there are no Canadian standards for the education and practice of support personnel in occupational therapy. CAOT is working with the Canadian Physiotherapy Association to develop accreditation standards for support personnel education programs, which often combine preparation for graduates to choose work in either profession. CAOT believes a key component of this accreditation program will be the requirement for a qualifications recognition process that will assess a worker's competency in relation to job requirements. The feasibility of developing a qualifications recognition process to assess and formally recognize the competency of occupational therapy support personnel, is currently under investigation (Klaiman, 2006).

Most occupational therapy support personnel with formal education have dual/combined training to work both as an occupational therapist and physiotherapist assistant, or rehabilitation assistant in occupational therapy and physiotherapy. This dual/combined education strategy mirrors the period from the 1920s to 1970s, when professional occupational therapy and physiotherapy education were combined at the University of Toronto, McGill University, the University of Alberta, and the University of British Columbia (Friedland, 2003). The argument for efficiency in dual/combined training is based on the same arguments used for almost 50 years to defend combined professional education for occupational therapy and physiotherapy. As Friedland (2003) notes, combined/dual training disadvantaged occupational therapy, given the emphasis of programs on physical rehabilitation, not mental health and other areas of occupational therapy, and the high number of graduates who then chose physiotherapy.

Support personnel in occupational therapy are most frequently employed to manage equipment and supplies (e.g., wheelchairs) implement routine programs with individuals and groups (e.g., monitoring self-care routines in long-term care) and do office administration. Occupational therapists supervise their work and are responsible and liable for issues of safety and quality with clients. Occupational therapy support personnel are responsible to provide appropriate levels of competent service as assigned by occupational therapists.

We know that the positive inclusion of support personnel is optimized through professionalism, good communication, and collaborative problem solving (Blechert, Christiansen, & Kari, 1987; Dillon, 2001; Glantz & Richman, 1997; Pucetti, 1988). Good workforce planning strives to avoid role confusion and overly restrictive limitations, two frequently cited sources of conflict when professionals and support personnel work together (Hayes, 1994; Huber, Blegen, & McCloskey, 1994; Painter & Akroyd, 1998; Workman, 1996). Good planning also strives to avoid the inappropriate use of support personnel, which can result in lower standards, poorer outcomes, and ineffective service planning (Pong, 1997).

Support personnel and professionals who work well together consider themselves to be partners, and speak of teamwork and complementary roles, rather than hierarchical relationships (Jung, Sainsbury, Grum, Wilkins, & Tryssenaar, 2002). Having clear boundaries, understanding each other's knowledge base, and appreciating respective roles are identified as the basis of successful relationships (Jung et al., 2002). Written guidelines are available from regulatory and professional associations and outline supervisory responsibilities for occupational therapists working with support personnel. These include identifying appropriate tasks to assign, developing a supervision plan, and monitoring and evaluating task assignment (CAOT, 2003b; College of Occupational Therapists of British Columbia, 2004).

14.7 Demand for and utilization of Canada's occupational therapy workforce

Analysis of utilization complements the analysis of supply for occupational therapy workforce planning. The demand for, and utilization of, occupational therapy is extremely difficult to assess. Variations in demand and utilization will be influenced by a combination of service differences across and between provinces, and different provincial definitions of demand.

To illustrate the complexity, occupational therapy demand and utilization may be high in resource-rich, urban services where occupational therapy is better known, funds are available, teams define the need for occupational therapy, and collective efforts to advance the profession are more influential. Conversely, demand and utilization may also be high in rural, remote, or other low service resource areas, if other professions are absent and occupational therapists are proactive in developing the profession.

One strong variable in demand and utilization is the energy and ingenuity of individual occupational therapists. Occupational therapists who can sustain the scope of occupational therapy and who are sufficiently connected with management and policy makers, are well positioned to advocate for necessary funding, policy, and legislative support. While occupational therapists continually use advocacy skills with and for their clients, those who utilize their advocacy and other political skills in promoting the profession will likely have an impact on demand and utilization (Duncan et al., 2005; Jacobs, 1999; Kronenberg & Pollard, 2005; O'Shea, 1979). Demand and utilization may in fact be influenced by occupational therapists who use the politically-grounded advocacy strategies outlined in section IV: using evidence to profile the profession, and demonstrate our effectiveness as well as cost-benefits, using innovation to find funding, policy, and legislative supports, and providing workforce data to illustrate where access to occupational therapy exists, is lacking, or is entirely absent.

Typically, the prevalence of disability within the general population is a major indicator of demand for occupational therapy. However, provincial, occupational therapy regulatory organization data across the 10 provinces indicate that the per-capita distribution and utilization of occupational therapists in Canada, varies greatly and is not directly proportional to disability rates (CIHI, 2006; Statistics Canada, 2002) (see table 14.3). Québec has the lowest disability rate and the highest utilization of occupational therapists in Canada; conversely, Nova Scotia, with the highest disability rate, is below the Canadian average in its utilization of occupational therapists. Health and community service systems in these two provinces are different, as are the funding mechanisms. Public and government attitudes to hospital-based, medical services differ. Access to occupational therapy education is likely a factor. Nova Scotia's low rate of occupational therapy utilization appears to be directly related to the absence of occupational therapy in Atlantic Canada until Dalhousie University opened an Atlantic Region School in 1982. The higher utilization rates in the other three Atlantic

Table 14.3 Disability rates compared with rates of occupational therapists per 100,000 population*

Province	Disability rate in 2001 (Statistics Canada, 2002)	Occupational therapists per 100,000 population (Canadian Institute for Health Information [CIHI], 2006)
Nova Scotia	17.1	30.2
Saskatchewan	14.5	21.5
New Brunswick	14.4	31.8
Prince Edward Island	14.3	25.3
Manitoba	14.2	37.6
British Columbia	14.0	32.1
Ontario	13.5	31.1
Alberta	12.5	37.0
Newfoundland and Labrador	12.3	28.3
Québec	8.4	41.1
Canada	12.4	34.0

*Rates are for Canada's 10 provinces, not the territories, due to limited availability of reliable data as occupational therapists are not regulated in the territories.
CIHI (2006); Statistics Canada (2002)

provinces — New Brunswick, Newfoundland and Labrador, and Prince Edward Island — appear to be the result of advocacy efforts and government policies.

Other important data used to assess demand and utilization of occupational therapy might be the age structures of the population, particularly the proportion of children, adolescents, and seniors: these are age groups who are known to face what may be difficult occupational transitions. Useful data are prevalence rates for chronic diseases, such as chronic cardiac, neurodegenerative, psychiatric, or respiratory diseases. Those living with chronic disease can be enabled to live a fuller life, possibly with less medical expense, when guided to adapt or modify their environment, abilities and routines, and when policies and funding support community participation by all members. The prevalence of people with severe and persistent mental illness indicates the potential to utilize occupational therapy to address homelessness, unemployment, stigma, addictions, crime, and the general suffering of this target population.

Information on per capita ratios is difficult to use to determine demand and utilization without more data collection and analysis. We know that in the past 20 years, the average per capita utilization and availability of occupational therapists has more than tripled. In 1984, Health and Welfare Canada reported the rate of occupational therapists as 9.1 per 100,000 population. The ratio has grown in 20 years to 35.0 occupational therapists per 100,000 (CAOT, 1989; CIHI, 2006).

Modelling to compare national and international utilization of occupational therapy will be difficult because the education, responsibilities, roles, positions, and salary levels of occupational therapists differ around the world. An important advance was made with publication of the revised *World Federation of Occupational Therapists' Minimum Standards* (2002), which benchmark educational standards for the accreditation of occupational therapy education worldwide. An outstanding international effort is being made to harmonize European education through "tuning initiatives" to define common learning outcomes for occupational therapy education at the bachelor's, master's, and doctoral levels (Council of Occupational Therapists for European Countries, 2005). At present, data from the Scandinavian, national occupational therapy organizations, including Iceland, report by far the highest rates of occupational therapy utilization. Their ratios are between 70 and 90 occupational therapists per 100,000 population (Council of Occupational Therapists for European Countries, 2005), whereas the highest ratio reported by CIHI (2006) for Canada was 41.1 in Québec.

While disability rates, economies, education and health, and funding structures, service delivery models, and other factors all complicate the comparison, it appears that the occupational therapy workforce in Canada has made progress in the last 20 years and has considerable scope to develop. This observation is consistent with Canadian labour market reports, which call for a drastic increase in the number of occupational therapists (Human Resources and Skills Development Canada, 2005).

14.8 Supply and utilization of the occupational therapy workforce in Québec

The workforce in Québec is presented as a special case because this province holds a historic place in the founding of Canada. Québec is Canada's only officially Francophone province and currently reports the highest per-capita availability of occupational therapists in Canada, with over one quarter of the Canadian occupational therapy workforce (28.5%) employed in that province (CIHI, 2005a, 2006; Statistics Canada, 2005a).

The development of occupational therapy in Québec merits particular discussion because of the size of the occupational therapy workforce serving this province. Although universities in Québec already produce one third of Canadian, occupational therapy graduates (ACOTUP, 2006), there are documented shortages of occupational therapists in the province. The Québec government is exploring options to increase workforce capacity, including the development of two new educational programs. One program has been accepted at l'Université de Sherbrooke; another one is being considered for l'Université du Québec à Trois-Rivières (Québec Santé et Services sociaux, 2002).

French-speaking occupational therapists work with the over one million Francophones living in Québec and other provinces, particularly New Brunswick, Ontario, Manitoba, Alberta, and British Columbia (Citizenship and Immigration Canada, 2005). New Brunswick is Canada's only officially bilingual province and does much to cultivate Francophone service delivery, including occupational therapy.

The evolution of occupational therapy education and practice in Québec, parallels the development of the profession in the rest of Canada in many ways (see figures 14.1 and 14.3). In the mid 1970s, the ministère de l'Éducation du Québec was concerned about the relevance of maintaining education in occupational therapy at the university level. Today, the scope of occupational therapy is such that Québec, like the other Canadian provinces, has agreed to implement a master's entry-level degree. While this move is not unique to Québec, it represents one of the most important changes in the profession in the province within the last 30 years.

Since the 1980s, using innovation and ingenuity, occupational therapists in Québec continue to resolve occupational challenges with clients, using a range of activities/occupations, environmental modifications, and learning strategies to help the same diverse clients that have been discussed throughout the book. The heartbeat of occupational therapy continues to be a comprehensive approach centred on the process of activity or occupation. As with Anglophone Canada, the term *occupation* is problematic in that the general public and funding bodies equate occupation with work or a hobby.

Human activity (occupation), as an influencing factor of physical and mental health, and a key enabler in rehabilitation, is now recognized in Québec to be the core of occupational therapy. Great advances were made toward such recognition when the federal and Québec governments invested in a community-based approach to the organization of Québec health services. Within this approach, occupational therapists have spearheaded resource plans for maintaining the ability of persons with disabilities to live in their own environments. Occupational therapists in Québec are also advancing the use of activity and occupation among people without disabilities, by fostering a balance of work, leisure, and activities of daily living. There is considerable attention to the use of activity and rest for both health promotion and the prevention of illness. Developments in community-based services have coincided with the ongoing emergence of private practice occupational therapy. The profession in Québec will need to ensure that the body of knowledge about human occupation and enablement is well-used in practice, is applied in context, and is well researched to play a political role in the ongoing development of services in health settings, communities, and other areas.

14.9   Retention and career development

The retention and career development of occupational therapists is a workforce planning issue, closely linked with job satisfaction. Individuals who are satisfied with their work are more likely to stay in their position, remain in their chosen career, develop a career path for growth, and serve as a positive role model for others entering the field. Female occupational therapists with less than 20 years in the profession and who work directly with clients, report the highest levels of satisfaction with their work, particularly citing a sense of pride and achievement in enabling their clients to attain their goals (Moore, Cruickshank, & Haas, 2006). Autonomy and positive interaction with work colleagues also are reported to provide job satisfaction for occupational therapists (Jenkins, 1991; Rugg, 1999).

Involvement in professional development activities is a well known strategy for the retention of health professionals. Despite the challenges of on-line learning, new technologies, such as Internet-based courses, provide opportunities for continuing professional development (Hollis & Madill, 2006; Hunter & Nicol, 2002; Townsend, Le-May Sheffield, Stadnyk, & Beagan, 2006).

Retention in occupational therapy needs serious attention. The major losses to the occupational therapy workforce are from males, new graduates, and experienced practitioners who move into management, policy, education, or research positions without retaining their occupational therapy registration or identity. Some may leave because of workplace dissatisfaction, possibly with diminishing feelings of effectiveness and professional identity (Irvine & Graham, 1994).

Failure to successfully manage conflicts also undermines retention. Some factors are poor supervision, high workloads, low levels of professional recognition and a lack of congruence between work and personal values (Moore et al., 2006). Career development may require conflict resolution. For example, new graduates may become discouraged when their visions of an ideal career in occupational therapy conflict with the realities in the workplace (Kasar & Muscari, 2000). Academic faculty and fieldwork practicum preceptors may need to assist students in balancing idealism with the reality of workplace demands on this rapidly changing profession (Wilkins & Rosenthal, 2001). Disillusionment may still occur unless new graduates, often burdened with large financial debts, find ready employment in satisfying positions.

Role differentiation and identity may be exacerbated when occupational therapists find themselves working in positions with generic titles (e.g., case manager, intake worker, counsellor, manager, policy analyst). Important influences for managing such conflicts include role modelling by experienced practitioners, participation in occupational therapy conferences, membership and involvement in professional organizations, and participation in research and teaching (Molyneux, 2001). Retention of new graduates and seasoned practitioners requires access to continuing education and advancement, and the further development of occupational therapy as a vibrant, influential profession.

14.10 Occupational therapy partners in interprofessional contexts

CAOT offers associate membership for support personnel, clients, friends of the profession, and representatives of various agencies, government departments, and businesses; these are all potential partners in interprofessional and interdisciplinary contexts. Dickinson's message (see section IV) signals the importance of collaborating with occupational therapy clients or consumers[4] as partners. He reinforces Bonnie Sherr Klein's reminder (see case 1), who called on occupational therapists to develop partnerships with consumers. Consumer voices are sometimes present in occupational therapy literature, largely when they are brought into a professional presentation or publication. Some publications, such as the *Rehabilitation Digest*, have mandates to publish both professional and consumer writing.

To promote occupational therapy partnerships with consumers and others, section II reminds occupational therapists that enablement begins by ensuring that clients have a voice in all decision making and practice, and that enablement requires collaboration with people, rather than doing things to or for them. Section III illustrates client-therapist partnerships in the Canadian Practice Process Framework. Throughout the book, the *Canadian Occupational Performance Measure* (COPM) (Law et al., 2005) has been cited as an evaluation and outcomes measurement tool that involves clients as partners in identifying their priority, occupational performance issues.

Partnerships with professional colleagues are also important in positioning occupational therapy. Current trends suggest that there will be ongoing interest in developing interprofessional practices to ensure that Canadians can access a broad range of health-related services in a coordinated and timely manner. While the notion of interprofessional education as a foundation for interprofessional practice is good common sense, there have been a multitude of attitudinal, structural, and professional barriers (Gilbert, 2005). One barrier is to find space to coordinate educational time schedules. Another is to educate faculty who have little experience in the design and delivery of interprofessional curricula. Since educational accreditation standards expect students to develop profession-specific competencies, there is a need to define cross competencies for interprofessional practice (Oandasan & Reeves, 2005). The importance of interprofessional education has been recognized by the federal government, with funds to develop a framework for interprofessional education (Oandasan & Reeves,

---

[4] The business meaning of consumer or client is recognized here.

2005). While concerns for professional autonomy and identity need clear attention, there are real opportunities to educate our partners about occupational therapy. We can strengthen advocacy voices when we join with others.

Two national initiatives are good examples of occupational therapy partners in inter-professional collaborations. The Enhancing Interdisciplinary Collaboration in Primary Care Initiative (2006) and the Canadian Collaborative Mental Health Initiative (Gagné, 2005), were federally-funded projects in which CAOT was a national partner. Both projects engaged occupational therapists across Canada. Professional and consumer organizations developed visions, strategies, and resources to support collaboration as a means to high-quality primary care and mental health. Enhancing interdisciplinary collaboration is consistent with our occupational model and the social determinants of health. It will, however, necessitate further advocacy to integrate occupational therapy into primary care funding in areas of prevention, health promotion, and population health (Scriven & Atwal, 2004).

Occupational therapists and support personnel can expect to become more involved in interprofessional relationships outside the traditional boundaries of health services. Opportunities beyond health services exist in environments where Canadians carry out their daily occupations. For example, disability management, in which occupational therapy plays a part, has emerged as a comprehensive, workplace-based approach to reduce work disabilities and their related human, social, and economic costs (Williams & Westmorland, 2002). Occupational therapists involved with disability management programs define and deliver their services in collaboration with other health professions and support personnel, as well as with a broad range of payers.

Other potential occupational therapy partners are individual and organizational stakeholders such as labour unions, insurance companies, human resources depart-ments, and employee assistance programs. With each new partner, occupational ther-apists need to demonstrate their commitment to occupation-based, client-centred enablement within the context of complex practice relationships.

14.11 Stakeholder strategies in occupational therapy workforce planning

The evolution of ideas and education programs has radically transformed workforce planning in occupational therapy, paralleling the radical transformation of the pro-fession itself. The addition of new Canadians through immigration and the growth of support personnel are adding new energy and ideas to the profession.

Our history in Canada shows a female-dominated profession, transforming from a two-year educational requirement to master's-level credentials, and from biomedical to multiple contexts. Our knowledge has expanded beyond the biomedical model and the diversional use of activity, to an occupational model and occupational enablement (Polatajko, 2001). Questions about the supply and utilization of occupational therapists now require analysis of practice in a huge range of settings and conditions across the mosaic of practice in Canada. Canadian provincial registrars, such as Eugene, and many stakeholders are involved in workforce planning. Each is faced with questions about the supply and utilization of occupational therapists who practice with a multitude of diverse types of clients in a wide range of settings and systems. Furthermore, occupational therapists are engaged in education, research, and policy development, as well as in traditional clinical, consulting, and management positions. Supply and utilization are difficult to track given that, rather than being called occupational therapists, some positions may be called case manager, researcher, or another title.

The strategy to accelerate workforce planning for leadership in enabling occupation in this chapter has so far addressed supply, demand, utilization, retention, career development, and partnerships. Challenges in funding, professional identity, and market competition suggest that a major growth strategy involving multiple stakeholders is urgently needed. To that end, a Canadian Occupational Therapy Workforce Integration Project has developed recommendations with occupational therapy organizations and government agencies (see table 14.4) (von Zweck, 2006). The three-pronged growth strategy proposed in the introduction to chapter 14 is to increase supply, retain experienced practitioners, and develop a clear identity with the public and new alliances. These aims are congruent with the national workforce integration project.

The first two objectives of the project are to build capacity in the profession and make its identity known to others. The stakeholders for these objectives are all occupational therapists, regulatory and professional organizations, scholars, union members, government personnel, and the media/public. Other objectives are to improve public and private access to the profession by increasing both the numbers and the funding base of the profession. The stakeholders identified in table 14.5 all have different perspectives and interests in being involved.

Table 14.4   Recommendations from the Canadian Occupational Therapy Workforce Integration Project

1. Coordinate and centralize registration requirements and processes for working as an occupational therapist

2. Improve national certification examination access, preparation resources, and assistance

3. Provide clear and accessible information to help international graduates work in Canada

4. Increase access to academic upgrading and language training to help international graduates meet registration requirements

5. Help international graduates become linked with employers, occupational therapists, and professional resources

6. Advocate for the need for internationally-educated occupational therapists in Canada

7. Promote a diverse workforce for quality occupational therapy services

— *By Claudia von Zweck (2006)*

Many of the priority stakeholder issues listed in table 14.6 will build the profession's capacity, and clarify the identity as a means to increase the supply and utilization of this profession. The strategy highlights initiatives for occupational therapists to take with each stakeholder.

Table 14.5   Occupational therapy stakeholders

Stakeholder group	Stakeholder interests
Clients or consumers	The ultimate stakeholders, those whom the profession serves; have interests in effectiveness and satisfaction and will relay positive and negative experiences
The public	Citizens and the media with interests as potential clients or consumers with the profession and interests in public knowledge of the profession
Colleagues and partners	Professional and non-professional stakeholders with interests in occupational therapy as part of teams, groups, collaborations, partnerships
Governments	Public bodies with interests to create and implement public policies and legislation that influence access to the profession and demand accountability, through processes such as funding of programs and professional registration, e.g., for enabling occupation
Businesses and corporations	Private funding bodies with interests in efficiency and cost-benefit toward economic, not social indicators of success; they influence private access to the profession and have high demands for economic accountability; occupational therapy businesses are stakeholders who balance economic and professional interests
Employers and unions	Funders and organizations with interests in management and labour practices that influence occupational therapy supply, utilization, retention, and career development; interests are in managing, coordinating, grouping, and streamlining occupational categories
Occupational therapists	Professional self-interest to advance the clinical, management, consulting, education, research, policy, and other forms of practice; specific interests may be in regulation, professional promotion, evaluation of the profession, development of theories and practice models, etc.

The occupational therapy workforce in Canada could grow significantly by both increasing the number of admissions to existing educational programs, and the number and locations of educational programs in Canada. Access to occupational therapy can also be improved by actions to support retention and career development in occupational therapy.

Even more powerful would be to increase universality of access and utilization of occupational therapy across Canada (see text box 14.1). Many parts of Canada offer poor access to occupational therapy, particularly outside major centres in resource-rich provinces. Many types of occupational therapy services are available in only a handful of places, such as the few new initiatives in addictions, primary health care, or corrections. Many long-standing services in some sectors are not available across Canada, such as the availability of occupational therapy in schools in some provinces but not others. Occupational therapy mental health services are quite uneven: acute care hospital services tend to offer occupational therapy, but occupational therapy is absent in many community mental health programs. Whereas there may be policy positions in some provinces, there may be no voices for occupational therapy in the policy arenas of other provinces. Advances in the use of occupational therapy have been made in some diagnostic-based services, such as arthritis services; however, there is little consistency in access to occupational therapy in services for children with learning disabilities or attention deficit disorders. Services for seniors

Positioning occupational therapy for leadership

Table 14.6 Occupational therapy workforce planning: A strategy to develop leadership in enabling occupation

Stakeholder	Occupational therapists' leadership initiatives
Clients and consumers	• Build alliances to raise client and consumer awareness of an occupational perspective of health, well-being and justice, and occupation as a health benefit • Enable clients and consumers to identify, analyze, document, and publicize their occupational challenges and issues
The public	• Build media and other alliances to raise public awareness of an occupational perspective of health, well-being and justice, and occupation as a health benefit • Profile "wait times" and advocate with others to increase access through public and private insured services • Prompt media to promote good news stories and occupational therapy as a career
Colleagues and partners	• Build alliances to raise colleagues' and partners' awareness of an occupational perspective of health, well-being and justice, and occupation as a health benefit • Advocate to include occupational therapy as a team collaborator
Government	• Build alliances to raise government awareness of an occupational perspective of health, well-being and justice, and occupation as a health benefit • Create policies, funding, and legislation to integrate occupation-based enablement in government priorities to meet population needs through diverse programs and initiatives • Implement an integrated, occupational therapy, human resource strategy • Advocate for senior positions with the job title and requirements of a registered occupational therapist
Businesses and corporations	• Build alliances to raise business awareness of an occupational perspective of health, well-being and justice, and occupation as a health benefit • Develop private occupational therapy businesses that demonstrate ethical, cost-effective, socially conscious, environmentally-sustainable practices
Employers and unions	• Build alliances to raise employer and union awareness of an occupational perspective of health, well-being and justice, and occupation as a health benefit • Target meaningful health outcomes relating to occupation and quality of life in service and workforce planning • Advocate for policies and funding to support enabling occupation • Advocate for senior positions with the job title and requirements of a registered occupational therapist • Advocate to recruit and retain occupational therapists, negotiate employee benefit packages that include time and resources such as Internet access, and financial support for evidence-based decision making and continuing education • Advocate to include occupational therapy as an insured benefit in extended health plans for employees
All occupational therapists – with many stakeholders	• Build alliances to increase scholarship and evidence on an occupational perspective of health, well-being and justice, and occupation as a health benefit • Make the title occupational therapy visible and explicit in all communications; for example, brochures, signs, media releases, referral and service documents • Mentor new graduates, internationally educated occupational therapists, and those on interprofessional teams • Supervise and mentor occupational therapy support personnel • Raise awareness of gender stereotypes and other diversity issues associated with occupations and occupational therapy • Develop national, regional, and local networks to develop occupational therapy leadership in health and other sectors

Continued ...

Continued ...

Table 14.6 Occupational therapy workforce planning: A strategy to develop leadership in enabling occupation

Stakeholder	Occupational therapists' leadership initiatives
Occupational therapists in senior positions	• Retain professional registration to build alliances and increase scholarship and evidence on an occupational perspective of health, well-being and justice, and occupation as a health benefit • Advocate for senior positions to use the job title occupational therapists or to include occupational therapy as an eligible profession in job searches • Retain active links with occupational therapy to mentor occupational therapy leadership development
Occupational therapy support personnel	• Advocate for clear educational content, credential recognition, and union support for occupational therapy support workers
Occupational therapy regulators and professional organizations	• Build alliances to raise awareness of an occupational perspective of health, occupational determinants of health, and occupation as a health benefit • Coordinate competency development with university programs and facilitate workforce mobility, recruitment, and retention • Define occupational therapy broadly for retention and growth to improve access to occupational therapy in Canada and the world

tend to include occupational therapy, but utilization may be mostly for consultation on technical equipment and devices. Some insurers are recognizing occupational therapy as an insured service, but others are yet to be convinced.

Many questions remain to understand what attracts mostly women and few men to the profession. We also need to know why some stay in occupational therapy while others move on. Retention requires clear attention to typical initiatives, including mentoring, continuing professional development, providing adequate resources and equipment, and respecting the dissemination of new knowledge by recent graduates

Text box 14.1

Reflections on access to occupational therapy

How universal is access to occupational therapy in your community? Who is without occupational therapy services that you would expect to be available? How is occupational therapy known and portrayed in the media where you live? Would everyone in your community relate to the profession as portrayed, or would some not see its relevance to society?

How do you feel when you see occupational therapy advertised or reported in your community? How does the image of the profession speak to the diversity of people, social classes, races, and other differences that you know are present in the community? What are you seeing? What would you like to do about what you see — rejoice in occupational therapy as a positive force in society? Make changes in the profession? Or both?

— By Brenda Beagan

(Moore et al., 2006; Townsend et al., 2006). Vertical integration of occupational therapy human resources would identify, interconnect, and coordinate professionals and support personnel who comprise the occupational therapy workforce.

A small profession needs to carefully nurture future leaders and take advantage of being able to move quickly on new initiatives. Diverse groups, such as the Association of Canadian Occupational Therapy University Programs (ACOTUP), the Association of Canadian Occupational Therapy Regulatory Organizations (ACOTRO), the Professional Alliance of Canada (PAC), the Canadian Occupational Therapy Foundation (COTF), and CAOT might build a shared strategic vision and plan for future initiatives.

Chapter 14 is a guide for Eugene and others to accelerate workforce planning through data collection, critical analysis, and collaboration with key stakeholders. Working strategically, occupational therapy leaders might organize regular education and strategic planning sessions to include the array of occupational therapy human resources, employers, union representatives, government personnel, and members of the public. One strategy might be to gather together the occupational therapy leaders in each province, possibly sparking discussion around the suggestions proposed in table 14.6.

Occupational therapy is a profession in transformation. There is an explosion of knowledge and new practices for enabling occupation. Occupational therapy can build on a strong history of bringing groups together to transform the profession. The smallness of this profession can be used as a strategic springboard. We can launch a dramatic growth strategy by educating more occupational therapists, retaining those who enter the profession, and welcoming occupational therapists who come to Canada from elsewhere. We can also launch a concerted campaign to increase access and the consistency of availability of occupational therapy across services and locations in Canada. Canadian occupational therapists have opportunities to develop cohesiveness, clarity, and vision to make the best contribution possible to the everyday lives of Canadians and others around the world.

Leadership in enabling occupation is ultimately in our hands and those who work with the profession to improve access and availability to occupational therapists for all Canadians. Together, we can advance an occupational therapy vision of health, well-being, and justice for all, through occupation.

EPILOGUE & GLOSSARY

Epilogue

"The future belongs to those who believe in the beauty of their dreams."

Does occupational therapy have a fixed view of its future, or are there alternatives? The challenge, as Ashis Nandy[1] has pointed out, is to keep open the options of dissent. Dissent can be seen as a problem for the creation of more efficiency, or dissent can be seen as crucial information about one's future – the voice of dissent is helping us choose a different evolutionary possibility.

(Inayatullah, 2006[2])

Dear reader

An epilogue is written to take a moment for reflection. One might ask, what has been learned by reading *Enabling Occupation II: Advancing an Occupational Therapy Vision of Health, Well-Being, & Justice through Occupation*? We anticipate that, as readers, you will have learned about the core domain and competence and the constituent practice mosaic of this broad-reaching profession. We further anticipate that, as a reader, you will have been challenged to engage in the transformational agenda this book lays out. We also anticipate that as you finish reading this book you will note, as we have, that there is much more to be said — some of this has been left for another day.

The core domain and competence of occupational therapy

We, the primary authors, with over 60 contributing authors from across Canada, have written *Enabling Occupation II* to challenge Canadians and others around the world to tell everyone that occupational therapy rests on two foundations: occupation and enablement. We hope that you also tell everyone that the driving force for occupational therapists is a vision of health, well-being, and justice in occupations, accomplished through engagement in occupations.

We organized the book as both a study and practice guide. Two sections embrace the two foundations: occupation and enablement. A third section uses practice cases and exemplars to illustrate the integration of occupational enablement, also referred to as occupation-based enablement or enabling occupation. The final section offers four strategies to position occupational therapy for leadership in enabling occupation in Canada and around the world.

Enabling Occupation II offers practice guidelines to make sense of the breadth of diverse and seemingly unconnected expressions of practice that create our practice mosaic. We urge occupational therapists everywhere to practice as members of a Canadian and world community known for the common thread of our concern for

---

[1] Ashis Nandy, *Tradition, Tyranny, and Utopias*, Delhi, Oxford University Press, 1987. Also see, Ashis Nandy, "Bearing Witness to the Future," *Futures*, Vol 28, Nos. 6/7, 1996, 636-639.

[2] Sohail Inayatullah, Professor, Tamkang University, Taiwan; Adjunct Professor, University of the Sunshine Coast, Australia; www.metafuture.org, Mooloolaba. S.inayatullah@qut.edu.au.

occupation and our competence in enablement. To show the profession's common thread in action, real cases have been used to illustrate where primary health care, health promotion, and environmental change might bring occupation and enablement into the realm of public health, healthy public policy, and community planning. Other cases illustrate our traditional and best known work in rehabilitation and mental health programs in hospitals, rehabilitation centres, schools, correctional institutions, and clinics. Still other cases illustrate new initiatives with new public and private funding sources where an occupational perspective and enablement may offer new solutions in situations such as delayed or disrupted child development, youth at-risk, addictions, workplace safety and accommodations, obesity across the lifespan, immigrant occupations, and living a meaningful old age.

In juxtaposing vision and actual practice, challenges have been boldly confronted, not sidestepped. Idealism has been celebrated as the source of energy to realize the vision. One of the marks of being an enablement practitioner is tireless optimism. Hence, the potential for disillusionment in everyday practice has been acknowledged without discouragement. Instead, occupational therapists have been encouraged to take a "*carpe diem*" stance, to "seize the day" and to transform their practice, transform the settings where they work with clients, and transform their communities and societies toward a vision of health, well-being, and justice through occupation. Occupational therapy clinicians, managers, consultants, educators, policy makers, and researchers are encouraged to imbue their practice with the trademark of five essential elements: recognizing occupational challenges; responding through client-centred enablement; enabling asset-based, occupational solutions; drawing on a multidisciplinary knowledge base on occupation and enablement; and engaging others in abductive reasoning to seek the best possible solutions in light of complex occupational experiences and contexts.

Whether you are an occupational therapist or an interested reader, and you are asked for details about the book, you might say that section I proclaims that occupational therapists look at the world through an occupational lens. It profiles our occupational perspective to serve society within and well beyond health services. Section II embraces the language, ideas, values, and skills of enablement that are the common core that binds this profession's diverse forms of practice with a broad range of clients from individuals and families to organizations and populations. It aligns the collaborative power relations of enablement with client-centred practice and with world movements that are democratic, participatory, action-based, and critically reflective. Section III presents cases and discussion for occupational therapists to transform occupational therapy and the contexts of practice. It illustrates a new eight-point practice process which adds the entry, setting the stage, and exit stages to typical processes. The final section IV integrates four strategies to position occupational therapy for enabling occupation in Canada and around the world. It proposes an integrated, multistakeholder strategy to improve the quality of occupational therapy through greater attention to scholarship, evidence and accountability, and to improve access to occupational therapy through the innovative use of funding opportunities and careful workforce planning.

Finally, you might profile *Enabling Occupation II* as Canada's "triple model" guidelines. An expanded Canadian Model of Occupational Performance and Engagement (CMOP-E) guides the focus of concern on occupation; the first ever Canadian Model of Client-Centred Enablement (CMCE) guides the focus of competence in enablement; and a new Canadian Practice Process Framework (CPPF), guides the process of practice through action points and alternative pathways with any client from individuals to populations.

Challenges and opportunities

The Canadian Association of Occupational Therapists is to be congratulated for championing and publishing these new guidelines. *Enabling Occupation II* lays out a transformational agenda for practice thorough the voices of the two primary authors, 63 contributing authors, and the national advisory panel. This collective national voice calls occupational therapists everywhere to both focus our traditional practices on occupation and enablement and to expand beyond the traditional arenas and modes of practice. The agenda to transform practice presented in the book offers challenges and creates opportunities.

Enabling Occupation II challenges the practitioner to embrace an occupational perspective in enabling the occupational participation of their clients and to seize the opportunity to transform their practice, transform the settings where they work with clients, and transform their communities and societies to enable health, well-being, and justice through occupation.

Albeit the juxtaposition of vision and practice presented is restricted to exemplars drawn from front-line practice, the challenge is not solely directed at the front, line practitioner. *Enabling Occupation II* challenges the profession as a whole. As envisioned in this book, occupational therapy encompasses the full spectrum of professional roles. Accordingly, the profession of occupational therapy is a mosaic comprised of all manner of practice roles including: clinicians, consultants, educators, managers, policy makers, and researchers. With *Enabling Occupation II* the entire profession is called to take up the challenge and create a practice imbued with the five essential elements that underlie the mosaic. Most importantly, student occupational therapists, who, by their very status in the profession, represent its future, are asked to take up the challenge, embrace the transformational agenda and make everyday practice and everyday life around the world more inclusive and just.

Recognizing that no profession exists in isolation, the vision of *Enabling Occupation II* necessitates that occupational therapists fully engage our stakeholders if we are to be truly client-centred. Accordingly, practitioners are challenged to seek opportunities to bridge the divide that separates practice from consumer, to use their enabling skill set, not only to enable their clients' occupational goals but also to enable all stakeholders to engage with us as we work to realize our occupational vision. Further, *Enabling Occupation II* challenges all stakeholders of occupational therapy including consumers, funders, administrators, regulatory bodies, and national associations, to insist on being engaged with us in enabling everyone to realize health, well-being, and justice through occupation. As a translational profession, occupational therapy has great potential to enable integrated approaches to bridge separate "silos." Our occupational perspective and enablement approaches can link health services and everyday life, environmental strategies to promote health, well-being and justice, and strategies to address the health of persons.

In the tradition of an epilogue, we encourage you, the reader, individually or in groups, to engage in critical reflection and consider how you might meet the challenges and seize the opportunities of *Enabling Occupation II*. In the spirit of client-centred enablement we offer the following suggestions for reflection and share with you the reflections of colleagues and stakeholders from around the country.

Reflections

Suggestions for readers:

Consider, individually, or in small groups:

- How you will become comfortable in the discourse of occupation and enablement;
- After reading the book, how you will respond to the question: What do occupational therapists do;
- What you might put in your "basket" of exemplars to illustrate the mosaic of occupational therapy.

In partnership with colleagues and stakeholders:

- Reflect on the question: If I envision an expansive future for occupational therapy, what might I do this week? This month? Over the next year?
- Consider your actions: Write out a commitment to change statement[2] and enact it.

For another day

Enabling Occupation II will likely leave you with questions. There is so much more to say about occupational therapy, our vision, and our practice mosaic. You have read a snapshot of current occupational therapy with clients. You have been challenged to consider what a focus on occupation and enablement mean for occupational therapy clients or consumers, or for occupational therapy managers, policy analysts, educators, and researchers.

Those who know occupational therapy from the inside, so to speak, as clients or consumers, may find this book of interest. Much more could be said to guide clients to participate in client-centred practice. What might you expect of an occupational therapist? What boundaries do occupational therapists put around client-centred practice and why? How can you voice your own interests and concerns in systems that may not support such client activism?

Students of occupational therapy will have many questions for another day. How might you bridge the natural idealism of university education with the realities of everyday practice? What career options are open to you with your occupational and

---

[2] Commitment to change statements have been shown to relate significantly to actual changes in practice (e.g., Wakefield, J., Herbert, C.P., Maclure, M., Dormuth, C., Wright, J.M, Legare, J., et al. (2003). Commitment to change statements can predict actual change in practice. *The Journal of Continuing Education in the Health Professions, 23*, 81-93).

enablement perspective? Are job options likely to open in new areas when funding is not easily available, even if the need for occupational therapists is there?

Occupational therapy administrators, managers, and regulators will find section IV most useful to advance the quality of practice, improve access to occupational therapy and ensure the development of standards that protect the public. Educators may find the brief introduction to occupational therapy education and the profile of graduates interesting. Researchers will likely have views on the comments to support greater integration of scholarship and evidence in practice.

Possibly the work for another day will be to write guidelines for occupational therapy management. What, for instance, might be helpful in developing workload measurement policies, program information, program evaluation, and staff development initiatives? How might one spark strategic planning to make occupation and enablement explicit, and visible to higher management and funders? What strategies might be helpful to capture the interest and support of funding agents when presenting an occupational perspective and enablement approaches? How might a manager engage staff at all levels in becoming more occupation-based and attentive to effective enablement?

One can also imagine guidelines being written for academic occupational therapy programs. A central question is: How do you develop the ideal curriculum so as to prepare graduates for enabling occupation? It is clear that the new master's level curricula cannot educate students in every possible practice skill, nor will students learn everything in fieldwork. What might be the core educational experiences that transform students into confident, capable occupational therapy graduates? Academic practice includes some form of scholarship from simple program evaluation to complex, externally funded, multidisciplinary, international projects. What guidelines would help occupational therapy academics to investigate nationally and internationally significant questions from an occupational and enablement perspective?

The realm of policy development and analysis, regulations, program management, and business development — all focused on enabling occupation — is for another day as well. It is clear that practices in enabling occupation require changes in the structure of systems and society. From our focus in health services on medical intervention and caregiving, occupational therapists need to develop more systems and funding structures to support occupation-based enablement.

All this and more has been left for another day.

Glossary

Glossary terms without references are new with this publication.

Abductive reasoning is to find the best explanation in a complex situation; it is "a matter of utilizing the principle of maximum likelihood in order to formalize a pattern of reasoning known as the 'inference to the best explanation'" (Fetzer, 1990, p. 103); to advance already existing conceptual ideas or theoretical understandings; or create new concepts that broaden current descriptions of phenomena (Aliseda, 2006).

Action is a set of voluntary movements or mental processes that form a recognizable and purposeful pattern, such as grasping, holding, pulling, pushing, turning, kneeling, standing, walking, thinking, remembering, smiling, chewing, winking, etc. (adapted from Polatajko et al., 2004; and Zimmerman et al., 2006).

Activity is the "execution of a task or action by an individual" (WHO, 2001, p. 193); a set of tasks with a specific end point or outcome that is greater than that of any constituent task, such as writing a report (adapted from Polatajko et al., 2004; and Zimmerman et al., 2006).

Activity limitations are problems in health functioning when an individual has difficulty executing activities (WHO, 2001, p. 193).

Adapt is a key occupational therapy enablement skill to make suitable to or fit for a specific use or situation (Answers.com), and to respond to occupational challenges (Schkade & Schultz, 1992) with all clients from individuals to populations given that "individuals continuously adapt their occupations" (Meltzer, 2001, p. 17). In the *Profile of Occupational Therapy Practice in Canada* (CAOT, 2007), this skill is part of the occupational therapy competency role as *change agent*.

Advocate is a key occupational therapy enablement skill enacted with or for people to raise critical perspectives, prompt new forms of power sharing, lobby or make new options known to key decision makers; to speak, plead, or argue in favour of (Houghton-Mifflin Company, 2004). In the *Profile of Occupational Therapy Practice in Canada* (CAOT, 2007), advocacy contributes to the occupational therapy competency role of change agent.

Body functions are the "physiological functions of body systems (including psychological functions)" (WHO, 2001, p. 193).

Body structures are "anatomical parts of the body such as organs, limbs and their components" (WHO, 2001, p. 193).

Canadian Model of Client-Centred Enablement (CMCE) is a visual metaphor for client-centred enablement, through occupation, illustrating occupational therapy's core competency in key and related enablement skills in a client-professional relationship (E. Townsend, H. Polatajko, G. Whiteford, J. Craik, & J. Davis, personal communication, July–December, 2006).

Canadian Model of Occupational Performance and Engagement (CMOP-E) is an extension of the 1997/2002 conceptual framework that describes occupational therapy's view of the dynamic, interwoven relationship between persons, environment, and occupation; engagement signals occupational therapy interests that include and extend beyond occupational performance over a person's lifespan (H. Polatajko, E. Townsend, & J. Craik, personal communication, July–December, 2006).

Canadian Practice Process Framework (CPPF) (2007) is a generic, occupational therapy framework that portrays the process of occupational enablement with clients from individuals to populations (J. Craik, J. Davis, H. Polatajko, & E. Townsend, personal communication, July–December, 2006).

Change means to take a different position, course, or direction (*Merriam-Webster*, 2003), or to experience a process of transition or transformation to a new, altered, or different state (Answers.com; Jonsson, in press) in order to maintain opportunities, to prevent losses, or to promote and develop opportunities (CAOT, 1991).

Clients in occupational therapy may be individuals, families, groups, communities, organizations, or populations who participate in occupational therapy services by direct referral or contract, or by other service and funding arrangements with a team, group, or agency that includes occupational therapy.

Client-centred enablement is based on enablement foundations and employs enablement skills in a collaborative relationship with clients who may be individuals, families, groups, communities, organizations, populations to advance a vision of health, well-being, and justice through occupation.

Client participation is an active concept characterized by involvement and engagement and is driven in part by biological needs to act, find meaning, and connect with others through doing (Wilcock, 2006).

Coach is a key occupational therapy enablement skill to develop and sustain "… an ongoing partnership designed to help clients produce fulfilling results in their personal and professional lives, improve their performance and enhance their quality of life" (International Coach Federation, 2006. In the *Profile of Occupational Therapy Practice in Canada* (CAOT, 2007), coaching is related to the competency roles of communicator and collaborator.

Collaborate is arguably *the* key enablement skill that involves power-sharing (Schaeffer, 2002) to work *with* clients, versus doing things to or for them in a joint intellectual effort or toward a common end (Answers.com) by sharing talents and abilities in mutual respect with genuine interest, acknowledgement of others, empathy, altruism, trust, and creative communication to achieve results that are greater than the sum of individual efforts (Linden, 2003), with awareness that professions operate hierarchically in a top-down manner based on the priority given to professional expertise over client experience (Freidson, 1970, 1986, 1994, 2001). In the *Profile of Occupational Therapy Practice in Canada* (CAOT, 2007), collaborate is directly mirrored in the competency role of *collaborator*.

Consult is a key enablement skill to exchange views and confer (Answers.com) throughout the practice process with a wide range of clients or in management, education, or research, with team members, community support personnel, social agencies, government personnel, business representatives, non-governmental organizations, consumer groups, special interest groups, and more. In the *Profile of Occupational Therapy Practice in Canada* (CAOT, 2007), consulting is part of the competency role of expert in enabling occupation.

Coordinate is a powerful and under-recognized key enablement skill through which occupational therapists integrate, synthesize and document information, link people with resources, manage teams with students and support personnel, facilitate interaction between government "silos" and otherwise harmonize and orchestrate initiatives by a broad range of stakeholders in a common action or effort (Houghton-Mifflin Company, 2004) in order to develop an accord, combine and adapt in order to attain a particular effect (Answers.com). In the *Profile of Occupational Therapy Practice in Canada* (CAOT, 2007), coordination is aligned with the leadership competency role to manage practice.

Competent occupational therapist. Competent is the word that reflects the minimal and ongoing performance expectation of practitioners. In the *Profile of Occupational Therapy in Canada,* For the Competent Practitioner, the performance expectations reflect the requisite knowledge, skills and abilities to meet performance expectations throughout their career (i.e. newly registered and lifelong practice) (CAOT, 2007).

Components of occupational performance refer to the affective, cognitive, and physical performance of individuals (CAOT, 1997a; 2002).

Culture is a set of values, beliefs, traditions, norms, and customs that determine or define the behaviour of a group of people (Wells, 1994); also "a shared system of meanings that involve ideas, concepts and knowledge and include the beliefs, values and norms that shape standards and rules of behaviour as people go about their everyday lives" (Dyck, 1998, p. 68) in a system of shared meanings and a dynamic process by which "meanings are ascribed to commonly experienced phenomena and objects" (Iwama, 2005, p. 8.).

Design/build is a traditional key occupational therapy enablement skill that encompasses the design and/or building of products, such as assistive technology or orthotics (McKee & Morgan, 1998), designs to adapt the built and/or emotional environment (Clark et al., 2001), and the design and implementation of programs and services (Rebeiro et al., 2001) by formulating a plan or strategy (Answers.com) and in some situations actually building the technology, program, or service. In the *Profile of Occupational Therapy Practice in Canada* (CAOT, 2007), design/build contributes to the competency role of change agent.

Disability is an "umbrella terms for impairment of body function or body structure, an activity limitation and/or a participation restriction" (WHO, 2001, p. 193).

Diversity has not been defined in occupational therapy; rather a joint statement on diversity by the five national occupational therapy organizations states: "the profession is stimulating discussion to identify which definition or definitions of diversity most effectively move the profession forward" (ACOTRO, ACOTUP, CAOT, COTF, PAC, 2006, p. 1).

Educate is a key occupational therapy enablement skill and one of the historic knowledge foundations of occupational therapy, drawing on philosophies and practices of adult and childhood education, notably experiential and behaviourial education that emphasize learning through doing (Dewey, 1900; Dewey & Bentley, 1949). In the *Profile of Occupational Therapy Practice in Canada* (CAOT, 2007), educate contributes to the competency role of change agent.

Empowerment refers to "personal and social processes that transform visible and invisible relationships so that power is shared more equally" (CAOT, 1997a, 2002, p. 180).

Enabling (verb) – Enablement (noun), focused on occupation, is the core competency of occupational therapy — what occupational therapists actually do — and draws on an interwoven spectrum of key and related enablement skills, which are value-based, collaborative, attentive to power inequities and diversity, and charged with visions of possibility for individual and/or social change.

Enabling occupation refers to enabling people to "choose, organize, and perform those occupations they find useful and meaningful in their environment" (CAOT, 1997a; 2002, p. 180).

Enablement continuum (EC) is the portrayal of a range of variations from ineffective to effective enablement, resulting from complex practice conditions and decisions that support or limit enablement (E. Townsend, G. Whiteford, & H. Polatajko, personal communication, July–December, 2006.

Enablement foundations (EF) are the interests, values, beliefs, ideas, concepts, critical perspectives, and concerns that inform and shape decision-making priorities in enabling occupation.

Enablement reasoning integrates narrative, conditional, clinical (positivistic), and other forms of reasoning; a component of occupational therapy professional reasoning, based on conceptual foundations, including values, beliefs and concepts, framed by the practice context with different clients in different situations, and influences the application of competence in key and related enablement skills, which are highly inter-related, dynamic, and evolving.

Engage/engagement is a historical cornerstone of occupational therapy and is the enablement skill to involve clients in doing, in participating, that is to say, in action beyond talk by involving others and oneself to become occupied (Answers.com). In the *Profile of Occupational Therapy Practice in Canada* (CAOT, 2007), occupational therapists engage others through the core competency role as *experts in enabling occupation.*

Environmental elements are "cultural, institutional, physical, and social forces that lie outside individuals, yet are embedded in individuals actions" (CAOT, 1997a; 2002, p. 180).

Environmental factors are "all aspects of the external or extrinsic world that form the context of an individual's life"; physical, social, and attitudinal (WHO, 2001, p. 193).

Evidence is a ground for a belief, that which tends to prove or disprove any conclusion (Brown, 1993). In health care, evidence is conceived in a scientific context and can be defined as "an observation, fact or organized body of information offered to support or justify inferences or beliefs in the demonstration of some proposition or matter at issue" (Upshur, 2001, p. 7). Evidence consists of many things besides research; evidence may include such things as clinical and other reasoning. Occupational therapists collect and use evidence generated from clients, the literature, their peers, and from reflecting on their own personal experiences (Dubouloz, Egan, Vallerand, & von Zweck, 1999).

Evidence-based practice includes experiential, qualitative, and quantitative evidence. "The occupational therapist provides knowledge of client, environment and occupational factors relevant to enabling occupation. Ideally, this evidence is derived from a critical review of the research literature, expert consensus and professional experience" (CAOT, ACOTUP, ACOTRO, & PAC, 1999, p. 267).

Expert in enabling occupation. Occupational Therapy Practitioners use evidence-based processes that focus on occupation – including self care, productive pursuits, and leisure - as a medium for action. Practitioners take client perspectives and diversity into account. Expert in Enabling Occupation is the central role, expertise and competence of an occupational therapy practitioner. Clients may include individuals, families, groups, communities, organizations or populations (CAOT, 2007).

Fit Chart illustrates the relationship of the components of occupational performance and engagement. (H. Polatajko & J. Craik, personal communication, July–December, 2006).

Frame of reference is the viewpoint, context, or set of assumptions within which a person's perception and thinking seem always to occur, and which constrains selectively the course and outcome of action (Atherton, 2002). Occupational therapy frames of reference are sets of interrelated theories, constructs, and concepts that determine how specific occupational challenges will be perceived, understood, and approached (Mosey, 1986), and that guide occupational therapists' decision making through the practice process.

Function refers "to the skill to perform activities in a normal or accepted way (Reed & Sanderson, 1983) and/or adequately for the required tasks of a specific role or setting (Christiansen & Baum, 1997) (CAOT, 1997a; 2002, p, 181).

Health is more than the absence of disease (WHO, 1986); from an occupational perspective, health includes having choice, abilities, and opportunities for engaging in meaningful patterns of occupation for looking after self, enjoying life, and contributing to the social and economic fabric of a community over the lifespan to promote health, well-being, and justice through occupation (adapted from CAOT 1997a; 2002).

Holism is a "view of persons as whole beings, integrated in mind, body, and spirit" (CAOT, 1997a; 2002, p. 181).

Impairments are "problems in body function or structure such as a significant deviation or loss" (WHO, 2001, p. 193).

Implementation is the "process of activating a plan, versus intervention which implies doing to or for people" (CAOT 1997a; 2002 p. 181).

Individual change involves stretching beyond former ways of thinking and doing, given time and openness to give voice to experiences of changing identity and to integrate new assumptions and perspectives, on a continuum and is interconnected with enabling social change.

Knowledge translation is the exchange, synthesis and ethically-sound application of knowledge (CIHR, 2002), disseminated through empirical research, peers, and continuing education (Craik, 2003).

Meaningful occupations are "chosen, performed and engaged in to generate experiences of personal meaning and satisfaction by individuals, groups, or communities" (CAOT, 1997a, 2002, p. 181).

Occupations are groups of activities and tasks of everyday life, named, organized, and given value and meaning by individuals and a culture; occupation is everything people do to occupy themselves, including looking after themselves (self-care), enjoying life (leisure), and contributing to the social and economic fabric of their communities (productivity); the domain of concern and the therapeutic medium of occupational therapy (CAOT, 1997a, 2002); a set of activities that is performed with some consistency and regularity; that brings structure and is given value and meaning by individuals and a culture (adapted from Polatajko et al., 2004; and Zimmerman et al., 2006).

Occupational adaptation is a response to occupational challenges (Schkade & Schultz, 1992) with all clients from individuals to populations given that "individuals continuously adapt their occupations" (Meltzer, 2001, p. 17).

Occupational alienation is the outcome when people experience daily life as meaningless or purposeless (Stadnyket al., in press).

Occupational analysis, previously known as activity or task analysis, requires competency to analyze and adapt the parts, steps, processes or components of an occupation. Occupational analysis is a form of assessment focused on occupation, and the competency to use that information is to consider and implement various forms of adaptation or transformation.

Occupational apartheid a willful exclusion of a group, "refers to the segregation of groups of people through the restriction or denial of access to dignified and meaningful participation in occupations of daily life on the basis of race, color, disability, national origin, age, gender sexual preference, religion, political beliefs, status in society or other characteristics. Occasioned by political forces, its systematic and pervasive social, cultural and economic consequences jeopardize health and wellbeing as experienced by individuals, communities and societies." (Kronenberg & Pollard, 2005, p. 67); a willful exclusion of a group (Rachel Thibeault, chapter 3).

Occupational behaviour is that aspect or class of human action that encompasses mental and physical doing.

Occupational balance/imbalance "is a temporal concept since it refers to allocation of time use for particular purposes and is based on the reasoning that human health and well-being require a variation in productive and leisure occupations" (Stadnyk et al., in press).

Occupational capacity is the actual or potential ability to engage in occupations.

Occupational change occurs by adding, abandoning or altering occupations through the use of adapting, restructuring, refraining and reconstruction strategies to (a) develop through occupational transitions across the life course, (b) monitoring occupational engagement, health and well-being, (c) restore occupational potential and performance, or (d) prevent occupational losses and deprivation, occupational alienation or other forms of occupational justice.

Occupational citizenship is optimal engagement as a fully integrated citizen in a just and inclusive society with entitlement for all people to participate, enabled by the opportunities and resources they require, in the occupations of everyday life that foster health and well-being.

Occupational competence refers to adequacy or sufficiency in an occupational skill, meeting all requirements of an environment; develops as a progression from novice to master in the performance of occupations; an iterative process repeated again and again with the addition of mastery in each new occupation.

Occupational deprivation is "a state of prolonged preclusion from engagement in occupations of necessity and/or meaning due to factors which stand outside of the control of the individual" (Whiteford, 2000, p. 201); the influence of an external circumstance that prevents a person from acquiring, using, or enjoying occupation over an extended period of time (Whiteford, 1997; Wilcock, 1996, 2006).

Occupational development is a systematic process of change in occupational behaviours across time, resulting from the growth and maturation of the individual in interaction with the environment; the constellation of occupations an individual accumulates across the life span, her or his life course occupational repertoire; marked by the changes in the specific occupations that an individual can and does perform over the course of life; governed by the principles underlying the occupational trajectories and transitions that occur across the life course, and the processes whereby these occur (Davis & Polatajko, 2006, p. 138).

Occupational disruption "may appear to be similar to occupational deprivation … but it refers to a temporary or transient disruption … and results from factors that are internal or individual, such as illness" (Whiteford, 2004, p. 223).

Occupational engagement to involve oneself or become occupied, to participate in occupation (Houghton Mifflin Company, 2004). Involvement for *being, becoming, and belonging,* as well as for performing or doing occupations (Wilcock, 2006).

Occupational enrichment is the "deliberate manipulation of environments to facilitate and support engagement in a range of occupations congruent with those that the individual might normally perform" (Molineux & Whiteford, 1999, p. 127).

Occupational grouping is a set of occupations grouped by a theme, primarily named by the individual or society (e.g., such as self-care, productivity, leisure) (Polatajko et al., 2004).

Occupational history is a record of how one progresses from one occupation to another, often due to a transitional event such as a marriage or divorce (Meltzer, 2001).

Occupational identity is "how an individual sees the self in terms of various occupational roles, an image of the kind of life desired" (Kielhofner, Mallinson, Forsyth, & Lai, 2001, p. 261).

Occupational issues (OI) are challenges to occupational engagement or to inclusive and just participation in occupations, including yet not limited to occupational performance issues, occupational alienation issues, occupational balance issues, occupational development issues, occupational deprivation issues, occupational marginalization issues.

Occupational justice/injustice. "Whilst social justice addresses the social relations and social conditions of life, occupational justice addresses what people do in their relationships and conditions for living" (Wilcock & Townsend, 2000, p. 84). Motivating this exploration is a utopian vision of an *occupationally just world* governed to enable all individuals to flourish in diverse ways by doing what they decide they can do that is most meaningful and useful to themselves and to their families, communities, and nations (Wilcock & Townsend, in press).

Occupational life course is the occupational repertoire that accumulates across the life course; an occupational life course narrative is the history of occupational experiences and transitions over the life course (Davis & Polatajko, 2006).

Occupational marginalization occurs when some social groups more than others are denied or restricted in making choices and decisions about their participation in everyday occupations, often resulting from invisible expectations, norms, and standards (Townsend & Wilcock, 2004).

Occupational mastery refers to competent occupational functioning (adapted from Schkade & Schultz, 1992).

Occupational participation refers to involvement in a life situation (WHO, 2001) through occupation.

Occupational pattern is the "regular and predictable way of doing; occurs when human beings organize activities and occupations" (Bendixon et al., 2006, p. 4).

Occupational performance is the "result of a dynamic, interwoven relationship between persons, environment, and occupation over a person's lifespan; the ability to choose, organize, and satisfactorily perform meaningful occupations that are culturally defined and age appropriate for looking after oneself, enjoying life, and contributing to the social and economic fabric of a community" (CAOT, 1997a; 2002, p. 181).

Occupational performance goal (OPG) is directed towards choosing, organizing, or performing a meaningful occupation. An OPG is essential for the initiation of an occupational therapy process. An OPG becomes relevant for occupational therapy when attaining the goal becomes a challenge.

Occupational performance issue (OPI) is "an actual or potential issue (or problem)" (Fearing and Clark, 2000, p. 184) in the "ability to choose, organize, and satisfactorily perform meaningful occupations" (CAOT, 1997a; 2002, p. 30). An OPI becomes relevant for occupational therapy when solutions to choosing, organizing, or performing an occupation become a challenge.

Occupational performance model (OPM) was a "1991 portrayal of the interacting elements of individual performance components, areas of occupational performance, and the environment" (CAOT, 1997a; 2002, p. 182).

Occupational performance process model (OPPM) is a seven-stage process of practice for focusing on occupational performance using client-centred approaches with individual, organization, and other clients (CAOT, 1997a; 2002; Fearing et al., 1997).

Occupational potential is what might be in future beyond what is in the present; a combination of capacity, opportunity, resources, and social structure that enable engagement in occupations by individuals, families, groups, communities, organizations, and populations to reach beyond an existing occupational status to a predictable or unpredictable occupational status.

Occupational reasoning is the component of occupational therapy professional reasoning which integrates *environmental*, conditional reasoning about the context of practice and client lives, and biomedical clinical reasoning, both narrative and empirical, about the body, persons, and clinical practice.

Occupational repertoire is "the set of occupations an individual has at a specific point in the life course" (Davis & Polatajko, 2006, p. 137).

Occupational role refers to the rights, obligations, and expected behaviour patterns associated with a particular set of activities or occupations, done on a regular basis, and associated with social cultural roles (adapted from Hillman & Chapparo, 1995, p. 88).

Occupational satisfaction the state of being satisfied or content with ones occupational performance or engagement.

Occupational science is the rigorous study of humans as occupational beings (Wilcock, 2006).

Occupational therapy is the art and science of enabling engagement in everyday living, through occupation; of enabling people to perform the occupations that foster health and well-being; and of enabling a just and inclusive society so that all people may participate to their potential in the daily occupations of life.

Occupational therapy support personnel are persons who are supervised by occupational therapists and who have formal or on-the-job training in the basic theory and methods of occupational therapy.

Occupational well-being is an experience in which people derive feelings of satisfaction and meaning from the ways in which they have orchestrated their occupational lives (Caron Santha & Doble, 2006; Doble et al., 2006).

Participation is "involvement in a life situation" (WHO, 2001, p. 193).

Participation restrictions are "problems an individual may experience in involvement in life situations" (WHO, 2001, p. 193).

Professional reasoning in occupational therapy is a synthesis of occupational reasoning and enablement reasoning, guiding critical reflection and actions with diverse clients in diverse contexts, incorporating narrative, conditional, positivist or other reasoning, and including while extending beyond clinical reasoning (Schön, 1983).

Proficient occupational therapist. Where practitioners demonstrate advanced abilities, their performance is called 'proficient' and where the practitioners demonstrate a recognized level of mastery, they are called 'experts'. The term proficient usually does not describe an occupational therapist in all contexts (e.g., area of practice, setting, etc); rather, a practitioner may be proficient in one or more areas and competent in the other areas. Proficient infers that the performance expectations for competent are met and exceeded (CAOT, 2007).

Quality of life from an occupational perspective, refers to choosing and participating in occupations that foster hope, generate motivation, offer meaning and satisfaction, create a driving vision of life, promote health, enable empowerment, and otherwise address the quality of life (adapted from CAOT, 1997a; 2002).

Role from an occupational perspective is a "culturally defined pattern of occupation that reflects particular routines and habits; stereotypical role expectations may enhance or limit persons' potential occupational performance" (CAOT, 1997a; 2002, p, 182).

Scholarship refers to organized inquiry that helps to produce theory and evidence from multiple research paradigms using a dynamic process to move between: (a) knowledge of a specific situation, (b) generalized theories regarding the complex process of engaging or re-engaging people in valued occupations; and (c) emerging knowledge. In client/clinical contexts, the process may include (d) how the client wishes to change or minimize change.

Service team Client-centred service teams include clients, professionals and other members/stakeholders. Teams work closely together at one site or are extended groups working across multiple settings and in the broader community (CAOT, 2007).

Social change lies on a continuum and is interconnected with individual change, looks beyond psychological or other individualized explanations for human behaviour, and targets social structures, systems, culture, and the built and natural environment.

Social construction, **social construct** or **social concept** is an institutionalized entity or artifact in a social system "invented" or "constructed" by participants in a particular culture or society that exists because people agree to behave as if it exists, or agree to follow certain conventional rules, or behave as if such agreement or rules existed (Answers.com).

Social justice is a "vision and an everyday practice in which people can choose, organize, and engage in meaningful occupations that enhance health, quality of life, and equity in housing, employment and other aspects of life" (CAOT 1997a; 2002, p. 182).

Specialize is a key enablement skill to use specific techniques in particular situations, examples being therapeutic touch and positioning, the use of neurodevelopmental techniques to enable children to participate in occupations, or psychosocial rehabilitation techniques to engage adults in their own empowerment. In the *Profile of Occupational Therapy Practice in Canada* (CAOT, 2007), specialize is a composite of enablement skills that contributes to the competency role of *expert in enabling occupation*.

Spirituality is sensitivity to the presence of spirit (McColl, 2000), a "pervasive life force, manifestation of a higher self, source of will and self-determination, and a sense of meaning, purpose and connectedness that people experience in the context of their environment" (CAOT, 1997a; 2002, p. 182); "spirituality resides in persons, is shaped by the environment, and gives meaning to occupations" (CAOT, 1997a; 2002, p. 33).

Task is a set of actions having an end point or a specific outcome; simple or compound actions involving tool use, such as printing a report (adapted from Polatajko et al., 2004; and Zimmerman et al., 2006).

Tool use enables the performance of compound tasks, which can be broken into task segments and units, where a task unit is an action involving tool use and a task segment is a set of task units (Polatajko et al., 2004).

Transformative learning is a process of getting beyond gaining factual knowledge alone to instead become changed by what one learns in some meaningful way. It involves questioning assumptions, beliefs and values, and considering multiple points of view, while always seeking to verify reasoning (Mezirow, 2000).

Visions of possibility are grounded in particular values, beliefs, and ideals about hope and the value and potential of persons to use diverse abilities to engage in life in mind, body, and spirit not limited to usual expectations in particular contexts.

Voluntary movement is a simple voluntary muscle or mental activation, such as flexion, extension, adduction, abduction, rotation, supination, pronation, blinking, memory, attention, focusing, scanning, etc. (adapted from Polatajko et al., 2004; and Zimmerman et al., 2006).

Well-being is experienced when people engage in occupations that they perceive: (a) are consistent with their values and preferences; (b) support their abilities to competently perform valued roles; (c) support their occupational identities; and (d) support their plans and goals (Caron Santha & Doble, 2006; Christiansen, 1999; Doble et al., 2006).

REFERENCES

Ås, D. (1982). Designs for large-scale time use studies of the 24-hour day. In Z. Staikov (Ed.), *It's about time: International research group on time budgets and social activities* (pp. 17-53). Sofia, Bulgaria: Institute of Sociology at the Bulgarian Academy of Sciences, Bulgarian Sociological Association.

Abberley, P. (1995). Disabling ideology in health and welfare – the case of occupational therapy. *Disability and Society, 10*(2), 221-232.

Alaszewski, A. (1979). Rehabilitation, the remedial therapy professions and social policy. *Social Science and Medicine, 13A*(4), 431-433.

Aldous, J., Mulligan, G. M., & Bjarnason, T. (1998). Fathering over time: What makes the difference? *Journal of Marriage and the Family, 60*(4), 809-820.

Aliseda, A. (2006). *Abductive reasoning: Logical investigations into discovery and explanation.* Dordrecht, The Netherlands: Springer Publishing Company.

Allsop, J., & Saks, M. (Eds.). (2002). *Regulating the health professions.* London: Sage Publications.

American Occupational Therapy Association (2002). Occupational therapy practice framework: Domain and process. *American Journal of Occupational Therapy, 56*(6), 609-639.

Andersen, M., Yaojun, L. I., Bechhofer, F., McCrone, D., & Stewart, R. (2000). Sooner rather than later? Younger and middle-aged adults preparing for retirement. *Ageing and Society, 20*, 445-466.

Answers.com. *Online dictionary.* Retrieved March 31, 2007 from http://www.answers.com/

Answers.com. (n.d.). *Organization.* Retrieved March 28, 2007 from http://www.answers.com/organizations

Archer-Heese, G., & Stratton Johnson, L. (2002). Current and future work-related occupational therapy services – a Canadian perspective. *Occupational Therapy Now, 4*(4), 22-25.

Armstrong, P., Armstrong, H., Bourgeault, I. L., Choiniere, J., Mykhalovskiy, E., & White, J. P. (2000). *Heal thyself: Managing health care reform.* Aurora, ON: Garamond Press.

Arnold, M. (1879). *Mixed essays.* London: Smith, Elder, & Co.

Aronson, J. (1999). Conflicting images of older people receiving care: Challenges for reflexive practice and research. In S. M. Neysmith (Ed.), *Critical issues for future social work practice with aging persons* (pp. 47-69). New York: Columbia University Press.

Ashe, B., Taylor, M., & Dubouloz, C. (2005). The process of change: Listening to transformation in meaning perspectives of adults in arthritis health education groups. *Canadian Journal of Occupational Therapy, 72*(5), 280-288.

Aspinwall, L. G., & Staudinger, U. M. (2003). *A psychology of human strengths: Fundamental questions and future directions for a positive psychology.* Washington, DC: American Psychological Association.

Association of Canadian Occupational Therapy Regulatory Organizations (2003). *Essential competencies of practice for occupational therapy in Canada* (2nd ed.). Toronto, ON: College of Occupational Therapists of Ontario. Retrieved February 4, 2009 from http://www.cotbc.org/documents/EssentialCompetencies_2ndEd_mar04_english.pdf

Association of Canadian Occupational Therapy Regulatory Organizations, Association of Canadian Occupational Therapy University Programmes, Canadian Association of Occupational Therapists & Professional Alliance of Canada (2006). Preliminary joint position statement on diversity. Retrieved March 20, 2007 from http://www.acotup-acpue.ca//PDF's/JointPositionStatementonDiversityFinalFebruary2007.pdf, or http://www.cotfcanada.org/download/JointPositionDiversity.doc

Association of Canadian Occupational Therapy University Programmes. (2006). *Canadian occupational therapy university programs.* Retrieved February 4, 2009 from http://www.caot.ca/pdfs/programprereqs.pdf

Atherton, J. S. (2002). *Tools: Frames of reference: On learning to "see."* Retrieved June 29, 2006 from http://www.doceo.co.uk/tools/frame.htm

Atkinson, A. M., & Hull, S. (2001). *Prince Edward Island advisory committee on health human resources: Health human resources supply and demand analysis.* Charlottetown, PEI, DMR Consulting. Retrieved February 4, 2009 from http://www.gov.pe.ca/photos/original/hss_nov162001_b.pdf

Aubin, G., Hachey, R., & Mercier, C. (1999). Meaning of daily activities and subjective quality of life in people with severe mental illness. *Scandinavian Journal of Occupational Therapy, 6*(2), 53-62.

Aubin, G., Hachey, R., & Mercier, C. (2002). La signification des activités quotidiennes chez les personnes souffrant de troubles mentaux graves. *Canadian Journal of Occupational Therapy, 69*(4), 218-228.

Ayres, J. (1972). *Sensory integration and learning disorders.* Los Angeles, CA: Western Psychological Services.

Backman, C. (2005). Outcomes and outcome measures: Measuring what matters is in the eye of the beholder. *Canadian Journal of Occupational Therapy, 72*(5), 259-264.

Bandura, A. (1986). *Social foundations of thought and action.* Upper Saddle River, NJ: Prentice Hall.

Baptiste, S. (2003). Culture as environment: Complexity, sensitivity and challenge. In L. Letts, P. Rigby, & D. Stewart (Eds.), *Using environments to enable occupational performance* (pp. 97-116). Thorofare, NJ: SLACK, Inc.

Baranowski, T., Perry, C. L., & Parcel, G. S. (1997). How individuals, environments, and health behavior interact: Social cognitive theory. In K. Glanz, F. M. Lewis, & B. Rimer (Eds.), *Health behavior and health education: Theory, research, and practice* (pp. 153-178). San Francisco, CA: Jossey-Bass Publishers.

Barbara, A., & Whiteford, G. (2005). The legislative and policy context of practice. In G. Whiteford & V. Wright-St. Clair (Eds.), *Occupation and practice in context* (pp. 332-348). Merrickville, NSW, Australia: Elsevier.

Barber, K. (Ed.). (2004). *Canadian Oxford dictionary* (2nd ed.). Toronto, ON: Oxford University Press.

Barer, M., Marmor, T., & Evans, R. (1994). *Why are some people healthy and others not?: The determinants of health of populations.* New York: Aldine de Gruyter.

Baril, R., Clarke, J., Friesen, M., Stock, S., & Cole, D. (2003). Management of return-to-work programs for workers with musculoskeletal disorders: A qualitative study in three Canadian provinces. *Social Science & Medicine, 57*(11), 2101-2114.

Barnes, K. J., & Turner, K. D. (2001). Team collaborative practices between teachers and occupational therapists. *American Journal of Occupational Therapy, 55*, 83-89.

Bartlett, D. J., MacNab, J., MacArthur, C., Mandich, A., Magill-Evans, J., Young, N. L., et al. (2006). Advancing rehabilitation research: An interactionist perspective to guide question and design. *Disability and Rehabilitation, 28*(19), 1169-1176.

Bates, D. G., & Plog, F. Y. (1990). *Cultural anthropology.* New York: McGraw-Hill.

Baum, C. M., & Christiansen, C. H. (2005). Person-environment-occupation-performance: An occupation-based framework for practice. In C. H. Christiansen, C. M. Baum, & J. Bass-Haugen (Eds.), *Occupational therapy: Performance, participation, and well-being* (pp. 243-266). Thorofare, NJ: SLACK, Inc.

Baum, C. M., & Edwards, D. F. (2001). *Activity card sort.* St. Louis, MO: Simon Enterprises Co.

Beagan, B. L. (2007). The impact of social class: Learning from occupational therapy students. *Canadian Journal of Occupational Therapy 74(2): 125-133.*

Beagan, B. L., & Kumas-Tan, Z. (2006). *Diversity issues in Canadian occupational therapy: A background discussion paper for the profession.* Unpublished manuscript. School of Occupational Therapy, Dalhousie University at Halifax, NS.

Beagan, B. L., Etowa, J., Acton, J., & Egbeyemi, J. (April 2006). Panel on social justice: Strong black women: Everyday racism and the daily occupations of black Nova Scotian women. American Occupational Therapy Association Annual Conference, Charlotte, NC, April 2006.

Beattie, M. (1992). *Codependent no more: How to stop controlling others and start caring for yourself.* Center City, MN: Hazelden. Retrieved March 26, 2007 from http://www.findarticles.com/p/articles/mi_m1000/is_n361/ai_9050108

Becker, G. (1997). *Disrupted lives: How people create meaning in a chaotic world.* Berkley, CA: University of California Press.

Beery, K. E., & Buktenica, N. A. (1989). *Developmental test of visual-motor integration* (3rd ed.). Cleveland, OH: Modern Curriculum Press.

Belcham, C. (2004). Spirituality in occupational therapy: Theory in practice? *British Journal of Occupational Therapy, 67*(1), 39-46.

Bendixon, H. J., Kroksmark, U., Magnus, E., Jakobsen, K., Alsaker, S., & Nordell, K. (2006). Occupational pattern: A renewed definition of the concept. *Journal of Occupational Science, 13*(1), 3-10.

Bhatti, M. (2006). 'When I'm in the garden I can create my own paradise': Homes and gardens in later life. *The Sociological Review, 54*(2), 318-341.

Bircher, A. U. (1975). On the development and classification of diagnoses. *Nursing Forum, 14*(1), 11-29.

Black, R. M. (2005). Intersections of care: An analysis of culturally competent care, client centered care, and the feminist ethic of care. *Work, 24*(4), 409-422.

Blain, J., & Townsend, E. A. (1993). Occupational therapy guidelines for client-centred practice: Impact study findings. *Canadian Journal of Occupational Therapy, 60*(5), 271-285.

Blechert, T. F., Christiansen, M. F., & Kari, N. (1987). Intraprofessional team building. *American Journal of Occupational Therapy, 41*(9), 576-582.

Bloom, B. S., Engelhart, M. D., Furst, E. J., Hill, W. H., & Krathwohl, D. R. (1956). *Taxonomy of educational objectives: The classification of educational goals. Handbook I – Cognitive domain.* New York: David McKay.

Bobath, B. (1990). *Adult hemiplegia evaluation and treatment* (3rd ed.). Oxford, UK: Butterworth-Heinemann.

Bonder, B., Martin, L., & Miracle, A. W. (2004). Culture emergent in occupation. *American Journal of Occupational Therapy, 58*(159), 168.

Bontje, P., Kinebanian, A., Josephsson, S., & Tamura, Y. (2004). Occupational adaptation: The experiences of older persons with physical disabilities. *American Journal of Occupational Therapy, 58,* 140-149.

Bootes, K., & Chapparo, C. J. (2002). Cognitive and behavioural assessment of people with traumatic brain injury in the work place: Occupational therapists' perceptions. *Work, 19*(3), 255-268.

Borel, L., Lija, M., Sviden, G. A., & Sadlo, G. (2001). Occupations and signs of reduced hope: An explorative study of older adults with functional impairments. *American Journal of Occupational Therapy, 55*(3), 311-316.

Boudreau, M. L. (2004). Update on tools for healthy living project. *OT Now, 6*(3). Retrieved March 21, 2007 from http://www.caot.ca/default.asp?pageid=1123

Bourdieu, P. (1984). *Distinction: A social critique on the judgement of taste.* London: Routledge.

Bourdieu, P., & Johnson, R. (1998). *Practical reason: On the theory of action.* Oxford, UK: Polity Press.

Bowman, J., & Llewellyn, G. (2002). Clinical outcomes research from the occupational therapist's perspective. *Occupational Therapy International, 9*(2), 145-166.

Bridle, M., & Hawkes, B. (1990). A survey of Canadian occupational therapy practice. *Canadian Journal of Occupational Therapy, 57*(3), 160-166.

Brintnell, S. (1985). Muriel Driver Memorial Lecture 1984: Career planning in occupational therapy. I want up, not out. *Canadian Journal of Occupational Therapy, 52*(5), 227-233.

Brintnell, T. D. (1988). Mysticism and skeptism: Obstacles to the culturalization of the certified occupational therapist. *Occupational Therapy in Health care, 5,* 169-179.

Brown, G. T. (1998). Male occupational therapists in Canada: A demographic profile. *British Journal of Occupational Therapy, 61*(12), 561-567.

Brown, L. (Ed.). (1993). *The new shorter Oxford English dictionary on historical principles* (Vol. 1). Oxford, UK: Oxford University Press.

Brunnstrom, S. (1970). *Movement therapy in hemiplegia: Neurophysiological approach.* New York: Harper & Row.

Brunt, J. H., Lindsey, E., & Hopkinson, J. (1997). Health promotion in the Hutterite community and the ethnocentricity of empowerment. *Canadian Journal of Nursing Research, 29*(1), 17-28.

Bryant, W., Clark, C., & McKay, A. (2004). Living in a glasshouse: Exploring occupational alienation. *Canadian Journal of Occupational Therapy, 71*(5), 282-289.

Burgers, J. S., Grol, R., Klazinga, N. S., Mäkelä, M., & Zaat, J. (2003). Towards evidence-based clinical practice: An international survey of 18 clinical guideline programs. *International Journal for Quality in Health Care, 15*(1), 31-45.

Burke, J. P., & Kern, S. B. (1996). Is the use of life history and narrative in clinical practice reimbursable? Is it occupational therapy? *American Journal of Occupational Therapy, 50*(5), 389-392.

Campbell, M., Copeland, B., & Tate, B. (1998). *Project Inter-seed: Learning from the health care experiences of people with disabilities.* BC: University of Victoria: Faculty of Human and Social Development

Camus, A. (1942). *Le mythe de sisyphe : Essai sur l'absurde.* Paris: Gallimard.

Canadian Association of Occupational Therapists. (1989). *Ratio of occupational therapists: Population.* Toronto, ON: CAOT Publications ACE.

Canadian Association of Occupational Therapists. (1991). *Occupational therapy guidelines for client-centred practice.* Toronto, ON: CAOT Publications ACE.

Canadian Association of Occupational Therapists. (1993). *Occupational therapy guidelines for client-centred mental health practice.* Toronto ON: CAOT Publications ACE.

Canadian Association of Occupational Therapists. (1997a). *Enabling occupation: An occupational therapy perspective.* Ottawa ON: CAOT Publications ACE.

Canadian Association of Occupational Therapists. (1997b). *Profile of occupational therapy practice in Canada.* Ottawa, ON: CAOT Publications ACE.

Canadian Association of Occupational Therapists. (2002). *Enabling occupation: An occupational therapy perspective* (Rev. ed.). Ottawa ON: CAOT Publications ACE.

Canadian Association of Occupational Therapists. (2003a). *CAOT position statement: Universal design and occupational therapy.* Retrieved December 15, 2006 from http://www.caot.ca/default.asp?pageid=622

Canadian Association of Occupational Therapists. (2003b). *Guidelines for the supervision of assigned occupational therapy service components.* Retrieved December 15, 2006 from http://www.caot.ca/default.asp?pageid=579

Canadian Association of Occupational Therapists. (2003c). *Project summary report: Profile of performance expectations for Canadian support personnel in occupational therapy.* Retrieved December 15, 2006 from http://www.caot.ca/pdfs/Project%20Summary% 20Report.pdf

Canadian Association of Occupational Therapists. (2004a). *CAOT position statement: Healthy occupation and disability management services.* Retrieved December 15, 2006 from http://www.caot.ca/default.asp?pageid=1114

Canadian Association of Occupational Therapists. (2004b). *CAOT position statement: Healthy occupations for children and youth.* Retrieved December 15, 2006 from http://www.caot.ca/default.asp?pageid=1138

Canadian Association of Occupational Therapists. (2004c). *Frequently asked questions by occupational therapists on entry-level education of occupational therapists in Canada.* Retrieved February 4, 2009 from http://www.caot.ca/pdfs/FAQS_Masters_ therapists%20rev%20April % 202008.pdf

Canadian Association of Occupational Therapists. (2004d). *Membership statistics.* Ottawa, ON: CAOT Publishing ACE.

Canadian Association of Occupational Therapists. (2005a). *CAOT position statement: Occupational therapy and driver rehabilitation.* Retrieved December 15, 2006 from http://www.caot.ca/default.asp?pageid=1353

Canadian Association of Occupational Therapists. (2005b). *Membership statistics.* Ottawa, ON: CAOT Publishing ACE.

Canadian Association of Occupational Therapists. (2006). *Membership statistics.* Ottawa, ON: CAOT Publishing ACE.

Canadian Association of Occupational Therapists. (2007). *Canadian Association of Occupational Therapists code of ethics* (Rev. ed.). Retrieved January 14, 2007 from http://www.caot.ca/default.asp?ChangeID=50&pageID=35

Canadian Association of Occupational Therapists. (2007). *Profile of occupational therapy practice in Canada.* Ottawa, ON: Author.

Canadian Association of Occupational Therapists, Association of Canadian Occupational Therapy University Programs, Association of Canadian Occupational Therapy Regulatory Organizations, & Presidents' Advisory Committee [CAOT, ACOTUP, ACOTRO, PAC].

(1999). Joint position statement on evidence-based occupational therapy. *Canadian Journal of Occupational Therapy, 66*(5), 267-269. Retrieved December 15, 2006 from http://www.caot.ca/ default.asp?pageid=156

Canadian Association of Occupational Therapists, Association of Canadian Occupational Therapy University Programs, Association of Canadian Occupational Therapy Regulatory Organizations, & Presidents' Advisory Committee [CAOT, ACOTUP, ACOTRO, PAC]. (2006). *OT Education Finder.* Retrieved March 31, 2007 from, http://www.caot.ca/default. asp?pageid=1296

Canadian Institute for Health Information. (2004). *Health Personnel Trends.* Retrieved March 28, 2007 from http://secure.cihi.ca/cihiweb/dispPage.jsp?cw_page=AR_21_E

Canadian Institute for Health Information. (2005a). *Number of health personnel in selected professions, by registration status 2005.* Retrieved November 28, 2006 from http://secure.cihi.ca/cihiweb/products/2005_Provincial_Profiles_Full_Report_e.pdf

Canadian Institute for Health Information. (2005b). *Supply, distribution and migration of Canadian physicians, 2004.* Retrieved March 21, 2007 from http://secure.cihi.ca/cihiweb/ dispPage.jsp?cw_page=PG_385_E&cw_topic=385&cw_rel=AR_14_E

Canadian Institute for Health Information. (2005c). *Workforce trends of registered nurses in Canada, 2004.* Retrieved March 21, 2007 from http://secure.cihi.ca/cihiweb/dispPage. jsp? cw_page=PG_396_E&cw_topic=396&cw_rel=AR_20_E

Canadian Institute for Health Information. (2006). *Health personnel trends in Canada: 1995 – 2004.* Ottawa, Ontario: Author. Retrieved March 27, 2007 from http://secure. cihi.ca/cihiweb/dispPage.jsp?cw_page=PG_399_E&cw_topic=399&cw_rel=AR_21_E

Canadian Institute of Health Research, (2002). *Knowledge translation framework.* Retrieved July 17 from http://www.cihr-irsc.gc.ca/about_cihr/organization/knowledge_kt_framework_ prelim_e.shtm

CanChild Centre for Childhood Disability Research. (2005). *Developmental coordination disorder – DCD.* Retrieved January 16, 2007 from http://www.canchild.ca/Default.aspx? tabid=504&SubIndId=69#SubZoom

Cara, E., & MacRae, A. (1998). *Psychosocial occupational therapy: A clinical practice.* Clifton Park, NY: Thomson Delmar Publishers.

Cardwell, T. (1966). President's address. *Canadian Journal of Occupational Therapy, 33,* 139-140.

Caretto, V., Topolski, K. F., Linkous, C. M., Lowman, D. K., Murphy, S. M. (2000). Current parent education on infant feeding in the neonatal intensive care unit: The role of the occupational therapist. *American Journal of Occupational Therapy 54(1)* 159-164.

Carlsson, G. (2004). Travelling by urban public transport: Exploration of usability problems in a travel chain perspective. *Scandinavian Journal of Occupational Therapy, 11,* 78-89.

Caron Santha, J., & Doble, S. (2006).Development and measurement properties of the Occupational Well-Being Questionnaire. *Canadian Association of Occupational Therapy Conference 2006*, Montreal, PQ, June 2006.

Case-Smith, J., & Cable, J. (1996). Perceptions of occupational therapists regarding service delivery models in school-based practice. *Occupational Therapy Journal of Research, 16*(1), 23-44.

Cassirer, E. (1923). *Substance and function & Einstein's theory of relativity.* New York: Dover.

Cavanagh, R. (2005). Anishinaabe teaching wand and holistic education. In P. Tripp, & L. Muzzin (Eds.), *Teaching as activism: Equity meets environmentalism* (pp. 235-255). Kingston, ON: McGill-Queen's University Press.

Champagne, F. (2002). The ability to manage change in health care organizations. *Discussion paper no. 39.* Commission on the State of Heath Care in Canada.

Chappell, I., Higham, J., & McLean, A. M. (2003). An occupational therapy work skills assessment for individuals with head injury. *Canadian Journal of Occupational Therapy, 70*(3), 163-169.

Chenoy E., Ehrenraut, K., Foster, M., Letts, L., McDougall, C., et al. (2003). *How can a community group evaluate the impact of a program aimed at making their local environment more "senior friendly?"* Unpublished report. Available from L. Letts, School of Rehabilitation Science, McMaster University, Hamilton, ON.

Chompsky, N. (1968). *Language and mind*. Brighton, UK: Harcourt, Brace & World.

Christiansen, C. H. (1996). Three perspectives on balance in occupation. In R. Zemke, & F. Clark (Eds.), *Occupational science: The evolving discipline* (pp. 431-451). Philadelphia: F. A. Davis Company.

Christiansen, C. H. (1999). Occupation as identity: Competence, coherence and the creation of meaning: 1999 Eleanor Clarke Slagle lecture. *American Journal of Occupational Therapy, 53*(6), 547-558.

Christiansen, C. H., & Baum, C. M. (1997). Person-environment occupation performance: A conceptual model for practice. In C.H. Christiansen, & C.M. Baum (Eds.), *Occupational therapy: Enabling function and well-being* (2nd ed., pp. 47-70). Thorofare, NJ: SLACK, Inc.

Christiansen, C. H., Baum, C. M., & Bass-Haugen, J. (Eds.). (2005). *Occupational therapy: Performance, participation and well-being* (3rd ed.). Thorofare, NJ: SLACK, Inc.

Christiansen, C. H., Clark, F., Kielhofner, G., & Rogers, J. (1995). Position paper: Occupation. *American Journal of Occupational Therapy, 49*(10), 1015-1018.

Christiansen, C., & Townsend, E. (2004). *Introduction to occupation: The art and science of living* (1st ed.). Upper Saddle River, NJ: Pearson Education, Inc.

Citizenship and Immigration Canada. (2002). *Canada's immigration law.* Retrieved December 30, 2006 from http://www.cic.gc.ca/english/pub/imm-law.html

Citizenship and Immigration Canada. (2005). *Francophone and Acadian community profile of Canada: Demographic vitality.* Retrieved December 30, 2006 from http://www.cic.gc.ca/english/francophone/Canada/demographic1.html

Clark, F. A. (1993). Occupation embedded in a real life: Interweaving occupational science and occupational therapy: 1993 Eleanor Clarke Slagle Lecture. *American Journal of Occupational Therapy, 47*(12), 1067-1078.

Clark, F. A. (2000). The concepts of habit and routine: A preliminary theoretical synthesis: Habits I conference. *Occupational Therapy Journal of Research, 20* (Suppl. 1), 123S-137S.

Clark, F. A., Azen, S. P., Carlson, M., Mandel, D., LaBree, L., Hay, J., et al. (2001). Embedding health-promoting changes into the daily lives of independently-living older adults: Long-term follow-up of occupational therapy intervention. *Journals of Gerontology: Psychological Sciences, 56B*(1), 60-63.

Clark, F. A., Azen, S. P., Zemke, R., Jackson, J., Carlson, M., Mandel, D., et al. (1997). Occupational therapy for independent-living older adults: A randomized controlled trial. *Journal of the American Medical Association, 278*(16), 1321-1326.

Clouston, T. (2003). Narrative methods: Talk, listening and representation. *British Journal of Occupational Therapy, 66*(4), 136-142.

Cockburn, L. (2001).Change, expansion and reorganization – CAOT during the 1970's. *Occupational Therapy Now, 3*(4), 3-6.

Cockburn, L., & Trentham, B. (2002). Participatory action research: Integrating community occupational therapy practice and research. *Canadian Journal of Occupational Therapy, 69*(1), 20-30.

Cockerill, R., Scott, E., & Wright, M. (1996). Interest among occupational therapy mangers in measuring workload for case costing. *American Journal of Occupational Therapy, 50*, 447-451.

Cohen, M., & Mynks, D. (1993). *Compendium of activities for assessing and developing readiness for rehabilitation.* Boston: Boston University.

Cohen, M. R., Anthony, W. A., & Farkas, M. D. (1997). Assessing and developing rehabilitation readiness. *Psychiatric Services, 48*(5) 644-646.

College of Occupational Therapists of British Columbia. (2004). *Assigning of service components to unregulated support personnel.* Retrieved December 30, 2006 from http://www.cotbc.org/documents/AssignServiceComponents_mar04.pdf

College of Occupational Therapists of Ontario. (2002a). *Principled occupational therapy practice.* Retrieved February 4, 2009 from http://www.coto.org/pdf/Principled_OT_pratice.pdf

College of Occupational Therapists of Ontario. (2002b). *Conscious decision-making in occupational therapy practice.* Retrieved February 4, 2009 from http://www.coto.org/pdf/Concsious_Decision-Making.pdf

Colussi, M. (1999). The community resilience manual: A new resource will link rural revitalization. Making Waves: Canada's Community Economic Development Magazine, 10(4), 10-14.

Connor-Schisler, A. (1996). *The effect of environmental change on daily occupations: A case study of Burundian refugees in Southwestern Ontario.* Unpublished doctoral dissertation, Department of Occupational Therapy, Faculty of Applied Health Sciences, University of Western Ontario.

Connor-Schisler, A. M., & Polatajko, H. J. (2002). The individual as mediator or the person-occupation-environment interaction: Learning from the experience of refugees. *Journal of Occupational Science, 9*(2), 82-92.

Cooper, B. A., & Day, K. (2003). Therapeutic design of environments for people with dementia. In L. Letts, P. Rigby, & D. Stewart (Eds.), *Using environments to enable occupational performance* (pp. 253-268). Thorofare, NJ: SLACK, Inc.

Cooper, N., Stevenson, C., & Hale, G. (1996). The biopsychosocial model. In N. Cooper, C. Stevenson, & G. Hale (Eds.), *Integrating perspectives on health* (pp. 1-17). Buckingham, UK: Open University Press.

Cooperrider, D. L., & Whitney, D. (1999). *Appreciative inquiry.* San Francisco, CA: Berrett-Koehler Communications.

Cooperrider, D. L., Whitney, D., & Stavros, J. M. (2003). *Appreciative inquiry handbook.* San Francisco, CA: Berrett-Koehler Publishers.

Corring, D., & Cook, J. (1999). Client-centred care means that I am a valued human being. *Canadian Journal of Occupational Therapy, 66*(2), 71-82.

Council of Occupational Therapists for European Countries. (2005). *Summary of the occupational therapy profession in Europe.* London: Author.

Cowell, J. W. (2005). Effective quality programs enable sustainability. Health Quality Council of Alberta, May 4, 2005 presentation from http://www.hqca.ca

Craik, C., Austin, C., & Schell, D. (1999). A national survey of occupational therapy managers in mental health. *British Journal of Occupational Therapy, 62*(5), 220-228.

Craik, J. (2003). Enhancing research utilization in occupational therapy. Unpublished master's thesis, Graduate Department of Rehabilitation Science, University of Toronto, Ontario.

Craik, J., & Rappolt, S. (2003). Theory of research utilization enhancement: A model for occupational therapy. *Canadian Journal of Occupational Therapy, 70*(5), 266-275.

Cranton, P. (Ed.). (1994). *Understanding and promoting transformative learning: A guide for educators of adults.* San Fransico, CA: Jossey Bass Publishers.

Creek, J. (2002). *Occupational therapy and mental health* (3rd ed.). London: Churchill Livingstone.

Crepeau, E. B. (2003). Analyzing occupation and activity: A way of thinking about occupational performance. In E. B. Crepeau, E. Cohn, & B. Boyt Schell (Eds.), *Willard and Spackman's occupational therapy* (10th ed.) (pp. 189-198). Philadelphia, PA: Lippincott, Williams & Wilkins.

Crowther, R. E., Marshall, M., Bond, G. R., & Huxley, P. (2001). Helping people with severe mental illness to obtain work: Systematic review. *British Medical Journal, 322*(7280), 204-208.

Cruess S., Johnston, S., & Cruess, R. (2004). Profession: A working definition for medical educators. *Teaching and Learning in Medicine, 16*(1), 74-76.

Csikszentmihalyi, M. (1990). *Flow: The psychology of optimal experience.* New York: Harper & Row.

Csikszentmihalyi, M. (1993). *The evolving self.* New York: Harper.

Csikszentmihalyi, M. (1997). *Finding flow: The psychology of engagement with everyday life.* New York: Basic Books.

Csikszentmihalyi, M. (2003). *Good business: Leadership, flow, and the making of meaning.* London: Penguin Books Ltd.

Csikszentmihalyi, M., & Larson, R. (1987). Validity and reliability of the experience-sampling method. *Journal of Nervous and Mental Disease, 175*(9), 526-536.

Cusick, A., & McCluskey, A. (2000). Becoming an evidence-based practitioner through professional development. *Australian Occupational Therapy Journal, 47*(4), 159-170.

Danahar, G., Schirato, J., & Web, J. (2000). *Understanding Foucault.* Crows Nest, NSW, Australia: Allen & Unwin.

Dannefer, D., & Unlenberg, P. (1999). Paths of the life course: A typology.In V.L. Bengston, & K.

Warner Schaie (Eds.), *Handbook of theories of ageing* (pp. 306-326), New York: Springer.

Darragh, A. R., Sample, P. L., & Krieger, S. R. (2001). Tears in my eyes "cause somebody finally understood": Client perceptions of practitioners following brain injury. *American Journal of Occupational Therapy, 55*(2), 191-199.

Davis, J. A., & Polatajko, H. J. (2006). The occupational development of children. In S. Rodger, & J. Ziviani (Eds.), *Occupational therapy with children: Understanding children's occupations and enabling participation* (pp. 136-157), Oxford, UK: Blackwell Science.

Davis, J. A., & Polatajko, H. J. (in press). Occupational development. In C. Christiansen, & E. A. Townsend (Eds.), *An introduction to occupation: The art and science of living* (2nd ed.). Upper Saddle River, NJ: Pearson Education.

Degeling, P., Maxwell, S. E., Kennedy, J., & Coyle, B. (2003). Medicine, management, and modernisation: A "danse macabre"? *British Medical Journal, 326*(7390), 649-652.

Denton, M. A., Kemp, C. L., French, S., Gafni, A., Joshi, A., Rosenthal, C., et al. (2004). Reflexive planning for later life. *Canadian Journal on Aging* (Suppl. 1), S71-S82.

Department of National Health and Welfare (DNHW) & Canadian Association of Occupational Therapists (CAOT). (1983). *Guidelines for the client-centred practice of occupational therapy* (Cat. No. H39-33/1983E). Ottawa, ON: Author.

Department of National Health and Welfare (DNHW), & Canadian Association of Occupational Therapists (CAOT). (1986). *Intervention guidelines for the client-centred practice of occupational therapy* (Cat. H39-100/1986E). Ottawa, ON: Author.

Department of National Health and Welfare (DNHW), & Canadian Association of Occupational Therapists (CAOT). (1987). *Toward outcomes measures in occupational therapy* (Cat. H39-114/1987E). Ottawa, ON: Author.

Desrosiers, J., Noreau, L., Robichaud, L., Fougeyrollas, P., Rochette, A., Viscogliosi, C. (2004). Validity of the assessment of life habits (LIFE-H) in older adults. *Journal of Rehabilitation Medicine, 36*(4), 177-182.

Desrosiers, J. (2005). Participation and occupation. Muriel Driver Lecture 2005. *Canadian Journal of Occupational Therapy, 72*(4), 195-203.

Dewey, J. (1900). *The school and society.* Chicago: University of Chicago Press.

Dewey, J. & Bentley, A. F. (1949). *Knowing and the known.* Boston, MA: Beacon Press.

DiCenso, J. (Ed.). (1990). *Hermeneutics and the disclosure of truth: A study in the work of Heidegger, Gadamer, and Ricoeur.* Charlottesville: The University Press of Virginia.

Dickinson, E. (1990). From madness to mental health: A brief history of psychiatric treatments in the UK from 1800 to the present. *British Journal of Occupational Therapy, 53*(10), 419-424.

Dillon, T. H. (2001). Practitioner perspectives: Effective intraprofessional relationships in occupational therapy. *Occupational Therapy in Health Care, 14,* 59-48.

Dictionary.com. (n.d.-a). *Communities.* Retrieved March 28, 2007 from http://dictionary.reference.com/browse/communities

Dictionary.com. (n.d.-b). *Capacity.* Retrieved March 14, 2006 from http://dictionary.reference.com/browse/capacity

Dictionary.com (n.d.-c) *Individual.* Retrieved March 28, 2007 from http://dictionary.reference.com/browse/individuals

Dictionary.com. (n.d.-d). *Populations.* Retrieved from http://dictionary.reference.com/browse/ populations

Do Rozario, L. (1997). Shifting paradigms: The transpersonal dimensions of ecology and occupation. *Journal of Occupational Science: Australia, 4*(3), 112-118.

Doble, S. (2002). *Report of the professional issue forum on universal design for growing through occupation.* Retrieved March 21, 2007 from http://www.caot.ca/default.asp? pageid=577

Doble, S., Cameron, F., Diggins, C., Downer, A., Higgins, A., Hobson, S., Justason, T., Kumas, Z., Maldrae, R., St. John, D., & Watkins, L. (2002). Examination of the construct validity of the Occupational Well-Being Questionnaire (OWBQ). First Canadian Occupational Science Symposium, Halifax, NS, May 2002.

Doble, S., Caron Santha, J., Theben, J., & Knott, L., Lall-Phillips, J. (2006). The Occupational Well-Being Questionnaire: The development of a valid outcome measure. World Federation of Occupational Therapy Congress 2006. Sydney, Australia, July 2006.

Donabedian, A. (1966). Evaluating the quality of medical care. *Milbank Memorial Fund*

Quarterly: Health and Society, 44(3; pt. 2), 166-203.

Donabedian, A. (1994). *Explorations in quality assessment and monitoring: Volume 1 – the definition of quality and approaches to its assessment.* Ann Arbour, MI: Health Administration Press.

Donaldson, L. J. (2001). Professional accountability in a changing world. *Postgraduate Medical Journal, 77*(904), 65-57.

Dreiling, D., & Bundy, A. (2003). A comparison of consultative model and direct-indirect intervention with preschoolers. *American Journal of Occupational Therapists, 57*(5), 566-569.

Dressler, J., & MacRae, A. (1998). Advocacy, partnerships and client-centred practice in California. *Occupational Therapy in Mental Health, 14*(1/2), 35-43.

Driver, M. (1968). A philosophic view of the history of OT in Canada. *Canadian Journal of Occupational Therapy, 35*(2), 53-60.

Drummond, M., O'Brien, B., Stoddart, G., & Torrance, G. (1997). *Methods for the economic evaluation of health care programmes* (2nd ed.). UK: Oxford University Press.

Dubouloz, C., Chevrier, J., & Savoie-Zajc, L. (2001). Processus de transformation chez un groupe de personnes cardiaques suivies en ergothérapie pour une modification de leur équilibre du fonctionnement occupationnel. *Revue canadienne d'ergothérapie, 68*(3), 171-85.

Dubouloz, C., Egan, M., Vallerand, J., & von Zweck, C. (1999). Occupational therapists' perceptions of evidence-based practice. *American Journal of Occupational Therapy, 53*(5), 445-453.

Dubouloz, C., Laporte, D., Hall, M., Ashe, B., & Smith, C. D. (2004). Transformation of meaning perspectives in clients with rheumatoid arthritis. *American Journal of Occupational Therapy, 58*(4), 398-407.

Dubouloz, C., Vallerand, J., Lachaine, C., Castonguay, A., Gingras, C., & Rabow, R. (2002). Processus de transformation des perspectives de sens chez un groupe de quatre personnes atteintes de la sclérose en plaques: Le définition de soi. *REFLETS: Revue ontaroise d'intervention sociale et communautaire, 8*(1), 28-46.

Dudgeon, B., & Greenberg, S. (1998). Preparing students for consultation roles and systems. *American Journal of Occupational Therapy, 52*, 801-809.

Duggan, R. (2005). Reflection as a means to foster client-centred practice. *Canadian Journal of Occupational Therapy, 72*(2), 103-112.

Duncan, M., Buchanan, H., Lorenzo, T. (2005). Politics in occupational therapy education: a South African perspective. In F. Kronenber, S. Simo Algado, & N. Pollard (Eds.), *Occupational therapy without borders: Learning from the spirit of survivors* (pp 390-401). London: Churchill Livingston.

Dunlop, W. J. (1933). A brief history of occupational therapy. *Canadian Journal of Occupational Therapy, 1*, 6-11.

Dunn, W. (1988). Models of occupational therapy service provision in the school system. *American Journal of Occupational Therapy, 42*(11), 718-723.

Dunn, W. (1997). Implementing neuroscience principles to support habilitation and recovery. In C. H. Christiansen, & C. M. Baum (Eds.), *Occupational therapy: Enabling function and well-being* (2nd ed., pp. 182-233). Thorofare, NJ: SLACK, Inc.

Dunn, W., Brown, C., & McGuigan, A. (1994). The ecology of human performance: A framework for considering the effect of context. *American Journal of Occupational Therapy, 48*(7), 595-607.

Dunn, W., Brown, C., & Younstrom, M. (2003). Ecological model of occupation. In P. Kramer, J. Hinojosa, & C. B. Royeen (Eds.), *Perspectives on human occupation: Participation in life* (pp. 222-262). Philadelphia: Lippincott Williams & Wilkins.

Dunton, W. R. Jr. (1919). *Reconstruction therapy.* Philadelphia: W. B. Saunders.

Dürckheim, K. G. (1974). *La percée de l'être ou les étapes de la maturité.* Paris: Le Courrier du livre.

Duxbury, L., Higgins, C., & Johnson, K. (1999). *An examination of the implications and costs of work-life conflict in Canada.* Ottawa: Ontario: Department of Health.

Duxbury, L., & Higgins, C. (2001). *Work-life balance in the new millennium: Where are we? where do we need to go?* Retrieved December 21, 2006 from http://www.cprn.org/en/doc.cfm?doc=52

Dyck I. (1998). Multicultural society. In D. Jones S. E. Blair, & J. T. Hartery (Eds.), *Sociology and occupational therapy: An integrated approach* (pp. 67-80). London: Harcourt Brace.

Dyck, I., & Jongbloed, L. (2000). Women with multiple sclerosis and employment issues: A focus on social and institutional environments. *Canadian Journal of Occupational Therapy, 67*(5), 337-346.

Egan, M., Dubouloz, C., von Zweck, C., & Vallerand, J. (1998). The client-centred evidence-based practice of occupational therapy. *Canadian Journal of Occupational Therapy, 65*(3), 136-143.

Egan, M., Hobson, S., & Fearing, V. G. (2006). Dementia and occupation: A review of the literature. *Canadian Journal of Occupational Therapy, 73*(3), 132-140.

Egan, M., & Swedersky, J. (2003). Spirituality as experienced by occupational therapists in practice. *American Journal of Occupational Therapy, 57*(5), 525-533.

Eklund, M. (2004). Satisfaction in daily occupations: A tool for client evaluation in mental health care. *Scandinavian Journal of Occupational Therapy, 11*(3), 136-142.

Elder, H. W., & Rudolph, P. M. (1999). Does retirement planning affect the level of retirement satisfaction? *Financial Services Review, 9,* 117-127. Retrieved March 22, 2007 from http://www.rmi.gsu.edu/FSR/abstracts/Vol_08/Volume%208%20Number% 202/V8-2%20A5.pdf

Emerson, H., Cook, J., Polatajko, H., & Segal, R. (1998). Enjoyment experiences as described by persons with schizophrenia: A qualitative study. *Canadian Journal of Occupational Therapy, 65*(4), 183-192.

Emmons, R. A. (2003). Personal goals, life meaning, and virtue: Wellsprings of a positive life. In C. L. M. Keyes, & J. Haidt (Eds.), *Flourishing. Positive psychology and the life well-lived* (pp. 105-128). Washington, DC: American Psychological Association.

Engel, G. L. (1977). The need for a new medical model: A challenge for biomedicine. *Science, 196*(4286), 129-135.

Enhancing Interdisciplinary Collaboration in Primary Care. (2006). *Primary care: A framework that fits.* Retrieved February 4, 2009 from http://www.eicp.ca/en/who/default.asp

Epp, J. (1986). *Achieving health for all: A framework for health promotion.* Ottawa, ON: Health and Welfare Canada.

Ernest, M. (1972). *The changing role of the occupational therapist.* Vancouver: University of British Columbia.

Evans, J. (2004). Bodies matter: Men, masculinity, and the gendered division of labour in nursing. *Journal of Occupational Science, 11*(1), 12-22.

Evans, R. G. (2000). Canada: How the system works. *Journal of Health Politics, Policy and Law, 25*(5), 889-899.

Evans, R. G., Barer, M. L., & Marmor, T. R. (Eds.) (1994). *Why are some people healthy and others not? The determinants of health of populations.* New York: Aldine de Gruyter.

Farnworth, L., & Whiteford, G. (2002). Debate and dialogue: Professional necessity and responsibility. *Australian Occupational Therapy Journal, 49*(3), 113-114.

Fast, J., Eales, J., & Keating, N. (2001). *Economic impact of health, income security and labour policies on informal caregivers of frail seniors.* Edmonton, AB: Department of Human Ecology.

Fay, B. (1987). *Critical social science: Liberation and its limits.* Ithaca, NY: Cornell University Press.

Fearing, V. G., & Clark, J. (2000). *Individuals in context: A practical guide to client centered practice.* Thorofare, NJ: SLACK, Inc.

Fearing, V. G., Law, M., & Clark, M. (1997). An occupational performance process model: Fostering client and therapist alliances. *Canadian Journal of Occupational Therapy, 64*(1), 7-15

Fetzer, J. K. (1990). *Artificial intelligence: Its scope and limits.* Dordrecht, The Netherlands: Kluwer Academic Publishers.

Fidler, G. S., & Fidler, G. W. (1978). Doing and becoming: Purposeful action and self-actualization. *American Journal of Occupational Therapy, 32*(5), 305-310.

Fieldhouse, J. (2000). Occupational science and community mental health: Using occupational risk factors as a framework for exploring chronicity. *British Journal of Occupational Therapy,*

63(5), 211-217.

Finnie, R., Lascenes, E., & Sweetman, A. (2005). *Who goes? The direct and indirect effects of family background on access to post-secondary education.* Ottawa, ON: Statistics Canada. Retrieved March 22, 2007 from http://www.statcan.ca/bsolc/english/bsolc?catno= 11F0019MIE2005237

Fisher, A. G. (1994). Development of a functional assessment that adjusts ability measures for task simplicity and rater leniency. In M. Wilson (Ed.), *Objective measurement II: Theory into practice* (pp. 145-175). Norwood, NJ: Ablex.

Fisher A. G., Liu, Y., Velozo, C. V., & Pan, A. W. (1992) Cross-cultural assessment of process skills. *American Journal of Occupational Therapy, 46,* 876-885.

Fitzgerald, M. H., Mullavey-Obryne, C., & Clemson, L. (1997). Cultural issues from practice. *Australian Occupational Therapy Journal, 44,* 1-22.

Ford, M., McKee, P., & Szilagyi, M. (2004). A hybrid thermoplastic and neoprene thumb metacarpophalangeal joint orthosis. *Journal of Hand Therapy, 17*(1), 64-68.

Forsyth, K., & Kielhofner, G. (2003). Model of human occupation. In P. Kramer, J. Hinojosa, & C. B. Royeen (Eds.), *Perspectives on human occupation: Participation in life* (pp. 45-86). Philadelphia: Lippincott Williams & Wilkins.

Foucault, M. (1972). Two lectures. In C. Gordon (Ed.), *Power/knowledge: Selected interviews and other writings 1972-1977* (pp. 78-108). London: Harvester Press.

Frank, G. (1992). Opening feminist histories of occupational therapy. *American Journal of Occupational Therapy, 46*(11), 989-999.

Frank, A. W. (2001). Can we research suffering? *Qualitative Health Research, 11*(3), 353-362.

Frankish, C., Moulton, G., Quantz, D., Carson, A. J., Casebeer, A. L., Eyles, J. D., et al. (2007). Addressing the non-medical determinants of health: A survey of Canada's health region. *Canadian Journal of Public Health, 98*(1), 41-47.

Frankl, V. E. (1962). *Man's search for meaning.* Boston: Beacon Press.

Frankl, V. E. (1985). *The unheard cry for meaning.* New York: Washington Square Press.

Frederickson, B. (2003). The value of positive emotions. *America Scientist, 91*(4), 330-335.

Freeman, A. R., McWilliam, C. L., MacKinnon, J. R., Rappolt, S. G., & DeLuca, S. (June, 2006). *Health care professionalism: How occupational therapists enact their accountability obligations.* Poster presented at the Canadian Association of Occupational Therapists Conference, Montreal, PQ.

Freidson, E. (1970). *Profession of medicine; a study in the sociology of applied knowledge.* Chicago: University of Chicago Press.

Freidson, E. (1986). *Professional powers: A study of the institutionalization of formal knowledge.* Chicago: University of Chicago Press.

Freidson, E. (1994). *Professionalism reborn. Theory, prophecy and policy.* Cambridge: Polity Press.

Freidson, E. (2001). *Professionalism: The third logic.* Chicago: The University of Chicago Press.

Freire, P. (1970). *Pedagogy of the oppressed.* New York: The Continuum Publishing Company.

French, S. (1991). What's so great about independence? In J. Swain, V. Finkelstein, S. French, & M. Oliver (Eds.), *Disabling Barriers – Enabling environments* (pp. 44-48). London: Sage Publications.

Freudenberg, N., Eng, E., Flay, B., Parcel, G., Rogers, T., & Wallerstein, N. (1995). Strengthening individual and community capacity to prevent disease and promote health: In search of relevant theories and principles. *Health Education Quarterly, August,* 290-303.

Friedland, J. (2001). Knowing from whence we came: Reflecting on return-to-work and interpersonal relationships. *Canadian Journal of Occupational Therapy, 68*(5), 266-271.

Friedland, J. (2003). Why crafts? Influences on the development of occupational therapy in Canada from 1890 to 1930. *Canadian Journal of Occupational Therapy, 70*(4), 204-212.

Friedland, J., & Davids-Brumer, N. (2007). From education to occupation: The story of Thomas Bessell Kidner. *Canadian Journal of Occupational Therapy, 74*(1), 27-37.

Friedland, J., & Rais, H. (2005). Helen Primrose LeVesconte: Occupational therapy clinician, educator, and maker of history. *Canadian Journal of Occupational Therapy, 72*(3), 131-141.

Fromm, E. (1962). *Beyond the chains of illusions.* New York: Simon and Schuster.

Gage, M., & Polatajko, H. (1995). Naming practice: The case for the term client-driven. *Canadian*

Journal of Occupational Therapy, 62(3), 115-118.

Gagné, M.A. (2005). *Advancing the agenda for collaborative mental health care*. Mississauga, ON: Canadian Collaborative Mental Health Initiative. Retrieved on March 22, 2007 from www.ccmhi.ca

Gaines, R., Missiuna, C., Egan, M., & McLean, J. (2006). *Promoting inter-disciplinary identification and improved service delivery for children with developmental coordination disorder and their families. In progress.* Toronto, ON: Ontario Ministry of Health and Long-term Care for Primary Health Care Transition Fund Projects Ontario. Retrieved March 22, 2007 from http://www.dcd-uk.org/seminar4c.html

Galheigo, S. M. (2005). Occupational therapy and the social field: Clarifying concepts and ideas, In F. Kronenberg, S. Simo Algado, & N. Pollard (Eds.), *Occupational therapy without borders* (pp. 87-89). London: Elsevier Churchill Livingstone.

Gallew, H. A., & Mu, K. (2004). An occupational look at temporal adaptation: Night shift nurses. *Journal of Occupational Science, 11*(1), 23-30.

Garfinkel, M., & Blumenthal, E. (2001). Co-active coaching and HIV. *Aids Alert, 16*(8), 105-108.

Geertz, C. (1973). *The interpretation of cultures: Selected essays.* New York: Basic Books.

Gerlach, A. (2005). Celebrating the strengths of aboriginal consumers: Community consultation and partnerships. *Occupational Therapy Now, 5*(6), 15-17.

Gibson, L., Strong, J., & Wallace, A. (2003). Functional capacity evaluation as a performance measure: Evidence for a new approach for clients with chronic back pain. *Australian Journal of Occupational Therapy, 21*(3), 207-215.

Giddens, A. (1987). *Sociology: A brief but critical introduction* (2nd ed.). Philadelphia: Harcourt Bruce Jovanovich.

Giddens, A. (1991). *Modernity and self-identity: Self and society in the late modern age.* New York: Standford University Press.

Gilbert, J. V. (2005). Interprofessional learning and higher education structural barriers. *Journal of Interprofessional Care, 19*(Suppl. 1), 87-106.

Gillen, G. (2000). Improving activities of daily living performance in an adult with ataxia. *American Journal of Occupational Therapy, 54*(1), 89-96.

Glantz, C. H., & Richman, N. (1997). OTR-COTA collaboration in home health: Roles and supervisory issues. *American Journal of Occupational Therapy, 51*, 446-452.

Goffman, E. (1961). *Asylums: Essays in the social situation of mental patients and other inmates.* New York: Doubleday.

Goldberg, B., Brintnell, E. S., & Goldberg, J. (2002). The relationship between engagement in meaningful activities and quality of life in persons disabled by mental illness. *Occupational Therapy in Mental Health, 18*(2), 17-44.

Goldberg, M. (1998). *The art of the question.* New York: John Riley & Sons.

Golledge, J. (1998). Distinguishing between occupation, purposeful activity and activity, part 1: Review and explanation. *British Journal of Occupational Therapy, 61*(3), 100-105.

Government of Canada. (1982). *Canadian Charter of Rights and Freedoms, Constitution Act, part I.* Ottawa, ON: Supply and Services Canada. Retrieved March 31, 2007 from http://laws.justice.gc.ca/en/Const/annex_e.html#I

Government of Canada. (1984). *Canada Health Act.* Ottawa, ON: Supply and Services Canada.

Government of Canada. (1976-77). *Canadian Human Rights Act.*, c. 3, s. 1. Retrieved June 19, 2007 from http://laws.justice.gc.ca/en/ShowFullDoc/cs/H-6///en

Governments of Canada, Ontario, Quebec, Nova Scotia, New Brunswick, Manitoba, et al. (2005). *Blueprint on aboriginal health: A 10 year transformative plan.* Ottawa: Health Canada. Retrieved February 4, 2009 from http://www.hc-sc.gc.ca/hcs-sss/alt_formats/hpb-dgps/pdf/pubs/2005-blueprint-plan-abor-auto/plan-eng.pdf

Government of Nova Scotia (1999). Freedom of information and protection of privacy act, S.N.S. 1993, c.5, s.12 as am by S.N.S. (2nd sess.), c.11, s.8. Retrieved February 4, 2009 from http://www.canlii.net/ns/laws/sta/1993c.5/20080616/whole.html

Gowan, N., & Strong, S. (2002). The expanding world of occupational therapy. *Occupational Therapy Now, 4*(5), 9-13.

Grant A. (2003). The impact of life coaching on goal attainment, metacognition and mental health. *Social Behaviour and Personality, 31*(3), 253-264.

Gray, J. M. (1998). Putting occupation into practice: Occupation as ends, occupation as means. *American Journal of Occupational Therapy, 52*(5), 354-364.

Greenberg, E. S., Grunberg, L., & Moore, S. (2003). *The changing workplace, alcohol problems and well-being: Findings from our research program and reflections on their meaning.* Smithers symposium on alcohol and the workplace. Retrieved March 22, 2007 from http://www.colorado.edu/ibs/pubs/pec/pec2003-0005.pdf

Grenfell, M., & James, D. (Eds.). (1998). *Bourdieu and education: Acts of practical theory.* London: Falmer Press.

Griffin, S. (2001). Occupational therapists and the concept of power: A review of the literature. *Australian Occupational Therapy Journal, 48*(1), 24-34.

Gritzer, G., & Arluke, A. (1985). *The making of rehabilitation.* Los Angeles, CA: University of California Press.

Grue, L., & Laerum, K. T. (2002). "Doing motherhood": Some experiences of mothers with physical disabilities. *Disability & Society, 17*(6), 671-683.

Grunberg, L., Moore, S., Anderson-Connolly, R., & Greenberg, E. (1999). Work stress and self-reported alcohol use: The moderating role of escapist reasons for drinking. *Journal of Occupational Health Psychology, 4*(1), 29-36.

Guest, D. E. (2002). Perspectives on the study of work-life balance. *Social Sciences Information, 41*(2), 255-279.

Habermas, J. (1995). *The philosophical discourse of modernity: Twelve lectures* (F. Lawrence, Trans.). Cambridge: Massachussets Institute of Technology Press.

Hadikin, R. (2001). Co-active coaching: An introduction. *Practicing Midwife, 4*(7), 36-37.

Haertl, K., & Minato, M. (2006). Daily occupations of persons with mental illness: Themes from Japan and America. *Occupational Therapy in Mental Health, 22*(1), 19-32.

Hagedorn, R. (2000). *Tools for practice in occupational therapy: A structured approach to core skills and processes.* Toronto, Ontario: Harcourt Publishers.

Hall, E. M. (1980). *Canada's National-Provincial Health Program for the 1980's: A Commitment for Renewal.* Ottawa, ON: Government of Canada.

Hall, H., & Buck, M. M. C. (1915). *The work of our hands: A study of occupations for invalids.* New York: Moffat, Yard and Company.

Hall, R. H. (1968). Professionalization and bureaucratization. *American Sociological Review, 33*(1), 92-104.

Hamilton, N., & Bhatti, T. (1996). *Population health promotion: An integrated model of population health and health promotion.* Retrieved February 4, 2009 from http://www.phac-aspc.gc.ca/ph-sp/php-psp/index-eng.php

Hamilton, T. B. (2004). Occupations and places. In C. Christiansen, & E. A. Townsend (Eds.), *Introduction to occupation: The art and science of living* (pp. 173-196). Upper Saddle River, NJ: Prentice Hall.

Hammell, K. W. (2004a). Deviating from the norm: A skeptical interrogation of the classificatory practices of the ICF. *British Journal of Occupational Therapy, 67*(9), 408-411.

Hammell, K. W. (2004b). Dimensions of meaning in the occupations of daily life. *Canadian Journal of Occupational Therapy, 71*(5), 296-305.

Hammell, K. W. (2007). Reflections on…a disability methodology for the client-centred practice of occupational therapy. *Canadian Journal of Occupational Therapy, 74*(2), Early on-line edition.

Hannam, D. (1997). More than a cup of tea: Meaning construction in an everyday occupation. *Journal of Occupational Science: Australia, 4*(2), 69-74.

Hanson, S., & Pratt, G. (1988). Reconceptualizing the links between home and work in urban geography. *Economic Geography, 64*(4), 300-321.

Harrison, K. (2000). Put it to practice. Students enable clinicians' understanding of the occupational performance process model. *Occupational Therapy Now, 2*(5), 16-18.

Harvey, A., & Pentland, W. (2004). What do people do? In C. Christiansen & E.A. Townsend (Eds), *An introduction to occupation: The art & science of living* (1st ed.). Upper Saddle River, NJ:Pearson Education. p 63-90.

Hasselkus, B. (2002a). From the desk of the editor. Keeping body and soul together. *American Journal of Occupational Therapy, 56*(4), 367-368.

Hasselkus, B. (2002b). *The meaning of everyday occupation*. Thorofare, NJ: SLACK, Inc.

Hasselkus, B.R., & Rosa, S.A. (1997). The meaning of occupation. In C. Christiansen, & C. Baum (Eds.), *Occupational therapy: Achieving human performance needs in daily living* (2nd ed., pp 363-377). Thorofare, NJ: SLACK, Inc.

Hayes, P. M. (1994). Team building: Bringing RNs and NAs together. *Nursing Management, 25*(5), 52-54.

Hays, S. (1994). Structure and agency and the sticky problem of culture. *Sociological Theory, 12*(1), 57-72.

Head, B. J. (2005). *Moving evidence into practice: Enabling research utilization and knowledge transfer.* Unpublished master's thesis, School of Occupational Therapy, Dalhousie University, Halifax, Nova Scotia.

Health Canada & Interdepartmental Committee on Aging and Seniors Issues. (2002). *Canada's aging population.* Ottawa, ON, Canada: Minister of Public Works and Government Services Canada.

Health Professions Regulatory Advisory Council. (2006). *Regulation of health professions in Ontario: New directions.* Retrieved March 22, 2007 from http://www.health.gov.on.ca/ english/ public/ pub/ministry_reports/new_directions/new_directions.pdf

Helander, E. (1992). *Prejudice and dignity: An introduction to community-based rehabilitation.* New York: United Nations Development Programme.

Hemmingsson, H., & Jonsson, H. (2005). An occupational perspective on the concept of participation in the international classification of functioning, disability and health – some critical remarks. *American Journal of Occupational Therapy, 59*(5), 569-576.

Hemmingsson, S., Egilson, E., Hoffman, O., & Kielhofner, G. (2005). *The School Setting Interview* (Version 3.0). University of Illinois, Chicago: MOHO Clearinghouse.

Hendrickson-Gracie, K., Staley, D., & Neufeld-Morton, I. (1996). When worlds collide: Resolving value differences in psychosocial rehabilitation. *Psychiatric Rehabilitation Journal, 20*(1), 25-31.

Hendry, F., & McVittie, C. (2004). Is quality of life a healthy concept? Measuring and understanding life experiences of older people. *Qualitative Health Research, 14*(7), 961-975.

Hillman, A., & Chapparo, C. J. (1995). An investigation of occupational role performance in men over sixty years of age, following a stroke. *Journal of Occupational Science, 2*(3), 88-99.

Hirdes, J. P., & Carpenter, G. I. (1997). Health outcomes among the frail elderly in communities and institutions: Use of the minimum data set (MDS) to create effective linkages between research and policy. *Canadian Journal on Aging, Canadian Public Policy Special Supplement,* 53-69.

Hocking, C. (2001). Implementing occupation-based assessment. *American Journal of Occupational Therapy, 55*(4), 463-468.

Hocking C. & Ness N.E. (2002). *Revised Minimum Standards for the Education of Occupational Therapists.* Perth, Australia: World Federation of Occupational Therapists. Retrieved March 23, 2007 from http://www.wfot.org/faq.asp?name= Education

Hoffman, K., & Duponte, J. (1992). *Community health centres and community development.* Ottawa, ON: Health and Welfare Canada.

Holland, S. K., Greenberg, J., Tidwell, L., & Newcomer, R. (2003). Preventing disability through community-based health coaching. *Journal of the American Geriatrics Society, 51*(2), 265-269.

Hollis, V., & Madill, H. (2006). Online learning the potential for occupational therapy education. *Occupational Therapy International, 13*(2), 1-78.

Hollis V., Madill, H., Darrah J., Warren, S., & Rivard, A. (2006) Winners and losers: Occupational therapists' and physical therapists' experiences of community based rehabilitation services. *International Journal of Therapy and Rehabilitation, 13*(1), 7-13.

Holm, M. B., Rogers, J. C., & Stone, R. G. (2003). Person-task-environment interventions: A decision-making guide. In E. B. Crepeau, E. Cohn, & B. A. Boyt Schell (Eds.), *Willard & Spackman's occupational therapy* (10th ed., pp. 460-490). Philadelphia, PA: Lippincott Williams & Wilkins.

Holstein, J. A., & Gubrium, J. F. (2000). *Constructing the life course.* Dix Hills, NY: General Hall.

Hopkins, H., & Smith, H. (Eds.). (1988). *Willard and Spackman's occupational therapy* (7th ed.). Philadelphia, PA: J.B. Lippincott.

Houghton Mifflin Company. (2004). *The American heritage® dictionary of the English language* (4th ed.). Retrieved September 2, 2006 from http://www.answers.com

Howard, B. S., & Howard, J. R. (1997). Occupation as spiritual activity. *American Journal of Occupational Therapy, 51*(10), 181-185.

Howland, G. W. (1933). Editorial. *Canadian Journal of Occupational Therapy, 1*(1), 4-5.

Howland, G. W. (1944). President's address. *Canadian Journal of Occupational Therapy, 11*(1), 3.

Howland, G. W. (1986). Occupational therapy across Canada. *Canadian Journal of Occupational Therapy, 53*, 18-26.

Huber, D. G., Blegen, M. A., & McCloskey, J. C. (1994). Use of nursing assistants: Staff nurse opinions. *Nursing Management, 25*(5), 64-69.

Human Resources and Skills Development Canada. (2005). *Occupational therapists (NOC 3143)*. Retrieved August 30, 2005 from http://www.labourmarketinformation.ca

Human Resources and Social Development Canada. (2007). *Overview of understanding the early years*. Retrieved March 22, 2007 from http://www.hrsdc.gc.ca/en/hip/sd/300_UEYInfo.shtml

Humphris, D., Littlejohns, P., Victor, C., O'Halloran, P., & Peacock, J. (2000). Implementing evidence-based practice: Factors that influence the use of research evidence by occupational therapists. *British Journal of Occupational Therapy, 63*(11), 516-222.

Humphry, R. (1995). Families who live in chronic poverty: Meeting the challenge of family centered services. *American Journal of Occupational Therapy, 49*(7), 687-693.

Humphry, R. (2002). Young children's occupational behaviors: Explicating developmental processes. *American Journal of Occupational Therapy, 56*(2), 171-179.

Hunsley, T. (2006). Work life balance in an aging population. *Horizons, 8*(3), 3-13.

Hunter, E., & Nicol, M. (2002). Systematic review: Evidence of the value of continuing professional development to enhance recruitment and retention of occupational therapists in mental health. *British Journal of Occupational Therapy, 65*(5), 207-215.

Illich, I., Zola, I. K., McNight, J., Caplan, J., & Shaiken, H. (1977). *Disabling professions*. London: Marion Boyer.

Inayatullah, S. (2006). Futures of occupational therapy and occupational therapists. Keynote Lecture, Sydney, Australia: World Federation of Occupational Therapists Congress, July

International Coach Federation. (2006). *What is coaching?* Retrieved December 22, 2006 from http://www.coachfederation.org/ICF/For+Coaching+Clients/What+is+a+Coach/

International Labour Organisation, Bureau of Statistics. (2004). ISCO-88. Retrieved March 22, 2007 from http://www.ilo.org/public/english/bureau/stat/isco/isco88/index.htm

International Organization for Standardization. (1998). *8549-1: Prosthetics and orthotics - vocabulary, part 1: General terms for external limb prostheses and external orthoses*. Geneva, Switzerland: Author.

Irvine, R., & Graham, J. (1994). Deconstructing the concept of professions: A prerequisite to carving a niche in a changing world. *Australian Occupational Therapy Journal, 41*(1), 9-18.

Irwin, J. D., & Morrow, D. (2003). Health promotion theory in practice. An analysis of co-active coaching. *International Journal of Evidence-Based Coaching & Mentoring, 3*(1), 29-38.

Isaacowitz, D. M., Vaillant, G. E., & Seligman, M. (2003). Strengths and satisfaction across the adult lifespan. *International Journal of Aging and Development, 57*(2), 181-201.

Iwama, M. (2003). The issue is – toward culturally relevant epistemologies in occupational therapy. *American Journal of Occupational Therapy, 57*(5), 582-588.

Iwama, M. (2005). Occupation as a cross-cultural construct. In G. Whiteford, & V. Wright-St. Clair (Eds.), *Occupation & practice in context*. Marickville, NSW: Churchill Livingstone.

Iwama, M. (2006a). The Kawa (river) model: Client centred rehabilitation in cultural context. In S. Davis (Ed.), *Rehabilitation: The use of theories and models in practice (pp. 147-168)*. Oxford, UK: Churchill Livingstone Elsevier.

Iwama, M. (2006b). *The Kawa model: Culturally relevant occupational therapy*. Edinburgh, Scotland: Churchill Livingstone Elsevier.

Iwarrson, S., Isacsson, A., Persson, D., & Schersten, B. (1998). Occupation and survival: A 24-

year follow-up study of an aging population. *American Journal of Occupational Therapy, 52*(1), 65-70.

Iwarsson, S., & Slaug, B. (2001). *The enabler website: Providing tools for professional assessments of accessibility problems in the environment.* Retrieved January 14, 2007 from www.enabler.nu

Jackson, J., Carlson, M., Mandel, D., Zemke, R., & Clark, F. (1998). Occupation in lifestyle redesign: The Well Elderly Study Occupational Therapy Program. *American Journal of Occupational Therapy, 52*(5), 326-336.

Jackson, T., Mitchell, S., & Wright, M. (1989). The community development continuum. *Community Health Studies, 13*(1), 66-73.

Jacobs, K. (Ed.). (1999). *Quick reference dictionary for occupational therapy* (2nd ed.). Thorofare, NJ: SLACK, Inc.

Jantzen, A. C. (1963). Some strengths of occupational therapy. *Canadian Journal of Occupational Therapy, 30*(1), 21-25.

Jarman, J. (2004) Interdisciplinary perspectives on classifying human activity. In C. Christiansen, & E. A. (Eds.) *Introduction to Occupation: The art and science of living* (pp. 47–61). Upper Saddle River, NJ: Prentice Hall.

Jenkins, M. (1991). The problems of recruitment: A local study. *British Journal of Occupational Therapy, 54*(12), 449-452.

Jette, A. M., Haley, S. M., & Kooyoomjian, J. T. (2003). Are the ICF activity and participation dimensions distinct? *Journal of Rehabilitation Medicine, 35*(3), 145-149.

Johansson, U., & Bernspang, B. (2001). Predicting return to work after brain injury using occupational therapy assessments. *Disability & Rehabilitation, 23*(11), 474-480.

Johnson, S. E. (1996). Activity analysis. In A. Turner, M. Foster, & S. E. Johnson (Eds.), *Occupational therapy and physical dysfunction: Principles, skills, and practice* (4th ed., pp. 101-124). New York: Churchill Livingstone.

Jones, O. (2006). Politically aware or politically active? *OT Practice, 11*(5), 6.

Jongbloed, L. (1996). Factors influencing employment status of women with multiple sclerosis. *Canadian Journal of Rehabilitation, 9*(4), 213-222.

Jongbloed, L. (2003). Disability policy in Canada: An overview. *Journal of Disability Policy Studies, 13*(4), 203-209.

Jongbloed, L., & Crichton, A. (1990). A new definition of disability: Implications for rehabilitation practice and social policy. *Canadian Journal of Occupational Therapy, 57*(1), 32-38.

Jongbloed, L., & Wendland, T. (2002). The impact of reimbursement systems on occupational therapy practice in Canada and the United States of America. *Canadian Journal of Occupational Therapy, 69*(3), 143-152.

Jonsson, H. (in press). Occupational transitions in retirement. In C. Christiansen, & E. A. Townsend, *Introduction to occupation: The art and science of living,* (2nd Ed). Upper Saddle River, NJ: Pearson Education.

Jonsson, H., Borell, L., & Sadlo, G. (2000). Retirement: An occupational transition with consequences for temporality, balance and meaning of occupations. *Journal of Occupational Science, 7*(1), 29-37.

Jonsson, H., Kielhofner, G., & Borell, L. (1997). Anticipating retirement: The formation of narratives concerning an occupational transition. *American Journal of Occupational Therapy, 51*(1), 49-56.

Joseph, D., Griffin, M., Hall, R., & Sullivan, E. (2001). Peer coaching: An intervention for individuals struggling with diabetes. *The Diabetes Educator, 27*(5), 703-710.

Jung, B., Sainsbury, S., Grum, R. M., Wilkins, S., & Tryssenaar, J. (2002). Collaborative fieldwork education with student occupational therapists and student occupational therapist assistants. *Canadian Journal of Occupational Therapy, 69(2),* 95-104.

Kampa-Kokesch, S., & Anderson, M. Z. (2001). Executive coaching: A comprehensive review of the literature. *Consulting Psychology Journal, 53*(4), 205-229.

Kang, C. (2003). A psychospiritual integration frame of reference for occupational therapy. Part 1: Conceptual foundations. *Australian Occupational Therapy Journal, 50*(2), 92-103.

Kaplan, R. S., & Norton, D. P. (1992). The balanced scorecard – measures that drive performance. *Harvard Business Review, January-February*, 71-79.

Karasek, R., & Theorell, T. (1990). *Healthy work: Stress, productivity, and the reconstruction of working life.* New York: Basic Books.

Kasar, J., & Muscari, M. E. (2000). A conceptual model for the development of professional behaviours in occupational therapists. *Canadian Journal of Occupational Therapy, 67*(1), 42-50.

Kegan, R. (1982). *The evolving self: Problem and process in human development.* Cambridge, MA: Harvard University Press.

Kegan, R. (1994). *In over our heads. The mental demands of modern life.* Cambridge, MA: Harvard University Press.

Kegan, R., & Lahey, L. L. (2001). *How the way we talk can change the way we work.* San Franscisco, CA: Jossey-Bass Publishers.

Kemmis, B., & Dunn, W. (1996). Collaborative consultation: The efficacy of remedial and compensatory interventions in school contexts. *American Journal of Occupational Therapy, 50*(9), 709-717.

Kemp, C. L., Rosenthal, C., & Denton, M. (2005). Financial planning for later life: Subjective understandings of catalysts and constraints. *Journal of Aging Studies, 19*(3), 273-290.

Kennedy, L. (1997). The role of the occupational therapist in personal injury litigation—Part 1. *The Expert Witness Newsletter, 2*(3), 1-4.

Kerlinger, F. N. (1979). *Behavioral research: A conceptual approach.* New York: Holt, Rinehart, & Winston.

Kerlinger, F. N. (1986). *Foundations of behavioral research.* New York: Holt, Rinehart, & Winston.

Keys, C. L. M., & Haidt, J. (Eds.). (2003). *Flourishing: Positive psychology and the life well-lived.* Washington, DC: American Psychological Association.

Khan, S. (1991). *Organizing: A guide for grassroots leaders* (Rev. ed.). Washington, DC: National Association of Social Workers.

Kiefer, C. (2000). *Health work with the poor: A practical guide.* London: Rutgers.

Kielhofner G. (1980). A model of human occupation part three: Benign and vicious cycles. *American Journal of Occupational Therapy, 34*, 731-737.

Kielhofner, G. (1995). Introduction to the model of human occupation. In G. Kielhofner (Ed.), *A model of human occupation: Theory and application* (2nd ed., pp. 1-7). Baltimore, MD: Williams & Wilkins.

Kielhofner, G. (1997). *Conceptual foundations of occupational therapy.* Philadelphia: F.A. Davis Company.

Kielhofner, G. (Ed.). (2002). *A model of human occupation: Theory and application* (3rd ed.). Baltimore, MD: Lippincott, Williams & Wilkins.

Kielhofner, G. (June, 2002). *Challenges and directions for the future of occupational therapy.* Keynote presentation, World Federation of Occupational Therapists Congress June, 2002, Stockholm, Sweden.

Kielhofner, G., Castle, L., Dubouloz, C., Egan, M., Forsyth, K., Melton, J., et al. (2006). Participatory research for the development and evaluation of occupational therapy: Research-practitioner collaboration. In G. Kielhofner (Ed.), *Research in occupational therapy: Methods of inquiry for enhancing practice* (pp. 643-655). Philadelphia PA: F. A. Davis.

Kielhofner, G., Mallinson, T., Forsyth, K., & Lai, J. (2001). Psychometric properties of the second version of the occupational performance history interview (OPHI-II). *American Journal of Occupational Therapy, 55*(3), 260-267.

Kindig, D., & Stoddart, G. (2003). What is population health? *American Journal of Public Health, 93*(3), 380-383.

Kinebanian, A. (1992). Cross-cultural occupational therapy: A critical reflection. *American Journal of Occupational Therapy, 46*(8), 751-757.

King, G., Law, M., King, S. A.,P., Hanna, S., Kertoy, M., & Rosenbaum, P. A., (2004). *Children's assessment of participation and enjoyment (CAPE) and preferences for activities of children (PAC).* San Antonio, TX: Harcourt Assessment, Inc.

Kinsella, A. (2001). Reflections on reflective practice [Abstract]. *Canadian Journal of Occuaptional Therapy, 68*(3) 195-198.

Kirby, B. (2002). *The health of Canadians: The federal role. Final report. Volume 6. Recommendations for reform.* The Standing Senate Committee for Social Affairs, Science and Technology. Retrieved February 4, 2009 from http://www.parl.gc.ca/37/2/parlbus/ commbus/ senate/com-e/soci-e/rep-e/repoct02vol6-e.htm

Kirsh, B. (1996). A narrative approach to addressing spirituality in occupational therapy: Exploring meaning and purpose. *Canadian Journal of Occupational Therapy, 63*, 55-61.

Kirsh, B., Cockburn, L., & Gewurtz, R. (2005). Best practice in occupational therapy: Program characteristics that influence vocational outcomes for persons with serious mental illnesses. *Canadian Journal of Occupational Therapy, 72(5)*, 265-279.

Kirsh, B., & Tate, E. (2006). Developing a comprehensive understanding of the working alliance in community mental health. *Qualitative Health Research, 16*(8), 1054-1074.

Kirsh, B., Trentham, B., & Cole, S. (2006). Diversity in occupational therapy: Experiences of consumers who identify themselves as minority group members. *Australian Occupational Therapy Journal, 53*(4), 302-313.

Kivel, B. D., & Kleiber, D. A. (2000). Leisure in the identity formation of lesbian/gay youth: Personal, but not social. *Leisure Sciences, 22*(4), 215-232.

Klaiman, D. (2006). Qualification recognition framework underway for support personnel. *Occupational Therapy Now, 8*(3), 25.

Klinger, L. (2005). Occupational adaptation: Perspectives of people with traumatic brain injury. *Journal of Occupational Science, 12*(1), 9-16.

Klinger, L., Baptiste, B., & Adams, J. (2004). Life care plans: An emerging area for occupational therapists. *Canadian Journal of Occupational Therapy, 71*(2), 88-99.

Kluckhuhn, F. R., & Srodtbeck, F. L. (1961). *Variations in value orientations.* Evanston, IL: Row, Peterson, & Company.

Knowles, M. (Ed.). (1973). *The adult learner: A neglected species.* Houston: Gulf Publishing.

Knowles, M., Holton, E., & Swanson, R. (Eds.). (1998). *The adult learner: The definitive classic in adult education and human resource development.* Houston: Gulf Publishing.

Kohn, M. L. (1976). Occupational structure and alienation. *The American Journal of Sociology, 82*(1), 111-130.

Kolb, D. A. (1984). *Experiential learning. Experience as the source of learning and development.* Englewood, NJ: Prentice Hall.

Krathwohl, D. R., Bloom, B. S., & Masia, B. B. (1964). *Taxonomy of educational objectives: The classification of educational goals. Handbook II – Affective domain.* New York: Holt, Rinehart, & Winston.

Kravitz, R. L., Duan, N., & Braslow, J. (2004). Evidence-based medicine, heterogeneity of treatment effects, and the trouble with averages. *Milbank Quarterly, 82*(4), 661-687.

Krefting, L. (1992). Strategies for the development of occupational therapy in the third world. *The American Journal of Occupational Therapy, 46*(8), 758-761.

Krefting, L. H., & Krefting, D. V. (1991). Cultural influences on performance. In C. Christiansen, & C. Baum (Eds.), *Occupational therapy: Overcoming human performance deficits* (pp. 102-122). Thorofare, NJ: SLACK, Inc.

Kretzman, J., & McKnight, J. (1997). Mapping community capacity. In M. Minkler (Ed.), *Community organizing and community building for health* (pp. 157-172). New Brunswick, NJ: Rutgers University Press.

Kroeker, P. T. (1997). Spirituality and occupational therapy in a secular culture. *Canadian Journal of Occupational Therapy, 64*(3), 122-126.

Kronenberg, F. (2005). The right to be blind without being disabled. In F. Kronenber, S. Simo Algado & N. Pollard (Eds.), *Occupational therapy without borders: Learning from the spirit of survivors* (pp 31-39). London: Elsevier Churchill Livingstone.

Kronenberg, F., & Pollard, N. (2005). Overcoming occupational apartheid: A preliminary exploration of the political nature of occupational therapy. In F. Kronenberg, S. Simo Algado, & N. Pollard (Eds.), *Occupational therapy without borders: Learning from the spirit of survivors,* (pp. 58-86). London: Elsevier Churchill Livingstone.

Krupa, T., Lagarde, M., & Carmichael, K. (2003). Transforming sheltered workshops into affirmative businesses: An outcome evaluation. *Psychiatric Rehabilitation Journal, 26*(4), 359-367.

Krupa , T., Radloff-Gabriel, D., Whippey, E., & Kirsh, B. (2002). Occupational therapy and assertive community treatment. *Canadian Journal of Occupational Therapy, 69*(3), 153-157.

Kuhn, T. (1970). *The structure of scientific revolutions.* Chicago: The University of Chicago Press.

Kuhn, T. (1996). *The structure of scientific revolutions* (3rd ed.). Chicago: The University of Chicago Press.

Kuhn, A. M., & Youngberg, B. J. (2002). The need for risk management to evolve to assure a culture of safety. *Quality & Safety in Health Care 11*, 158–162.

Kumas-Tan, Z., & Beagan, B. (2003). *Ethical tensions in the caring professions: A summary report of interviews with occupational therapists in Nova Scotia.* Unpublished manuscript. School of Occupational Therapy, Dalhousie University at Halifax, NS.

Kuper, A. (1999). *Culture: The anthropologists' account.* Cambridge, MA: Harvard University Press.

Labonte, R. (1993). *Health promotion and empowerment: Practice frameworks.* Toronto, ON. Centre for Health Promotion, University of Toronto.

Labonte, R. (1994). Health promotion and empowerment: Reflections on professional practice. *Health education quarterly, 21*(2), 253-268.

Laliberte Rudman, D. (2005). Understanding political influences on occupational possibilities: An analysis of newspaper constructions of retirees. *Journal of Occupational Science, 12*(3), 149-160

Laliberte Rudman, D., Cook, J., & Polatajko, H. (1997). The potential of occupation: A qualitative exploration of seniors' perspectives. *American Journal of Occupational Therapy, 51*(8), 640-650.

Laliberte Rudman, D., Hoffman, L., Scott, E., & Renwick, R. (2004). Quality of life for persons with schizophrenia: Validating an assessment that addresses consumer concerns and occupational issues. *Occupational Therapy Journal of Research, 24*(1), 13-21.

Laliberte Rudman, D., Yu, B., Scott, E., & Pajouhandeh, P. (2000). Exploration of the perspectives of persons with schizophrenia regarding quality of life. *American Journal of Occupational Therapy, 54*(2), 137-147.

Lalonde, M. (1974). *A new perspective on the health of Canadians: A working document.* Ottawa, ON,: Health and Welfare Canada.

Landry, D., & Mathews, M. (1998). Economic evaluation of occupational therapy: Where are we at? *Canadian Journal of Occupational Therapy, 65*(3), 160-167.

Lang-Étienne, A. (1983). L'approche globale: Poncif ou réalité. *Revue canadienne d'ergothérapie, 50*(5), 177-181.

Lang-Étienne, A. (1986). L'action et l'adhésion à l'existence. *le transfert, 10*(1), 14.

Larson, E. (n.d.). *Occupational science.* Retrieved March 13, 2007 from http://www.education.wisc.edu/occupational_science/researchlibrary/index.html

Larson, E., & Zemke, R. (2003). Shaping the temporal patterns of our lives: The social coordination of occupation. *Journal of Occupational Science, 10*(2), 80-89.

Lave, J., & Wenger, E. (1990). *Situated learning: Legitimate peripheral participation.* UK: Cambridge University Press.

Law, M. (1991). The environment: A focus for occupational therapy. *Canadian Journal of Occupational Therapy, 58*(4), 171-179.

Law, M. (1998). *Client-centred occupational therapy.* Thorofare, NJ: SLACK, Inc.

Law, M., Baptiste, S., Carswell, A., McColl, M. A., Polatajko, H., & Pollock, N. (2005). *Canadian occupational performance measure* (Rev. 4th ed.). Ottawa, Ontario: CAOT Publications ACE.

Law, M., Cooper, B., Strong, S., Stewart, D., Rigby, P., & Letts, L. (1996). The person-environment-occupation model: A transactive approach to occupational performance. *Canadian Journal of Occupational Therapy, 63*(1), 9-23.

Law, M., King, G., & Russell, D. (2005). Guiding therapist decisions about measuring outcomes in occupational therapy. In M. Law, C. Dunn, & W. Dunn (Eds.), *Measuring occupational performance supporting best practice in occupational therapy* (2nd ed., pp. 31-40). Thorofare, NJ: SLACK, Inc.

Law, M., & Pollock, N., Stewart, D. (2004). Evidence-based occupational therapy: Concepts and strategies. *New Zealand Journal of Occupational Therapy, 51*(1), 14-22.

Law, M., Steinwender, S., & Leclair, L. (1998). Occupation, health and well-being. *Canadian Journal of Occupational Therapy, 65*(2), 81-91.

Layder, D. (1994). *Understanding social theory.* Thousand Oaks, CA: Sage Publications.

Leclerc, F. (1972). *100 000 façons de tuer un homme. Song from the record L'alouette en colère* (Éditions Canthus ed.). The Netherlands: Philips Records.

Letts, L. (2003a). Enabling citizen participation of older adults through social and political environments. In L. Letts, P. Rigby, & D. Stewart (Ed.), *Using environments to enable occupational performance* (pp. 71-80). Thorofare, NJ: SLACK, Inc.

Letts, L. (2003b). Occupational therapy and participatory research: A partnership worth pursuing. *American Journal of Occupational Therapy, 57*(1), 77-87.

Letts, L., Fraser, B., Finlayson, M., & Walls, J. (1993). *For the health of it! Occupational therapy within a health promotion framework.* Ottawa, ON: CAOT Publications ACE.

LeVesconte, H. P. (1935). Expanding fields of occupational therapy. *Canadian Journal of Occupational Therapy, 3*(1), 4-13.

Levine R. E., & Brayley, C. R. (1991). Occupation as a therapeutic medium: A contextual approach to performance intervention. In C. Christiansen, & C. Baum (Eds.), *Occupational therapy: Enabling function and well-being* (2nd ed., pp. 591-631). Thorofare, NJ: SLACK, Inc.

Lewin, K. (1933). *Dynamic theory of personality.* New York: McGraw Hill.

Lewin, K. (1951). In D. Cartwright (Ed.), *Field theory in social science: Selected theoretical papers.* New York: Harper & Row.

Lewis, F. M., & Daltroy, L. H. (1990). How Causal Explanations Influence Health Behavior: Attribution Theory. In K. Glanz, F. M. Lewis, & B. K. Rimer (Eds.), *Health Education and Health Behavior: Theory, Research. and Practice* (pp. 92-114). San Francisco, CA: Jossey-Bass Publishers.

Library and Archives Canada (2006). Bonnie Sherr Klein Canadian Women in Film. Celebrity Women's Achievements. Retrieved September 25, 2006 from http//www.collections canada.ca/femmes/002026-704-e.html

Linden, R. (2003). The discipline of collaboration. *Leader to Leader, 29*, 41-47.

Litterst, T. A. (1992). Occupational therapy: The role of ideology in the development of a profession for women. *American Journal of Occupational Therapy, 46*(1), 20-25.

Little, B. R. (1983). Personal projects: A rationale and method for investigation. *Environment and Behavior, 15*(3), 273-309.

Llorens, L. A. (1986). Activity analysis: Agreement among factors in a sensory processing model. *American Journal of Occupational Therapy, 40*(2), 103-110.

Lotz, J. (1982). The moral and ethical basis of community: Development: Reflections on the Canadian experience. *Community Development Journal, 17*(1), 27-31.

Lovden, M., Ghisletta, P., & Linderberger, U. (2005). Social participation attenuates decline in perceptual speed in old and very old age. *Psychology and Aging, 20*(3), 423-434.

Lum, J., Williams, A. P., Rappolt, S., Landry, M., Deber, R., & Verrier, M. (2004). Meeting the challenge of diversity: Results for the 2003 survey of occupational therapists in Ontario. *Occupational Therapy Now, 6*(4), 13-17.

Lunt, A. (1997). Occupational science and occupational therapy: Negotiating the boundary between a discipline and a profession. *Journal of Occupational Science: Australia, 4*(2), 56-61.

Lynch, T. R., Morse, J. Q., Mendelson, T., & Robins, C. J. (2003). Dialectical behavior therapy for depressed older adults. *American Journal of Geriatric Psychiatry, 11*(1), 33-45.

Lyon, L. (1989). *The community in urban society.* Lexington, MA: D. C. Health.

Lysaght, R. M. (2004). Approaches to worker rehabilitation by occupational and physical therapists in the United States: Factors impacting practice. *Work: A Journal of Prevention, Assessment & Rehabilitation, 23*(2), 139-146.

MacRae, A., Falk-Kessler, J., Julin, D., Padilla, R., & Schultz, S. (1998). Occupational therapy models. In A. MacRae, & E. Cara (Eds.), *Psychosocial occupational therapy: A clinical practice* (pp. 97-136). Albany, NY: Delmar Publishing Inc.

Madill, H., Cardwell, M., Robinson, I., & Britnell, E. (1986). Old themes, new directions – occupational therapy in the 21st century. *Canadian Journal of Occupational Therapy, 53*, 38-44.

Magnani, L. (2001). *Abduction, reason, and science: Processes of discovery and explanation.* New York: Plenum Publishers.

Mandich, A., Polatajko, H. J., Miller, L., & Baum, C. (2004). *The paediatric activity card sort.*

Ottawa, ON, Canada: CAOT Publications ACE.

Mandich, A. D., Polatajko, H. J., & Rodger, S. (2003). Rites of passage: Understanding participation of children with developmental coordination disorder. *Human Movement Science, 22*(4-5), 583-595.

Mangione, C. M., Lee, P. P., Gutierrez, P. R., Spritzer, K., Berry, S., & Hays, R. D. (2001). Development of the 25-item National Eye Institute Visual Function Questionnaire (UFQ-25). Archives of Ophthalmology, 119, 1050-1058.

Manojlovich, M. (2006). *Building occupational therapy research capacity in Atlantic Canada.* School of Occupational Therapy, Dalhousie University, Nova Scotia. Retrieved January 26, 2007 from http://occupationaltherapy.dal.ca/Files/Building_Research_Capacity_final.pdf

Manuel, P. M. (2003). Occupied with ponds: Exploring the meaning, bewaring the loss for kids and communities of nature's small spaces. *Journal of Occupational Science, 10*(1), 31-39.

Martin, E. F. (1941). Occupational therapy treatment for cerebral palsies at the children's rehabilitation institute. *Canadian Journal of Occupational Therapy, 8*(2), 48-51.

Martini, R., Polatajko, H. J., & Wilcock, A. A. (1995). The proposed revision of the international classification of impairments, disabilities, and handicaps (ICIDH): A potential model for occupational therapy. *Occupational Therapy International, 2,* 1-21.

Marx, K. (1992). In R. Livingston, & G. Benton (Eds.), *Economic and philosophical manuscripts.* New York: Penguin Press.

Matthews, A. (2005). Mainstreaming transformative teaching. In P. Tripp, & L. Muzzin (Eds.), *Teaching as activism: Equity meets environmentalism* (pp. 95-105). Kingston, ON: McGill-Queen's University Press.

Mattingly, C. (1998). In search of the good: Narrative reasoning in clinical. *Medical Anthropology Quarterly, 12*(3), 273-297.

Mattingly, C., & Fleming, M. (1994). *Clinical Reasoning: Forms of inquiry in a therapeutic practice.* Philidelphia: F. A. Davis.

Matuk, L. Y., & Ruggirello, T. (2007). Culture connection project: Promoting multiculturalism in elementary schools. *Canadian Journal of Public Health, 98*(1), 26-29.

Maxwell, J. D., & Maxwell, M. P. (1979). Graduate education: The case of occupational therapy. *Canadian Journal of Occupational Therapy, 46,* 189-196.

Maxwell, J. D., & Maxwell, M. P. (1983). Inner fraternity and outer sorority: Social structure and the professionalization of occupational therapy. In A. Wipper (Ed.), *The sociology of work: Papers in honour of Osward Hall. Carleton library series number 129.* Ottawa, ON: University of Ottawa Press.

McColl, M. A. (1998). What do we need to know to practice occupational therapy in the community? *American Journal of Occupational Therapy, 52*(1), 11-19.

McColl, M. (2000). Muriel Driver Memorial Lecture: Spirit, occupation and disability. *Canadian Journal of Occupational Therapy, 67*(4), 217-228.

McColl, M. (Ed.) (2003). *Spirituality and occupational therapy.* Ottawa, ON: CAOT Publications ACE.

McColl, M. A., Carswell, A., Law, M., Pollock, N., Baptiste, S., & Polatajko, H. J. (2006). *Research on the Canadian occupational performance measure: An annotated resource.* Ottawa, ON: CAOT Publications ACE.

McComas, J., & Carswell, A. (1994). A model for action in health promotion: A community experience. *Canadian Journal of Rehabilitation, 7*(4), 257-265.

McCormack, G. (1987). Culture and communication in the treatment planning for occupational therapy with minority populations. *Occupational Therapy in Health Care, 4*(1), 17-36.

McGoldrick, M., & Carter, B. (2001). Advances in coaching: Family therapy with one person. *Journal of Marital and Family Therapy, 27*(3), 281-300.

McGuire, B. K., Crowe, T. K., Law, M., & VanLeit, B. (2004). Mothers of children with disabilities: Occupational concerns and solutions. *OTJR: Occupation, Participation and Health, 24,* 54-63.

McKay, A. (1974). A model for community integration through leisure planning and activity. *Canadian Journal of Occupational Therapy, 43*(2), 66-68.

McKee, P., & Morgan, L. (1998). *Orthotics in rehabilitation: Splinting the hand and body.*

Philadelphia, PA: F. A. Davis.

McKee, P., & Nguyen, C. (2007). Customized dynamic splinting: Orthoses that promote optimal function and recovery after radial nerve injury: A case report. *Journal of Hand Therapy, 20*(1), p. 73-88.

McKee, P., & Rivard, A. (2004). Orthoses as enablers of occupation: Client-centred splinting for better outcomes. *Canadian Journal of Occupational Therapy, 71*(5), 306-314.

McKeough, A., Davis, L., Forgeron, N., Marini, A., & Fung, T. (2005). Improving story complexity and cohesion. *Narrative Inquiry, 15*(2), 241-266.

McLain, L., McKinney, J., & Ralston, J. (1992). Occupational therapists in private practice. *American Journal of Occupational Therapy, 46*(7), 613-618.

McWilliam, R. A. (1995). Integration of therapy and consultative special education: A continuum in early intervention. *Infants and Young Children, 7*(4), 29-38.

McWilliam, R. A., & Scott, S. (2001a). *Individualizing inclusion in child care: Integrating therapy into the classroom.* Retrieved December 22, 2006 from http://www.fpg.unc.edu/~inclusion/IT.pdf

McWilliam, R. A., & Scott, S. (2001b). A support approach to early intervention: A three-part framework. *Infants and Young Children, 13*(4), 55-66.

Mee, J., & Sumsion, T. (2001). Mental health clients confirm the motivating power of occupation. *British Journal of Occupational Therapy, 64*(3), 121-128.

Meltzer, P. J. (2001). Using the self-discovery tapestry to explore occupational careers. *Journal of Occupational Science, 8*(2), 16-24.

Merriam-Webster. (2003). *Merriam-Webster's collegiate® dictionary* (11th ed.). Retrieved September 2, 2006 from http://www.m-w.com/dictionary

Meyer, A. (1922). The philosophy of occupational therapy. *Archives of Occupational Therapy, 1,* 1-10.

Meyer, A. (1977). The philosophy of occupational therapy. *American Journal of Occupational Therapy, 31*(10), 639-642.

Mezirow, J. (1990). How critical reflection triggers transformative learning. In J. Mezirow, & Associates (Eds.), *Fostering critical reflection in adulthood* (pp. 1-20). San Francisco, CA: Jossey-Bass Publishers.

Mezirow, J. (1991). *Transformative dimensions of adult learning.* San Francisco, CA: Jossey-Bass Publishers.

Mezirow, J. (1994). Understanding transformation theory. *Adult Education Quarterly, 44*(4), 222-232.

Mezirow, J. (1998). On critical reflection. *Adult Education Quarterly, 48*(3), 185-198.

Mezirow, J. A. (2000). *Learning as a transformation: Critical perspectives on theory in progress.* San Francisco: Jossey-Bass Publishers.

Mezirow, J., & Marsick, V. (1978). *Education for perspective transformation: Women's re-entry programs in community colleges.* New York: Center for Adult Education, Columbia University.

Mill, J. S. (1863). *Utilitarianism.* London: Parker, Son, & Bourn.

Millar, W. (1999). Older drivers: A complex public health issue. *Health Reports, 11*(2), 59-71.

Miller, A. (1992). *The untouched key: Tracing childhood trauma in creativity and destructiveness.* New York: Anchor-Press.

Moen, P. (1996). A life course perspective on retirement, gender and well-being. *Journal of Occupational Health Psychology, 1*(2), 131-144.

Mok, E. (2001). Empowerment of cancer patients: From a Chinese perspective. *Nursing Ethics, 8*(1), 69-76.

Molineux, M., & Whiteford, G. (1999). Prisons: From occupational deprivation to occupational enrichment. *Journal of Occupational Science, 6*(3), 124-130.

Molineaux, M. (2001). Occupation: Two sides of popularity. *Australian Occupational Therapy Journal, 48*(2), 92-95.

Molke, D. K., & Laliberte Rudman, D. (2003). Occupational science: Foundation and future. *Occupational Therapy Now, 5*(2), 10-11.

Molke, D. K., Laliberte Rudman, D., & Polatakjo, H. J. (2004). The promise of occupational science: A developmental assessment of an emerging academic discipline. *Canadian Journal of*

Occupational Therapy, 71(5), 269-280.

Moll, S., Huff, J., & Detwiler, L. (2003). Supported employment: Evidence for a best practice model in psychosocial rehabilitation. *Canadian Journal of Occupational Therapy, 70*(5), 298-310.

Molyneux, J. (2001). Interprofessional teamworking: What makes teams work well? *Journal of Interprofessional Care, 15*(1), 29-35.

Moore, K., Cruickshank, M., & Haas, M. (2006). Job satisfaction in occupational therapy: A qualitative investigation in urban Australia. *Australian Occupational Therapy Journal, 53*(1), 18-26.

Morice, A. (2006). *Les émeutes urbaines d'octobre-novembre 2005 en France: Comprendre avant de juger.* France: Éditions Canthus.

Morreim, E. H. (2001). *Holding health care accountable: Law and the new medical marketplace.* New York: Oxford University Press.

Morris, J. (1991). *Pride against prejudice: Transforming attitudes to disability.* London: Women's Press.

Morris, J. (1992). Personal and political: A feminist perspective on researching physical disability. *Disability, Handicap and Society, 7,* 157-166.

Mosey, A. C. (1986). *Psychosocial components of occupational therapy.* New York: Raven Press.

Mounter, C., & Ilott, I. (2000). Occupational science: Updating the United Kingdom journey of discovery. *Occupational Therapy International, 7*(2), 111-120.

Mullan, L. (2003). Reflections of a consultant occupational therapist. *Occupational Therapy Now, 5*(2). Retrieved March 22, 2007 from http://www.caot.ca/default.asp?ChangeID=65&page ID=587

Murray, H. A. (1947). *Explorations in personality: A clinical and experimental study of fifty men of college age* (Rev. ed.). New York: Oxford University Press.

Nagle, S., Cook, J., & Polatajko, H. J. (2002). I'm doing as much as I can: Occupational choices of persons with persistent mental illness. *Journal of Occupational Science, 9*(2), 72-81.

National Organization on Disability [NOD]. (2000). *NOD/ Harris surveys of Americans with disabilities.* Retrieved September 26, 2006 from http://www.nod.org/

Nelson, D. L. (1988). Occupation: Form and performance. *The American Journal of Occupational Therapy, 42*(10), 633-641.

Neufeld, P., & Kniepmann, K. (2001). Gateway to wellness: An occupational therapy collaboration with the National Multiple Sclerosis Society. *Occupational Therapy in Health Care, 13(3/4),* 67-84.

New Brunswick Department of Health and Wellness. (2002). *Health human resources supply and demand analysis final report.* Fredericton, New Brunswick: Fujitsu Consulting.

Newfoundland and Labrador Health Boards Association, & Department of Health and Community Services. (2003). *Newfoundland and Labrador health and community services human resource planning steering committee final report.* St. John's, Newfoundland: Department of Health and Community Services.

Niedhammer, I., Goldberg, M., & Leclerc, A. (1998). Psychological factors at work and subsequent depressive symptoms in the Gazel cohort. *Scandinavian Journal of the Work Environment and Health, 24*(3), 197-205.

Nochajski, S. M. (2001). Collaboration between team members in inclusive educational settings. *Occupational Therapy in Health Care, 15*(3/4), 101-112.

Nussbaum, M. C. (2003). Capabilities as fundamental entitlements: Sen and social justice. *Feminist Economics, 9*(2/3), 33-59.

Nussbaum, M. C. (2004). Beyond the social contract: Capabilities and global justice. *Oxford Development Studies, 32*(1), 3-18.

Nygard, L., Bernspang, B., Fisher, A. G., & Winblad, B. (1994). Comparing motor and process ability of persons with suspected dementia in home and clinic settings. *American Journal of Occupational Therapy, 48*(8), 689-696.

Oandasan, I., & Reeves, S. (2005). Key elements for interprofessional education. Part 1: The learner, the educator and the learning context. *Journal of Interprofessional Care, Supplement, 1,* 87-106.

O'Brien, P. A., Dyck, I., Caron, S., & Mortenson, P. (2002). Environmental analysis: Insights from sociological and geographical perspectives. *Canadian Journal of Occupational Therapy, 69*(4), 229-238.

Office for Disability Issues, Social Development Canada. (2005). *Advancing the inclusion of persons with disabilities 2005: A government of Canada report.* Ottawa: Author. Retrieved March 29, 2007 from http://www.hrsdc.gc.ca/en/gateways/nav/top_nav/program/odi.shtml

Olson P. (1995). Poverty and education in Canada. In R. Ghosh, & D. Ray (Eds.), *Social change and education in Canada* (2nd ed., pp.158-174). Toronto: Harcourt Brace.

O'Neill, P., & Trickett, E. J. (1982). *Community consultation.* San Francisco, CA: Jossey-Bass Publishers.

Ontario Hospital Association. (2003). *OHA consultation on health care human resources supply strategies for Ontario hospitals – Final report.* Toronto, ON: Ontario Hospital Association.

Ontario Human Rights Commission. (2006). *Age discrimination: Your rights and responsibilities.* Retrieved March 22, 2007 from http://www.ohrc.on.ca/en/issues/age/index_html/view

Orlinsky, D. E., Grawe, K., & Parks, B. K. (1994). Process and outcome in psychotherapy: Noch einmal. In A. E. Bergin, & S. L. Garfield (Eds.), *Handbook of psychotherapy and behavior change* (4th ed., pp. 270-376). New York: Wiley & Sons.

O'Shea, B. (1979). Me? Political? *Canadian Journal of Occupational Therapy, 46*(4), 143-145.

Oxford English Dictionary. (1989). Retrieved March 22, 2007 from http://www.askoxford.com/

Page, L. J. (2005). Coaching VERSUS or coaching AND? Adlerian applications for organizations and individuals. *Journal of Individual Psychology, 61,* 130-138.

Painter, J. (1990). Family intervention with the traumatically brain injured patient. *Occupational Therapy in Health Care, 7*(1), 69-85.

Painter, J., & Akroyd, D. (1998). Predictors of organizational commitment among occupational therapists. *Occupational Therapy in Health Care, 11*(2), 1-15.

Palisano, R. J., Tieman, B. L., Walter, S. D., Bartlet, D. J., Rosenbaum, P. L., Russell, D., et al. (2003). Effect of environmental setting on mobility methods of children with cerebral palsy. *Developmental Medicine and Child Neurology, 45,* 12-16.

Parham, L., & Mailloux, Z. (2001). Sensory integration. In J. Case-Smith (Ed.), *Occupational therapy for children* (pp. 329-382). St. Louis, MO: Mosby.

Passmore, A. (2003). The occupation of leisure: Three typologies and their influence on mental health in adolescence. *OTJR: Occupation, Participation and Health, 23*(2), 76-83.

Pearson, A., Wiechula, R., Court, A., & Lockwood, C. (2005). The JBI model of evidence-based healthcare. *International Journal of Evidence-based Healthcare, 3*(8), 207-215.

Pellegrino, E. D. (2002). Professionalism, profession and the virtues of the good physician. *Mount Sinai Journal of Medicine, 69*(6), 378-384.

Perkins, D. D., & Zimmerman, M. A. (1995). Empowerment theory, research and application. *American Journal of Community Psychology, 23*(5), 569-578.

Perlman, C., Weston, C., & Gisel, E. (2005). A web-based tutorial to enhance student learning of activity analysis. *Canadian Journal of Occupational Therapy 72(3),* 153-163.

Persson, D., Erlandsson, L., Eklund, M., & Iwarsson, S. (2001). Value dimensions, meaning, and complexity in human occupation: A tentative structure for analysis. *Scandinavian Journal of Occupational Therapy, 8*(1), 7-18.

Petrella, L., McColl, M. A., Krupa, T., & Johnston, J. (2005). Returning to productive activities: Perspectives of individuals with long-standing brain injury. *Brain Injury, 19*(9), 643-655.

Pierce, D. (2001). Occupation by design: Dimensions, therapeutic power, and creative process. *American Journal of Occupational Therapy, 55*(3), 249-259.

Pincus, T., Esther, R., DeWalt, D., & Callahan, L. (1998). Social conditions and self management are more powerful determinants of health than access to health care. *Annals of Internal Medicine, 129*(5), 406-411.

Piskur, B., Kinebanian, A., & Josephsson, S. (2002). Occupation and well-being: A study of some Slovenian people's experiences of engagement in occupation in relation to well-being. *Scandinavian Journal of Occupational Therapy, 9,* 63-70.

Polatajko, H. J. (1998) *A portrait of the occupational human.* Key note address of the 12th International Congress of the World Federation of Occupational Therapists, Montreal, Canada (May 31-June 5)

Polatajko, H. J. (1992). Muriel Driver Memorial Lecture: Naming and framing occupational ther-

apy: A lecture dedicated to the life of Nancy B. *Canadian Journal of Occupational Therapy,*
59, 189-200.

Polatajko, H. J. (1994). Dreams, dilemmas, and decisions for occupational therapy practice in a
new millennium: A Canadian perspective. *American Journal of Occupational Therapy,*
48(7), 590-594.

Polatajko, H. J. (2001). National perspective: The evolution of our occupational perspective: The
journey from diversion through therapeutic use to enablement. *Canadian Journal of*
Occupational Therapy, 68(4), 203-207.

Polatajko, H. J., Davis, J. A., Hobson, S., Landry, J. E., Mandich, A. D., Street, S. L. et al. (2004).
Meeting the responsibility that comes with the privilege: Introducing a taxonomic code for
understanding occupation. *Canadian Journal of Occupational Therapy, 71*(5), 261-264.

Polatajko, H. J., & Mandich, A. (2004). *Enabling occupation in children: The cognitive orientation*
to daily occupational performance (CO-OP) approach. Ottawa, Ontario: CAOT Publications
ACE.

Policy Research Initiative. (2005a). *New approaches for addressing poverty and exclusion.* Ottawa:
Author. Retrieved May 9, 2006 from http://policyresearch.gc.ca/page.asp?pagenm
=rp_ep_index

Policy Research Initiative. (2005b). *Social capital as a public policy tool: Project report.* Ottawa:
Author. Retrieved May 9, 2006 from http://policyresearch.gc.ca/doclib/SC_Synthesis_E.pdf

Pollard, N., Smart, P., & the Voices Talk and Hands Write Group. (2005). Voices talk and hands
write. In F. Kronenberg, S. Simo Algado, & N. Pollard (Eds.), *Occupational therapy without*
borders (pp. 287-301). London: Elsevier Churchill Livingstone.

Pollock, N. (1990). Occupational performance measures: A review based on the guidelines.
Canadian Journal of Occupational Therapy, 57(2), 77-81.

Pollock, N. (1993). Client-centered assessment. *American Journal of Occupational Therapy, 47*(4),
298-301.

Pond Clements, E. (2002). Return-to-work counseling. *Occupational Therapy Now, 4*(5). Retrieved
March 22, 2007 from http://www.caot.ca/default.asp?ChangeID=65&pageID=492

Pong, R. (1997). Towards developing a flexible workforce. *Canadian Journal of Radiography,*
Radiotherapy, Nuclear Medicine, 28(1), 11-26.

Pranger, T. (May, 2002). *Report of the professional issue forum on growing through occupation*
and active living, St. John, New Brunswick. Retrieved March 22, 2007 from
http://www.caot.ca/default.asp?pageid=576

Precin, P. (2002). *Client-centered reasoning, narratives of people with mental illness.* London:
Butterworth Heinemann.

Primeau, L. (1996). Work and leisure: Transcending the dichotomy. *American Journal of*
Occupational Therapy, 50(7), 569-577.

Pringle, E. (1996). Evidence-based practice: Exploring the implications for research within the
therapy professions. *British Journal of Therapy & Rehabilitation, 3*(12), 669.

Provident, J. M., Joyle-Gaguzis, K. (2005). Creating an occupational therapy level II fieldwork
experience in a county jail setting. *American Journal of Occupational Therapy, 59*(1) 101-
106.

Prochaska, J. O., & Velicer, W. F. (1997). The transtheoretical model of health behavior change.
American Journal of Health Promotion, 12(1), 38-48.

Public Health Agency of Canada. (2004). *The social determinants of health: An overview of the*
implications for policy and the role of the health sector. Retrieved February 4, 2009 from
http://www.phac-aspc.gc.ca/ph-sp/oi-ar/01_overview-eng.php

Pucetti, D. (1988). Supervision of the certified occupational therapy assistant: Developing a knowledge base and strategy. *Occupational Therapy in Health Care, 5*(2/3), 23-35.

Purdie, L., Zimmerman, D., Davis, J. A., & Polatajko, H. J. *Testing the validity of the taxonomic*
code of occupational performance. Manuscript submitted for publication.

Québec Santé et Services sociaux. (2002). *Planification de main-d'oeuvre dans le secteur de la*
réadaptation physique. Quebec City, PC: Author.

Quinsey, V. L., Coleman, G., Jones, B., & Altrows, I. F. (1997). Proximal antecedents of eloping
and reoffending among supervised mentally disordered offenders. *Journal of Interpersonal*
Violence, 12(6), 794-813.

Raeburn, J., & Rootman, I. (1998). *People-centred health promotion.* West Sussex, UK: John Wiley and Sons.

Raphael, D. (2004). Introduction to the social determinants of health. In D. Raphael (Ed.), *Social determinants of health: Canadian perspectives* (pp. 1-18). Toronto: Scholars' Press.

Raponi, R. A., & Kirsh, B. (2004). What can community support programs do to promote productivity? Perspectives of service users. *Canadian Journal of Community Mental Health, 23*(2), 81-94.

Rappaport, J. (1987). Terms of empowerment: Exemplars of prevention: Toward a theory for community psychology. *American Journal of Community Psychology, 15*(2) 121-145.

Rappolt, S. G. (2003). The role of professional expertise in evidence-based occupational therapy. *American Journal of Occupational Therapy, 57*(5), 589-593.

Rappolt, S., Williams, A. P., Lum, J., Deber, R., Verrier, M., & Landry, M. (2004). Clinical autonomy in occupational therapy practices: Results of a 2003 Ontario survey. *Occupational Therapy Now, 6*(3), 3-7.

Rebeiro, K. L. (1998). Occupation-as-means to mental health: A review of the literature, and a call for research. *Canadian Journal of Occupational Therapy, 65*(1), 12-19.

Rebeiro, K. L. (1999). The labyrinth of community mental health: In search of meaningful occupation. *Psychiatric Rehabilitation Journal, 23*(2), 143-152.

Rebeiro, K. L. (2001). Enabling occupation: The importance of an affirming environment. *Canadian Journal of Occupational Therapy, 68*(2), 80-89.

Rebeiro, K. L., & Cook, J. (1999). Opportunity, not prescription: An exploratory study of the experience of occupational engagement. *Canadian Journal of Occupational Therapy, 66*(4), 176-187.

Rebeiro, K. L., Day, D. G., Semeniuk, B., O'Brien, M. C., & Wilson, B. (2001). Northern initiative for social action: An occupation-based mental health program. *American Journal of Occupational Therapy, 55*(5), 493-500.

Reed, K. L., & Sanderson, S. N. (1983). *Concepts of occupational therapy* (2nd ed.). Baltimore, MD: Williams & Wilkins.

Registered Nurses Association of Ontario. (2005). *Risk assessment and prevention of pressure ulcers* (Rev. ed.). Toronto, ON: Author.

Rehabilitation Outcomes Measurement System Vendor Survey II. (1999). *Journal of Rehabilitation Outcomes Measurement, September*(1), 1-99.

Reid, D., Chiu, T., Sinclair, G., Wehrmann, S., Naseer, Z. (2006). Outcomes of an occupational therapy school-based consultation service for students with fine motor difficulties. *Canadian Journal of Occupational Therapy, 73*(4), 215-224.

Reid, D., Rigby, P., & Ryan, S. (1999). Functional impact of a rigid pelvic stabilizer on children with cerebral palsy who use wheelchairs: Users' and caregivers' perceptions. *Pediatric Rehabilitation, 3*(3), 101-118.

Reilly, M. (1962). Occupational therapy can be one of the greatest ideas of 20th century medicine. *American Journal of Occupational Therapy, 16*(1), 1-9.

Reilly, R. (2005) Strongest Dad in the World. *Sports Illustrated,* June 20, 2005. Time Inc.

Reitz, S. M. (1992). A historical review of occupational therapy's role in preventive health and wellness. *American Journal of Occupational Therapy, 46*(1), 50-55.

Reitzes, D. C., & Mutran, E. J. (2004). The transition to retirement: Stages and factors that influence retirement adjustment. *International Journal of Aging and Human Development, 59*(1), 63-84.

Restall, G., Ripat, J., & Stern, M. (2003). A framework of strategies for client-centred practice. *Canadian Journal of Occupational Therapy, 70*(2), 103-112.

Reynolds, P. D. (1971). *A primer in theory construction.* Indianapolis, IN: Bobbs-Merrill.

Richardson, J., Letts, L., Wishart, L., Stewart, D., Law, M., & Wojkowski, S. (2006). *Rehabilitation in primary care: National and international examples and training requirements.* Occupational Therapy, McMaster University, Hamilton, ON.

Rigby, P., Reid, D., Ryan, S., & Schoger, S. (2001). Effects of a wheelchair-mounted rigid pelvic stabilizer on caregiver assistance for children with cerebral palsy. *Assistive Technology, 13*(1), 2-11.

Riger, S. (1993). What's wrong with empowerment. *American Journal of Community Psychology, 21*(3), 279-292.

Ringaert, L. (2003). Universal design of the built environment to enable occupational performance. In L. Letts, P. Rigby, & D. Stewart (Eds.), *Using environments to enable occupational performance* (pp. 289-290). Thorofare, NJ: SLACK, Inc.

Roberts, C. A. (1962). Healing the sick – responsibility or privilege – for the patient or the professional therapist. *Canadian Journal of Occupational Therapy, 29*(1), 5-14.

Robins, C. S. (2001). Generating revenues: Fiscal changes in public mental health care and the emergence. *Culture, Medicine and Psychiatry, 25*(4), 457-466.

Robinson, I. M. (1942). Department of crafts. *Canadian Journal of Occupational Therapy, 9*(2), 61-67.

Robinson, I. M. (1981). The mists of time. *Canadian Journal of Occupational Therapy, 48*(4), 145-152.

Rogers, C. R. (1939). *The clinical treatment of the problem child.* Boston: Houghton Mifflin.

Rogers, C. R. (1951). *Client-centered therapy: Its current practice, implications and theory.* Boston: Houghton Mifflin.

Rogers, C. R. (1969). *Freedom to learn: A view of what education might become.* Columbus, OH: Charles Merrill.

Rogers, E. S., Chamberlin, J., Ellison, M. L., & Crean, T. (1997). A consumer-constructed scale to measure empowerment among users of mental health services. *Psychiatric Services, 48*(8), 1042-1047.

Rogers, J. C. (1983). Clinical reasoning: The ethics, science, and art. *American Journal of Occupational Therapy, 37*, 601-616.

Rogers, J., & Holm, M. (1994). Accepting the challenge of outcome research: Examining the effectiveness of occupational therapy practice. *American Journal of Occupational Therapy, 48*(10), 871-876.

Romanow, R. J. (2002). *Building on values: The future of health care in Canada.* Ottawa, ON: Commission on the Future of Health Care in Canada.

Rood, M. S. (1954). Neurophysiological reactions as a basis for physical therapy. *Physical Therapy Review, 34*(9), 444-449.

Rood, M. S. (1956). Neurophysiological mechanisms utilized in the treatment of neuromuscular dysfunction. *American Journal of Occupational Therapy, 10*, 220-225.

Rose, N. (1999). *Powers of freedom: Reframing political thought.* UK: Cambridge University Press.

Rosenbaum, P., Palisano, R., Walter, S., Russell, D., Wood, E., & Galuppi, B. (1996). *The gross motor function classification system.* Hamilton, ON: CanChild Centre for Childhood Disability Research.

Rosenfield, S. (1992). Factors contributing to the subjective quality of life of the chronic mentally ill. *Journal of health and Social Behaviour, 33*(4), 299-315.

Rosenstock, I. (1990). The health belief model: Explaining health behaviors through expectancies. In K. Glanz, F. Lewis, & B. Rimer (Eds.), *Health behavior and health education* (pp. 39-62). San Franciso, CA: Jossey-Bass Publishers.

Rothman, J., & Tropman, J. (Eds.). (1987). *Strategies of community organization.* Itasca, IL: F. E. Peacock Publishers.

Rotunda, R., & Doman, K. (2001). Partner enabling of alcoholics: Critical review and future directions. *American Journal of Family Therapy, 29*(4), 257-270.

Rowles, G. D. (2000). Habituation and being in place: Habits I conference. *Occupational Therapy Journal of Research, 20*(Suppl. 1), 52S-67S.

Royeen, C. B. (2003). Chaotic occupational therapy: Collective wisdom for a complex profession. *American Journal of Occupational Therapy, 57*(6), 609-624.

Rozier, C., Gilkeson, G., & Hamilton, B. (1992). Why students choose occupational therapy as a career. *American Journal of Occupational Therapy, 46*(7), 626-632.

Rugg. S. (1999). Factors influencing junior occupational therapists' continuity of employment: A review of the literature. *British Journal of Occupational Therapy, 62*(4), 151-156.

Ryan, R. M., & Deci, E. L. (2001). On happiness and human potential: A review of research on hedonic and eudaimonic well-being. In S. Fiske (Ed.), *Annual Review of Psychology* (pp. 141-160). Paolo Alto, CA: Annual Reviews.

Sackett, D. L., Rosenberg, W. M., Gray, J. A., Haynes, R. B., & Richardson, W. S. (1996). Evidence based medicine: What it is and what it isn't. *British Medical Journal, 312*(7023), 71-72.

Scaletti, R. (1999). A community development role for occupational therapists working with children, adolescents and their families: A mental health perspective. *Australian Occupational Therapy Journal, 46*(2), 43-51.

Schaeffer, J. (2002). *Community and communication in a diverse society.* Chicago: University of Chicago Press.

Schell, B. (2003). Clinical reasoning and occupation-based practice; changing habits. AOTA Continuing Education Article. *OT Practice 8*(18), 1-8.

Schellenberg, G. (2004). *The retirement plans and expectations of non-retired Canadians aged 45 to 59: Business and labour market analysis division research paper.* Ottawa, ON: Statistics Canada. Retrieved March 23, 2007 from http://dsp-psd.tpsgc.gc.ca/Collection/Statcan/11F0019MIE/11F0019MIE2004223.pdf

Schkade, J. K., & Schultz, S. (1992). Occupational adaptation: Toward a holistic approach for contemporary practice: Part 1. *American Journal of Occupational Therapy, 46*(9), 829-837.

Schmidt Hanson, C., Nabavi, D., & Yuen, H. (2001). The effect of sports on level of community integration as reported by persons with spinal cord injury. *American Journal of Occupational Therapy, 55*(3), 332-338.

Schön, D. A. (1983). *The reflective practitioner: How professionals think in action.* New York: Basic Books.

Schön, D. (1987). *Educating the reflective practitioner: Toward a new design for teaching and learning in the professions.* New York: Basic Books.

Schwartz, K. (1992). Occupational therapy and education: A shared vision. *American Journal of Occupational Therapy, 46*(1), 12-18.

Scriven, A., & Atwal, A. (2004). Occupational therapists as primary health promoters: Opportunities and barriers. *British Journal of Occupational Therapy, 67*(10), 424-429.

Seedhouse, D. (1997). *Health promotion: Philosophy, prejudice and practice.* London: John Wiley.

Segal, S. P., Silverman, C., & Temkin, T. (1995). Characteristics and service use of long-term members of self-help agencies for mental health clients. *Psychiatric Services, 46*(3), 269-244.

Selbee, L. K., & Reed, P. B. (2001). *Patterns of volunteering over the life cycle* (Catalogue No. 11-008). Ottawa, ON: Statistics Canada. Retrieved December 23, 2006 from http://dsp-psd.pwgsc.gc.ca/Collection-R/Statcan/11-008-XIE/0030111-008-XIE.pdf

Seligman, M. E. P. (2002). *Authentic happiness. Using the new positive psychology to realize your potential for lasting fulfillment.* New York: The Free Press.

Shafer, K. C., Kiebzak, L., & Dwoskin, J. (2003). Coaching: A new role for addictions. *Journal of Social Work Practice in Addictions, 3*(2), 105-112.

Shaw, L., & Polatajko, H. (2002). An application of the occupational competence model to organizing factors associated with return to work. *Canadian Journal of Occupational Therapy, 69*(3), 158-167.

Shimeld, A. (1971). Youth today and their influences on the practices of occupational therapy. *Canadian Journal of Occupational Therapy, 38*(1), 3-14.

Simó-Algado, S., Mehta, N., Kronenberg, F., Cockburn, L., & Kirsh, B. (2002). Occupational therapy intervention with children survivors of war. *Canadian Journal of Occupational Therapy, 69*(4), 205-217.

Sinetar, M. (1991). *Developing a 21st century mind.* New York: Villard Books.

Sinnott, J. (1994). Development and yearning: Cognitive aspects of a spiritual development. *Journal of Adult Development, 1*(2), 91-99.

Smith, D. (1987). *The everyday world as problematic: A feminist sociology.* Toronto, ON: University of Toronto Press.

Smith, D. (2005). *Institutional ethnography: A sociology for people.* Walnut Creek, CA: Alta Mira Press.

Snyder, C. R., & Lopez, S. J. (2002). *Handbook of positive psychology.* Oxford, UK: University Press.

Sökefeld, M. (1999). Debating self, identity, and culture in anthropology. *Current Anthropology, 40*(4), 417-447.

Stadnyk, R. (2005). *Personal contributions to the cost of nursing home care: Policy differences and their impact on community-dwelling spouses.* Unpublished doctoral thesis, University of Toronto, ON.

Stadnyk, R., Townsend, E. A., & Wilcock, A. A. (in press). Occupational justice. In C. Christiansen, & E. A. Townsend (Eds.), *Introduction to occupation: The art and science of living* (2nd ed.). Upper Saddle River, NJ: Prentice Hall.

Stamm, T. A., Cieza, A., Machold, K., Smolen, J. S., & Stucki, G. (2006). Exploration of the links between conceptual occupational therapy models and the international classification of functioning, disability and health. *Australian Occupational Therapy Journal, 53*(1), 9-17.

Stansfeld, S. A., Fuhrer, R., Head, J., Shipley, M. J., & Work, M. (1999). Work characteristics predict psychiatric disorder: Prospective results from the Whitehall II study. *Occupational and Environmental Medicine, 56*(5), 302-307.

Stark, S. L., & Sanford, J. A. (2005). Environmental enablers and their impact on occupational performance. In C. H. Christiansen, C. M. Baum, & J. Bass-Haugen (Eds.), *Occupational therapy performance, participation, well-being* (pp. 298-337). Thorofare, NJ: SLACK, Inc.

Statistics Canada. (2001). *Participation and activity limitation survey: A profile of disability in Canada, 2001.* Retrieved March 23, 2007 from http://www.statcan.ca/english/freepub/89-577-XIE/

Statistics Canada. (2002). *A profile of disability in Canada.* Retrieved March 23, 2007 from http://www.statcan.ca/english/freepub/89-577-XIE/index.htm

Statistics Canada. (2005a). *Population by year, by province and territory.* Retrieved February 4, 2009 from http://www40.statcan.gc.ca/l01/cst01/demo02a-eng.htm

Statistics Canada. (2005b). *Visible minority population, by province and territory. 2001 Census.* Retrieved February 4, 2009 from http://www40.statcan.gc.ca/l01/cst01/demo52a-eng.htm

Statistics Canada. (2005c). Average time spent on activities by sex. Retrieved February 4, 2009 from http://www40.statcan.ca/l01/cst01/famil36a-eng.htm

Statistics Canada. (2006). *Health human resources and education: Outlining information needs.* Retrieved February 4, 2009 from http://www.statcan.gc.ca/bsolc/olc-cel/olc-cel?catno=81-595-MIE2006041&lang=eng

Stein, J. G. (2001). *The cult of efficiency.* Toronto, ON: Anansi Press.

Stein, F., & Cutler, S. K. (2002). *Psychosocial occupational therapy: A holistic approach.* San Diego, CA: Singular Publishing Group.

Steultjens, E., Kekker, J., Bouter, L., Jellema, S., Bakker, E., & Et van den Ende, C. (2004). Occupational therapy for community dwelling elderly people: A systematic review. *Age and Aging, 33*(5), 453-460.

Stewart, D. (2002). The new ICF: International classification of functioning, disability and health. Concepts and implementation issues of occupational therapists. *Occupational Therapy Now, 4*(4), 17-21.

Stewart, M., Brown, J. B., Weston, W., McWhinney, I., McWilliam, C., & Freeman, T. (1995). *Patient centred medicine : Transforming the clinical method.* Thousand Oaks, CA: Sage Publications.

Stober, D., & Grant, A. (2006). *Evidence-based coaching handbook.* Hoboken, NJ: John Wiley & Sons.

Story, M. F., Mueller, J. L., & Mace, R. L. (1998). *The universal design file: Designing for people of all ages and abilities.* Raleigh: The Center for Universal Design, North Carolina State University.

Strong, S. (2002). Functional capacity evaluations: The good, the bad and the ugly. *Occupational Therapy Now, 4*(1), 5-9.

Sumsion, T. (1997). Environmental challenges and opportunities of client-centred practice. *British Journal of Occupational Therapy, 60*(2), 53-56.

Sumsion, T. (Ed.). (1999). *Client-centred practice in occupational therapy: A guide to implementation.* London: Churchill Livingstone.

Sumsion T. (2000). Barriers to client-centredness and their resolution. *Canadian Journal of Occupational Therapy, 67*(1), 15-21.

Sumsion, T. (2005). Facilitating client-centred practice: Insights from clients. *Canadian Journal of Occupational Therapy, 72*(1), 13-21.

Sumsion, T., & Smyth, G. (2000). Barriers to client-centredness and their resolution. *Canadian Journal of Occupational Therapy, 67*(1), 15-21.

Swedlove, F. (2006). Changing health care policy: Achieving equity in health care through policy change. *Occupational Therapy Now, 8*(5), 25-26.

Swee Hong, C., Pearce, S., & Withers, A. (2000). Occupational therapy assessments: How client-centred can they be? *British Journal of Occupational Therapy, 63*(7), 316-318.

Tague N.R. (2004). *The quality toolbox* (2nd ed.). Milwaukee, WI: ASQ Quality Press.

Taub, D. E., Blinde, E. M., & Greer, K. R. (1999). Stigma management through participation in sport and physical activity: Experiences. *Human Relations, 52*(11), 1469-1484.

The Center for Universal Design. (1997). *The principles of universal design.* Raleigh: The Center for Universal Design, College of Design, North Carolina State University.

Thibeault, R. (2002). Occupation and the rebuilding of civil society: Notes from the war zone. *Journal of Occupational Science, 9*(1), 38-47.

Timmermans, S., & Berg, M. (1997). Standardization in action: Achieving local universality through medical protocols. *Social Studies of Science, 27*(2), 273-305.

Toth-Cohen, S. (2000). Role perceptions of occupational therapists providing support and education for caregivers of persons with dementia. *American Journal of Occupational Therapy, 54*(5), 509-515.

Townsend, E. A. (1993). 1993 Muriel Driver Memorial Lecture: Occupational therapy's social vision. *Canadian Journal of Occupational Therapy, 60*(4), 174-184.

Townsend, E. A. (1996). Enabling empowerment: Using simulations versus real occupations. *Canadian Journal of Occupational Therapy, 63*(2), 114-128.

Townsend, E. A. (1998). *Good intentions overruled: A critique of empowerment in the routine organization of mental health services.* Toronto, ON: University of Toronto Press.

Townsend, E. A. (1999). Client-centred practice: Good intentions overruled. *Occupational Therapy Now, 1*(4), 8-10.

Townsend, E. A. (2002). Preface 2002. In Canadian Association of Occupational Therapists (Ed.), *Enabling occupation: An occupational therapy perspective* (Rev. ed., pp. xvii-xxxi). Ottawa, ON: CAOT Publications ACE.

Townsend, E. A. (2003). Reflections on power and justice in enabling occupation. *Canadian Journal of Occupational Therapy, 70*(2), 74-87.

Townsend, E. A., Birch, D. E., Langley, J., & Langille, L. (2000). Participatory research in a mental health clubhouse. *OTJR: Occupation, Participation & Health, 20*(1), 18-44.

Townsend, E. A., & Landry, J. (2005). Interventions in a social context: Enabling participation. In C. Christiansen, C. Baum, & J. Bass-Haugen (Eds.), *Occupational therapy: Performance, participation, and well-being* (pp. 495-517). Thorofare, NJ: SLACK, Inc.

Townsend, E. A., Langille, L., & Ripley, D. (2003). Professional tensions in client-centered practice: Using institutional ethnography to generate understanding and transformation. *American Journal of Occupational Therapy, 57*(1), 17-28.

Townsend, E. A., Le-May Sheffield, S., Stadnyk, R., & Beagan, B. (2006). Effects of workplace policy on continuing professional development: The case of occupational therapy in Nova Scotia, Canada. *Canadian Journal of Occupational Therapy, 73*(2), 98-108.

Townsend, E. A., Ryan, B., & Law, M. (1990). Using the World Health Organization's international classification of impairments, disabilities, and handicaps in occupational therapy. *Canadian Journal of Occupational Therapy, 57*(1), 16-25.

Townsend, E. A. & Whiteford, G. (2005). A participatory occupational justice framework: Population-based processes of practice. In F. Kronenberg, S. Simo Algado, & N. Pollard (Eds.), *Occupational therapy without borders: Learning from the spirit of survivors* (pp. 110-127). London: Elsevier Churchill Livingstone.

Townsend, E. A., & Wilcock, A. A. (2004a). Occupational justice and client-centred practice: A dialogue in progress. *Canadian Journal of Occupational Therapy, 71*(2), 75-87.

Townsend, E. A, & Wilcock, A. A. (2004b). Occupational justice. In C. Christiansen, & E. A.

Townsend (Eds.), *Introduction to occupation: The art and science of living* (pp. 243-273). Upper Saddle River, NJ: Prentice Hall.

Townson, M. (2001). *Pensions under attack.* Ottawa, ON: Canadian Centre for Policy Alternatives, and James Lorimer and Company.

Trafford, G. (1996). Joining a new culture and working within occupational therapy. *British Journal Occupational Therapy, 59*(6), 281-283.

Trentham, B., & Cockburn, L. (2005). Participatory action research: Creating new knowledge and opportunities for occupational engagement. In F. Kronenberg, S. Algado, & N. Pollard (Eds.), *Occupational therapy without borders: Learning from the spirit of survivors* (pp. 440-444). London: Elsevier Churchill Livingstone.

Trentham, B., Cockburn, L., & Shin, J. (2007). Health promotion and community development: An application of occupational therapy in primary health care. *Canadian Journal of Community Mental Health.*

Trombly, C. A. (1995). Occupation: Purposefulness and meaningfulness as therapeutic mechanisms. *American Journal of Occupational Therapy, 49*(10), 960-970.

Trombly, C. A. (1997). Purposeful activity. In C. A. Trombly (Ed.), *Occupational therapy for physical dysfunction* (pp. 237-254). Baltimore, MD: Lippincott Williams & Wilkins.

Tuohy, C. H. (2003). Agency, contract, and governance: Shifting shapes of accountability in the health care arena. *Journal of Health Politics, Policy and Law, 28*(2-3), 195-215.

Turner, B. S. (2000). *The history of the changing concepts of health and illness: Outline of a general model of illness categories.* In G. L. Albrecht, R. Fitzpatrick, & S. C. Scrimshaw (Eds.), Handbook of social studies in health and medicine (pp. 9-23). Thousand Oaks, CA: Sage Publications.

Unruh, A. M. (2004). "So... what do you do?" Occupation and the construction of identity. *Canadian Journal of Occupational Therapy, 71*(5), 290-295.

Unruh, A. M., Versnel, J., & Heintzman, P. (2001). *Application of evidence-based decision-making to the spirituality construct: Definitions and outcome measures.* Toronto, Canada: COTF. Retrieved March 23, 2007 from http://www.cotfcanada.org/download/review_unruh.pdf

Upshur, R. E. G. (2001). The status of qualitative research as evidence. In J. M. Morse, J. M. Swanson, & A. J. Kuzel (Eds.), *The nature of qualitative evidence* (pp. 5-27). Thousand Oaks, CA: Sage Publications.

Urbanowski, R. (2005). Transcending practice borders through perspective transformation. In F. Kronenberg, S. Simo Algado, & N. Pollard (Eds.), *Occupational therapy without borders* (pp. 302-313). London: Elsevier Churchill Livingstone.

Utsugi, M., Saijo, Y., Yoshioka E., Horikawa N., Sato T., Yingyan G., et al. (2005). Relationships of occupational stress to insomnia and short sleep in Japanese workers. *Sleep, 28*(6), 728-735.

Vaillant, G. (2002). *Aging well.* Boston, MA: Little, Brown & Company.

Vale, M. J., Jelinek, M. V., Best, J. D., Dart, A. M., Grigg, L. E., Hare, D. L., et al. (2003). Coaching patients on achieving cardiovascular health (COACH). *Archives of Internal medicine, 163*(22), 2775-2783.

Vale, M. J., Jelinek, M. V., Best, J. D., & Santamaria, J. D. (2002). Coaching patients with coronary heart disease to achieve the target cholesterol: A method to bridge the gap between evidence-based medicine and the "real world" – randomized controlled trial. *Journal of Clinical Epidemiology, 55*(3), 245-252.

Valkenburg, G., Achterhuis, H., & Nijhof, A. (2003). Fundamental shortcomings of evidence-based medicine. *Journal of Health Organization and Management, 17*(6), 463-471.

Voss, D. E., Ionta, M. K., & Myers, B. J. (1985). *Proprioceptive neuromuscular facilitation: Patterns and techniques* (3rd ed.). Philadelphia, PA: Harper & Row.

Wada, M., & Beagan, B. L. (2006). Values concerning employment-related and family-related occupations: Perspectives. *Journal of Occupational Science, 13*(2), 117-125.

Wakefield, J., Herbert, C. P., Maclure, M., Dormoth, C., Wright, J. M., Legare, J. et al. (2003). Commitment to change statements can predict actual change in practice. *The Journal of Continuing Education in the Medical Professions, 23,* 81-93.

Wallace, A. F. (1961). *Culture and personality.* New York: Random House.

Wallenbert, I., & Jonsson, H. (2005). Waiting to get better: A dilemma regarding habits in daily occupations after stroke. *American Journal of Occupational Therapy, 59*(2), 218-224.

Walker, K. F. (2001). Adjustments to managed health care: Pushing against it, going with it, and making the best of it. *American Journal of Occupational Therapy, 55*(2), 129-137.

Wagner, R. (1975). *The invention of culture.* Chicago, Il: University of Chicago Press.

Waring, M. (1988). *If women counted: A new feminist economics.* San Francisco, CA: Harper and Row.

Warren, A. (2002). An evaluation of the Canadian model of occupational performance and the Canadian occupational performance measure in mental health practice. *British Journal of Occupational Therapy, 65*(11), 515-521.

Watson, R. (2006). Being before doing: The cultural identity (essence) of occupational therapy. Australian *Occupational Therapy Journal, 53*(3), 151-158.

Weinblatt, N., & Avrech-Bar, M. (2001). Postmodernism and its application to the field of occupational therapy. *Canadian Journal of Occupational Therapy, 68*(3), 164-170.

Wells, S. (1994). Valuing diversity. In *A multicultural education and resource guide for occupational therapy educators and practitioners* (pp. 9-11). Bethesda, MD: American Association of Occupational Therapy.

Wennberg, J. E. (2004). Perspective: Practice variations and health care reform: Connecting the dots. *Health Affairs, October.* Retrieved December 20, 2006 from http://content.healthaffairs.org/cgi/content/abstract/hlthaff.var.140

Westmoreland, M. (2002). Disability management – A rose by any other name. *Occupational Therapy Now, 4*(1). Retrieved March 23, 2007 from http://www.caot.ca//default.asp?ChangeID=347&pageID=345

Westmoreland, M. (2003). *Disability management. Report of the Professional Issues Forum from the CAOT Conference May 2003.* Retrieved December 20, 2006 from http://www.caot.ca//default.asp?ChangeID=4&pageID=706

Whalen, S. S. (2002). How occupational therapy makes a difference in the school system: A summary of the literature. *Occupational Therapy Now, 4*(3), 15-18.

Whiteford, G. (1995). Other worlds and other lives: A study of occupational therapy student perceptions of cultural difference. *Occupational Therapy International, 2,* 291-313.

Whiteford, G. (1997). Occupational deprivation and incarceration. *Journal of Occupational Science: Australia, 4*(3), 126-130.

Whiteford, G. (2000), Occupational deprivation: global challenge in the new millennium. *British Journal of Occupational Therapy, 63*(5), 200-204.

Whiteford, G. (2004). When people cannot participate: Occupational Deprivation. In C. Christiansen, & E. A. Townsend, *Introduction to occupation: the art and science of living* (pp. 221-242). Upper Saddle River, NJ: Prentice Hall.

Whiteford, G. (2005). Knowledge, power, evidence: A critical analysis of key issues in evidence based practice. In G. Whiteford, & V. Wright-St. Clair (Eds.), *Occupation and practice in context* (pp. 34-50). Merrickville, NSW: Elsevier Australia.

Whiteford, G., & Fossey, E. (2002). Occupation: The essential nexus between philosophy, theory and practice. *Australian Occupational Therapy Journal, 49*(1), 1-2.

Whiteford, G., Townsend, E. A., & Hocking, C. (2000). Reflections on a renaissance of occupation. *Canadian Journal of Occupational Therapy, 67*(1), 61-69.

Whiteford, G., & Wright St-Clair, V. (Eds.). (2005). *Occupation & practice in context.* Marickville, NSW, Australia: Churchill Livingstone.

Whittmore, R., Chase, S., Mandie, C. L., & Roy, S. C. (2001). The content, integrity, and efficacy of a nurse coaching intervention in type 2 diabetes. *The Diabetes Educator, 27*(6), 887-898.

Wikepedia. (n.d.-a). *Family.* Retrieved March 28, 2007 from http://en.wikipedia.org/wiki/Family

Wikepedia. (n.d.-b). *Groups* (soc). Retrieved March 28, 2007 from http://en.wikipedia.org/wiki/Group_%28sociology%29

Wilcock, A. A. (1991). Occupational science. *British Journal of Occupational Therapy, 54*(8), 297-300.

Wilcock, A. A. (1993). A theory of the human need for occupation. *Journal of Occupational Science: Australia, 1*(1), 17-24.

Wilcock, A. A. (1996). *The relationship between occupation and health. Implications for occupational therapy and public health.* Adelaide, Australia: University of Adelaide.

Wilcock, A. A. (1998a). *An occupational perspective of health.* Thorofare, NJ: SLACK, Inc.

Wilcock, A. A. (1998b). Reflections on doing, being and becoming. *Canadian Journal of Occupational Therapy, 65*(5), 248-257.

Wilcock, A. A. (2001a). *Occupation for health: A journey from self health to prescription,* Vol. 1. London: British Association and College of Occupational Therapists.

Wilcock, A. A. (2001b). Occupational science: The key to broadening horizons. *British Journal of Occupational Therapy, 64*(8), 412-416.

Wilcock, A. A. (2002). *Occupation for health: A journey from prescription to self health,* Vol. 2. London: British Association and College of Occupational Therapists.

Wilcock, A. A. (2003). A science of occupation: Ancient or modern? *Journal of Occupational Science, 10*(3), 115-119.

Wilcock, A. A. (2006). *An occupational perspective on health* (2nd ed.). Thorofare, NJ: SLACK, Inc.

Wilcock, A. A., Chelin, M., Hall, M., Hamley, N., Morrison, B., Scriverner, L., et al. (1997). The relationship between occupational balance and health: A pilot study. *Occupational Therapy International, 4*(1), 17-30.

Wilcock, A. A., & Townsend, E. A. (2000). Occupational justice: Occupational terminology inter-active dialogue. *Journal of Occupational Science, 7*(2), 84-86.

Wilcock, A. A., & Townsend, E. A. (in press). Occupational Justice. In E. Crepeau, E. Cohn, & B. Schell (Eds.), *Willard and Spackman's occupational therapy* (11th ed.). Baltimore, MD: Lippincott Williams & Wilkins.

Wilkins, S., Pollock, N., Rochon, S., & Law, M. (2001). Implementing client-centred practice: Why is it so difficult to do? *Canadian Journal of Occupational Therapy, 68*(2), 70-79.

Wilkins, S., & Rosenthal, C. (2001). Career choices: A comparison of two occupational therapy practice groups. *Canadian Journal of Occupational Therapy, 68*(1), 29-40.

Williams, R. (1958). Moving from high culture to ordinary culture. In N. McKenzie (Ed.), *Convictions* (pp. 74-92). London: MacGibbon and Kee.

Williams, R., & Westmorland, M. (2002). Perspectives on workplace disability management: A review of the literature. *Work, 19*(1), 87-93.

Willows, N. D. (2005). Determinants of healthy eating in Aboriginal peoples in Canada: The current state of knowledge and research gaps. *Canadian Journal of Public Health, 96* (Suppl. 3), S32-S36.

Wiseman, J. O., Davis, J. A., & Polatajko, H. J. (2005). Occupational development: Why children do the things they do. *Journal of Occupational Science, 12*(1), 26-35.

Wood, W. (1996). Legitimizing occupational therapy's knowledge. *American Journal of Occupational Therapy, 50*(8), 626-634.

Woodside, H. (1976). Dimensions of the occupational behaviour model. *Canadian Journal of Occupational Therapy, 43*(1), 11-14.

Woodside, H. (1991). National perspective. The participation of mental health consumers in health care issues. *Canadian Journal of Occupational Therapy, 58*(1), 3-5.

Woodward, G., Manuel, D. & Goel, V. (2004). *Developing a balanced score card for public health.* Retrieved December 20, 2006 from http://www.ices.on.ca/file/Scorecard_report _final .pdf

Workman, B. A. (1996). An investigation into how the health care assistants perceive their role as "support workers" to the qualified staff. *Journal of Advanced Nursing, 23*(3), 612-619.

World Federation of Occupational Therapists (2002). *Minimum standards for the education of occupational therapists.* Retrieved March 28, 2007 from http://www.wfot.org/singleNews. asp?name=NOW%20AVAILABLE%20-%20Minimum%20Standards% 20for%20the%20 Education%20of%20Occupational%20Therapists%202002&id=6

World Health Organization. (1986). *Ottawa charter for health promotion.* Geneva, Switzerland: World Health Organization. Retrieved March 31, 2007 from http://www.euro.who.int/About WHO/Policy/20010827_2

World Health Organization. (2001). *International classification of functioning, disability and health.* Geneva, Switzerland: World Health Organization.

World Health Organization. (2002). *Towards a common language for functioning, disability and health: ICF.* Retrieved December 22, 2006 from http://www3.who.int/icf/beginners/bg.pdf

Wressle, E., & Samuelsson, K. (2004). Barriers and bridges to client-centred occupational therapy in Sweden. *Scandinavian Journal of Occupational Therapy, 11*(1), 12-16.

Wright-St. Clair, V. (2003). Storymaking and storytelling: Making sense of living with multiple sclerosis. *Journal of Occupational Science, 10*(1), 49-54.

Wright-St. Clair, V., & Seedhouse, D. (2005). The moral context of practice and professional relationships. In G. Whiteford, & V. Wright-St. Clair (Eds.), *Occupation & practice in context* (pp. 16-33). Marickville, NSW: Churchill Livingstone.

Yen, L., Edington, M. P., McDonald, T., Hirschland, D., & Edington, D. (2001). Changes in health risks among the participants in united auto workers – General Motors LifeSteps health promotion program. *American Journal of Health Promotion, 16*(1), 7-15.

Yerxa, E. J. (1967). Authentic occupational therapy: Eleanor Clarke Slagle Lecture. *American Journal of Occupational Therapy, 21*(1), 1-9.

Yerxa, E.J. (1980). Occupational therapy's role in creating a future climate of caring. *American Journal of Occupational Therapy, 34*, 529-534.

Yerxa, E. (1981). Basic or applied? A "developmental assessment" of occupational therapy research in 1981. *American Journal of Occupational Therapy, 35*, 820-821.

Yerxa, E. (1987). Research: The key to the development of occupational therapy as an academic discipline. *American Journal of Occupational Therapy, 41*, 415-419.

Yerxa, E. (1991a). Occupational therapy: An endangered species or an academic discipline in the 21st century? *American Journal of Occupational Therapy, 45*(8), 680-685.

Yerxa, E. J. (1991b). Seeking a relevant, ethical, and realistic way of knowing for occupational therapy. *American Journal of Occupational Therapy, 45*(3), 199-204.

Yerxa, E. J. (1992). Some implications of occupational therapy's history for its epistemology, values, and relation to medicine. *American Journal of Occupational Therapy, 46*, 79-83.

Yerxa, E. J. (1998). Health and the human spirit for occupation. *American Journal of Occupational Therapy, 52*(6), 412-418.

Yerxa, E. J., Clark, F., Frank, G., Jackson, J., Parham, D., Pierce, D., et al. (1989). An introduction to occupational science: A foundation for occupational therapy in the 21st century. *Occupational Therapy in Health Care, 6*(4), 1-17.

Yerxa, E. J., Clark, F., Frank, G., Jackson, J., Parham, D., Pierce, D., et al. (1990). An introduction to occupational science: A foundation for occupational therapy in the 21st century. In J. A. Johnson, & E. J. Yerxa (Eds.), *Occupational science: The foundation for new models of practice* (pp. 1-18). New York: Haworth Press.

Young, I. R. (1990). *Justice and the politics of difference.* Princeton, NJ: Princeton University Press.

Zemke, R., & Clark, F. (Eds.) (1996). *Occupational science: The evolving discipline.* Philadelphia, PA: F. A. Davis.

Zimmerman, D., Purdie, L., Davis, J., & Polatajko, H. (2006, June). Examining the face validity of the taxonomic code of occupational performance. Presented at the Thelma Cardwell research day, Faculty of Medicine, University of Toronto, ON. Retrieved March 28, 2007 from http://www.ot.utoronto.ca/research/research_day/documents/rd_06_proceedings.pdf

Zweck, von C. (2006). *Enabling the workforce integration of international graduates: Issues and recommendations for occupational therapy in Canada.* Ottawa, ON: CAOT Publications ACE. Retrieved March 23, 2007 from http://www.caot.ca/pdfs/wip/WIP%20Report.pdf

INDEX

Interprofessional, interdisciplinary, transdisciplinary 128, 168, 249, 284, 287, 305, 306, 318, 331, 333, 340, 349, 350

Just and inclusive society xxi, 2, 27, 89, 91, 101, 154, 155, 185, 241

Just-right-challenge 114, 117, 129

Kawa Model 29, 30, 32, 279

Knowledge translation 114, 160

Leadership, occupational therapy xvii, 1, 7, 8, 274, 275, 296, 298-300, 304, 306, 308, 312, 316, 327, 331, 337, 351, 353-355

Learning through doing 91, 113, 114, 124, 158, 333

Locality development 163, 164, 166, 168

Marketing, occupational therapy 325

Meaning perspective, schemes 141, 146-148, 158, 219, 220

Mediate, negotiate 82, 92, 93, 114, 117, 123, 129, 143, 251, 259, 284, 292

Medical model, biomedical model 33, 179, 274, 300, 350

Medical sponsorship, historical roots 334, 338

Mental health, disorders 72, 112, 123, 131, 142, 151, 184, 189, 190, 200, 201, 220, 293, 317-319, 321, 322, 326, 331, 333, 334, 347, 350, 352

Minimum Data Sets (MDS) 306

Model of Human Occupation (MOHO) 27-30, 60

Monitor, modify, CPPF action point 116, 128, 233-235, 249, 251, 271

Narrative reasoning 280

Non-governmental organization 93, 113, 121, 157, 158, 164, 169, 323

Norms, normative 43, 75, 76, 92, 103, 106, 107, 127

Occupation, domain of concern xxi, 6, 8, 10, 11, 16, 18, 23, 39, 64, 89, 126, 181, 186, 189

Occupation, means, ends, outcomes xvii, 29, 71, 72, 81, 82, 98, 100, 116, 121, 125, 128, 129, 130, 139, 149, 151, 155, 156, 163, 183, 186, 192, 195, 198, 227, 231- 233, 249, 250, 261, 262, 264, 265, 271, 289, 293, 299, 300, 303-305, 310, 324, 346, 353

Occupation, phenomenon 39, 40, 147

Occupation, vision 2, 3, 27, 90-92, 100-104, 110, 129, 137, 138, 143, 150, 157, 158, 164, 174, 224, 238, 274, 275, 301, 331, 340, 355

Occupation, time 15, 17, 21, 22, 28, 40, 44, 45, 47, 54, 55, 56, 61, 65, 67, 69, 70, 72, 73, 76, 119, 184, 197, 198, 207, 209, 240, 294, 309

Occupation, place, space 29, 30, 32, 46, 56, 65, 68, 74, 76, 77, 106, 122, 147, 200, 209, 240, 259

Occupation work, 19th century 91, 333

Occupations, necessity for survival 20, 42, 46, 58, 281, 303

Occupations, diversional, therapeutic use 2, 4, 15, 16, 174, 179, 180, 181, 184, 185-189, 191, 350

Occupational alienation 60, 77-79, 81, 82, 103, 181, 211, 212

Occupational analysis 8, 117, 125, 126, 128, 183, 186, 212, 232, 245

Occupational apartheid 77-79

Occupational behavior 3, 24, 26, 143, 149

Occupational balance, imbalance 6, 46, 47, 81, 82, 212

Occupational capacity 24, 26, 27, 28, 30, 42, 55, 57, 66, 93, 126, 204, 209-215, 218, 220, 230, 257, 264, 265, 270

Occupational challenge 41, 70, 102, 114, 145, 162, 180, 187, 206, 207, 210, 213

Occupational citizenship 53, 80, 91, 101

Occupational competence 29, 55, 193, 216, 246, 261, 266, 268

Occupational deprivation 26, 60, 65, 77, 79, 80, 81, 103, 104, 130, 155, 181, 211, 212, 219, 260

Occupational development 54, 55, 56, 90, 119, 130, 160, 267, 323